Statistics for Biology and Health

Series Editors
K. Dietz, M. Gail, K. Krickeberg, A. Tsiatis, J. Samet

Springer
New York
Berlin
Heidelberg
Barcelona
Hong Kong
London
Milan
Paris
Singapore
Tokyo

Statistics for Biology and Health

Hougaard: Analysis of Multivariate Survival Data.
Klein/Moeschberger: Survival Analysis: Techniques for Censored and Truncated Data.
Kleinbaum: Logistic Regression: A Self-Learning Text.
Kleinbaum: Survival Analysis: A Self-Learning Text.
Lange: Mathematical and Statistical Methods for Genetic Analysis.
Manton/Singer/Suzman: Forecasting the Health of Elderly Populations.
Salsburg: The Use of Restricted Significance Tests in Clinical Trials.
Therneau/Grambsch: Modeling Survival Data: Extending the Cox Model.
Zhang/Singer: Recursive Partitioning in the Health Sciences.

Terry M. Therneau
Patricia M. Grambsch

Modeling Survival Data: Extending the Cox Model

With 80 Illustrations

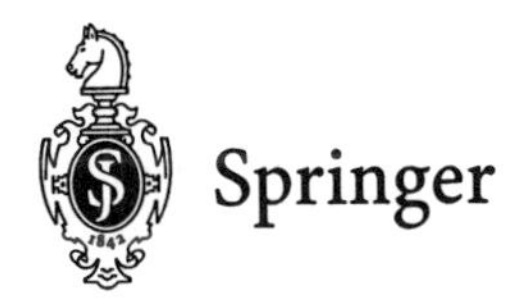

Terry M. Therneau
Department of Health Sciences Research
Mayo Clinic
200 First Street Southwest
Rochester, MN 55905
USA
therneau.terry@mayo.edu

Patricia M. Grambsch
Division of Biostatistics
School of Public Health
University of Minnesota
Minneapolis, MN 55455
USA
pat@biostat.umn.edu

Library of Congress Cataloging-in-Publication Data
Therneau, Terry M.
Modeling survival data : extending the Cox model / Terry M. Therneau, Patricia M. Grambsch.
p. cm. — (Statistics for biology and health)
Includes bibliographical references and index.
ISBN 0-387-98784-3 (alk. paper)
1. Medicine—Research—Statistical methods. 2. Medicine—Mathematical models.
3. Survival analysis (Biometry) I. Grambsch, Patricia M. II. Title. III. Series.
R853.S7 T47 2000
610'.7'27—dc21 00-030758

Printed on acid-free paper.

Production managed by MaryAnn Brickner; manufacturing supervised by Jacqui Ashri.
Camera-ready copy prepared from the authors' LaTeX files.
Printed and bound by Edwards Brothers, Inc., Ann Arbor, MI.
Printed in the United States of America.

9 8 7 6 5 4 3 2 1

ISBN 0-387-98784-3 SPIN 10660145

Springer-Verlag New York Berlin Heidelberg
A member of BertelsmannSpringer Science+Business Media GmbH

To Kathryn for her patience and support, to Victor for cracking the whip, and to Rex for nipping at our heels.

Preface

This is a book for statistical practitioners who analyse survival and event history data and would like to extend their statistical toolkit beyond the Kaplan-Meier estimator, log-rank test and Cox regression model to take advantage of recent developments in data analysis methods motivated by counting process and martingale theory. These methods extend the Cox model to multiple event data using both marginal and frailty approaches and provide more flexible ways of modeling predictors via regression or smoothing splines and via time-dependent predictors and strata. They provide residuals and diagnostic plots to assess goodness of fit of proposed models, identify influential and/or outlying data points and examine key assumptions, notably proportional hazards. These methods are now readily available in SAS and Splus.

In this book, we give a hands-on introduction to this methodology, drawing on concrete examples from our own biostatistical experience. In fact, we consider the examples to be the most important part, with the rest of the material helping to explain them. Although the notation and methods of counting processes and martingales are used, a prior knowledge of these topics is not assumed — early chapters give a not overly technical introduction to the relevant concepts.

SAS macros and S-Plus functions presented in the book, along with most of the data sets (all that are not proprietary) can be found on T. Therneau's web page at `www.mayo.edu/hsr/biostat.html`. It is our intention to also post any corrections or additions to the manuscript.

The authors would appreciate being informed of errors and may be contacted by electronic mail at

therneau.terry@mayo.edu

pat@biostat.umn.edu.

Both authors would like to acknowledge partial support from DK34238-14, a long term NIH grant on the study of liver disease. The influence of this medical work on both our careers is obvious from the data examples in this volume.

Terry Therneau
Patricia Grambsch
May 2000

Contents

1

Introduction

1.1 Goals

Since its introduction, the proportional hazards model proposed by Cox [35] has become the workhorse of regression analysis for censored data. In the last several years, the theoretical basis for the model has been solidified by connecting it to the study of counting processes and martingale theory, as discussed in the books of Fleming and Harrington [50] and of Andersen et al. [4]. These developments have, in turn, led to the introduction of several new extensions to the original model. These include the analysis of residuals, time-dependent coefficients, multiple/correlated observations, multiple time scales, time-dependent strata, and estimation of underlying hazard functions.

The aim of this monograph is to show how many of these can be approached using standard statistical software, in particular the S-Plus and SAS packages. As such, it should be a bridge between the statistical journals and actual practice. The focus on SAS and S-Plus is based largely on the authors' familiarity with these two packages, and should not be taken as evidence against the capabilities of other software products.

Several biases with respect to the two packages will become immediately evident to the reader, however, so we state them up front.

1. We find data set creation to be much easier with SAS; any serious manipulation, beyond the definition of simple yes/no variables, appears in that language.

2. Preparation of plots is much easier in S-Plus, all the figures were done in this way.

3. The important statistical computations are easy in both. The S-Plus output appears more frequently, however. Perhaps because of its historical roots which were focused on a terminal display as opposed to SAS's original printout orientation, the S-Plus output is in general much more compact (sometimes overly terse in fact). This is in itself neither good nor bad, but SAS output required more work, mostly removal of white space, in order to fit into the margins of a book column. Allow the authors some sloth.

4. Not every example needs to be shown both ways. Users of either package should have little difficulty in understanding/translating statements written in the other.

Each of these statements could be challenged, of course, and aficionados of both packages will likely send missives to the authors demonstrating the error of our ways. The computer code is *not* intended to demonstrate "clever" use of either package. It is the data sets and their insights which are exciting.

1.2 Overview

Chapters 2 to 4 lay the foundation for the methods. Chapter 2 deals with a simpler issue, the estimation of a survival curve without covariates. This is then used to illustrate a short overview of the mathematical details of *counting processes*. Only those few key results are given that are useful in the later exposition. Chapter 3 describes the basic Cox model, followed by an overview of the further flexibility that a counting process approach can provide, and Chapter 4 supplies an underpinning for the study and use of residuals.

Chapters 5, 6, and 7 use residuals to test the three basic aspects of a Cox model: the proportional hazards assumption, the appropriate choice of functional form of the covariates, and the influence of individual observations on the fit. The counting process formulation allows us to extend these methods to time-dependent covariate models as well.

Chapter 8 discusses one of the newer areas of application, the use of a Cox model for correlated survival data. Such data naturally arise when there are multiple observations per subject such as repeated infections, as well as correlated data from other sources such as familial studies. Because of its importance, and the many choices that are available in the setup of such problems, more examples are presented in this area than any of the other sections.

Chapter 9 explores a more recent innovation, the use of random effects or *frailty* terms in the Cox model. The practical utility of these models is not yet as well understood as the other areas, but it represents an exciting new area of application.

Chapter 10 discusses the computation of expected survival curves, based both on population based referents and on Cox models. These are important in the extrapolation of a given model to other subjects or populations of subjects.

The appendices give a short tutorial overview of the two packages, SAS and S-Plus, sufficient to help the reader of this book who is familiar with one and not the other. This is followed by documentation of the SAS macros and S-Plus functions used in the book that are not in the standard release of the packages, along with descriptions of many of the data sets. The code and data sets are available from the Section of Biostatistics Web server at `www.mayo.edu/hsr/biostat.html`. Last, there is documentation of a formal test/validation suite for the Cox model, residuals, and survival curves.

1.3 Counting processes

As we said above, the theoretical basis for the Cox model has been solidified in the last several years by connecting it to the study of counting processes and martingale theory. To give context to the counting process approach, we briefly review the familiar or "traditional" description of survival data. A concrete example is a clinical trial, such as the study conducted at Stanford University to assess the efficacy of maintenance chemotherapy in prolonging remission for patients suffering from acute myelogeneous leukemia (AML) [103]. Following induction therapy, patients who achieved complete remission were given a brief regimen of consolidation chemotherapy and then randomized to one of two groups. One group received a monthly course of maintenance chemotherapy, identical to the consolidation chemotherapy, and the other received no maintenance therapy. Both groups were then seen monthly for a thorough clinical evaluation to detect relapse from remission. Let T_i^* denote the time from consolidation therapy to relapse for the ith patient. We suppose that within each treatment group, the T_i^*s are iid with pdf $f_j(t)$, $j = 1, 2$; and survivor function

$$S_j(t) = \Pr_j(T^* > t).$$

The hazard function or instantaneous progression rate is

$$\begin{aligned} \lambda_j(t) &= \lim_{h \downarrow 0} \Pr_j(t \le T^* < t + h | T^* \ge t) \\ &= \frac{f_j(t)}{S_j(t)}. \end{aligned} \tag{1.1}$$

It gives the number of relapses per patient-month of followup time as a function of time since consolidation therapy. The study goal is to see whether maintenance therapy decreases the hazard. The investigators do not get to observe T_i^* for each patient. Some patients are still in remission when the study ends and all one knows is that T_i^* must be at least as great as the elapsed time. Let C_i^* denote the time from consolidation until the end of the study. This is the censoring time. In this particular study, C_i^* is known for every patient, but, in general, it might not be known when $T_i^* < C_i^*$. Let $T_i = \min(T_i^*, C_i^*)$, the followup time, and $\delta_i = I(\{T_i^* \le C_i^*\})$, the status, a 0/1 indicator which is 1 if T_i^* is observed and 0 if the observation is censored. What we actually observe is the pair (T_i, δ_i).

In a more general setting, T^* may be the time to any event of interest: time from diagnosis to death from a fatal illness, time from being put into service until failure for a machine, time from entering graduate school until the first paper is accepted at a refereed journal, and so on. C_i^* is the time from the same initiation point as T_i^* until observation of unit i (for purposes of the study) ceases. The C_i^*s may be random variables or predetermined constants. We suppose that each C_i^* is independent of the corresponding T_i^*. The observed data consist of pairs (T_i, δ_i) as well as covariates which may be vector-valued and/or time-varying, $X_i(t)$. The study goal is to estimate the hazard function and/or assess how the covariates affect it. The standard Cox proportional hazards model assumes a hazard function of the form

$$\lambda_i(t) = \lambda_0(t) e^{X_i(t)\beta},$$

where $\lambda_0(t)$ is an unspecified nonnegative function of time.

The counting process formulation replaces the pair of variables (T_i, δ_i) with the pair of functions $(N_i(t), Y_i(t))$, where

$$\begin{aligned} N_i(t) &= \text{the number of observed events in } [0,t] \text{ for unit } i \\ Y_i(t) &= \begin{cases} 1 & \text{unit } i \text{ is under observation and at risk at time } t \\ 0 & \text{otherwise.} \end{cases} \end{aligned}$$

This formulation includes right-censored survival data as a special case; $N_i(t) = I(\{T_i \le t, \delta_i = 1\})$ and $Y_i(t) = I(\{T_i \ge t\})$. It generalizes immediately to multiple events and multiple at-risk intervals, broadening the scope to more elaborate processes, such as nonstationary Poisson, Markov and other multistate, modulated renewal, and semi-Markov processes. This shifts the emphasis from modeling the hazard of a survival function to modeling the intensity or rate of a point process. Figure 1.1 shows the N and Y processes for four hypothetical subjects. The first two come from right-censored survival data and correspond to (T, δ) pairs of $(3, 0)$ and $(4, 1)$, respectively. The first subject is censored at time 3 and the second has an event at time 4. Subject 3 has multiple events, one at year .5 and another at year 2, and is followed to year 4. (The event in this case is not death, obviously.) Subject 4 is not at risk until year 2, and then experiences an event at year 3.

Note the right-continuity of $N(t)$ and the left-continuity of $Y(t)$. This distinction is important. $Y(t)$ is an example of a *predictable process*, a

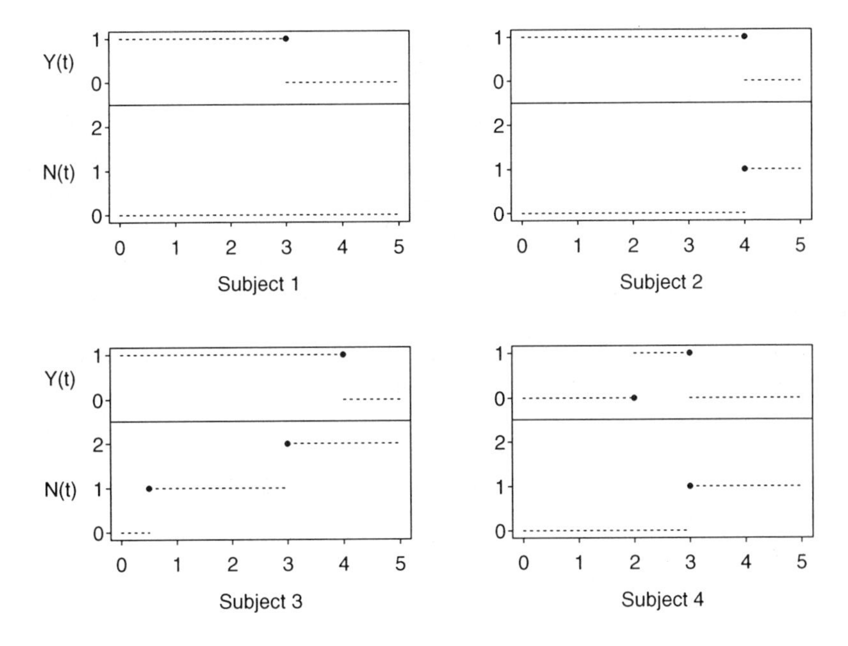

FIGURE 1.1: *N and Y processes*

process whose value at time t is known infinitesimally before t, at time $t-$ if not sooner. Placing this in the context of a gambling game, a roll of dice say, with t being the instant at which the throw is made, $Y_i(t)$ marks whether subject i is betting on this outcome; the wager can depend on the past in any way — perhaps every seventh bet is skipped due to superstition, or every third one after a win — but must be known before the throw. $N(t)$ is a counting process. Its value, the total number of wins, is updated precisely at time t.

A counting process is a stochastic process starting at 0 whose sample paths are right-continuous step functions with jumps of height 1. A predictable process is one whose value at any time t is known infinitesimally before t. Left-continuous sample paths are a sufficient (but not necessary) condition for predictability. Any deterministic function based on the past is a predictable process. These correspond in real models to the outcome and to the predictors.

When dealing with time-dependent covariates in a data set, it is sometimes difficult to decide what is a valid or invalid covariate process. The concept of predictability provides the answer, and can often be most clearly seen by relating the clinical question to a game of chance. Consider a large medical survival study on a fatal disease whose definitive diagnosis requires histological studies. Suppose that the records of the patients who die are carefully reviewed and those found to be wrongly diagnosed initially and thus ineligible are removed from analysis. A similar scrutiny can not be done on the censored patients, however, so all of them are included in the analysis. While this approach may seem reasonable, it will lead to biased results. First, $Y(t)$ is no longer a predictable process since a patient's inclusion in the study depends on the final outcome. Relating it to a gambling game, imagine a "fair" casino, patronage of which is limited to members of a fraternal organization. Worried about fraud, perhaps, the management has decided to review all cases where a patron had large winnings. For some, it is discovered that the subject's membership had lapsed; the gamblers are declared ineligible and are escorted from the casino *without their winnings.* This procedure obviously gives an unfair advantage ("bias") to the casino. Whether someone is "in the game" ($Y_i(t) = 1$) must be determined before recording the outcome ($N(t)$), if the game is to be fair. That is the essence of predictability.

Each subject also has a vector of covariates which may be time-dependent, $X_i(t)$. The covariate processes must also be predictable. Continuing the analogy, measuring a covariate simultaneously with the event is like placing a bet just as the ball comes to rest on a roulette wheel, something that no croupier would allow.

2

Estimating the Survival and Hazard Functions

This chapter gives an introduction to the simplest concept: estimating the survival curve when there are no covariates. Although simple, it forms a platform for understanding the more complex material that follows. We do it twice, once informally (although making use of counting process ideas) in Section 1, and then a second time with the connections to counting processes and martingales much more complete. Sections 2 and 3 first give an overview of the necessary theory and then apply it to the informal results of Section 1, both validating and extending them. Section 4 discusses the extension to tied data. The reader might want to focus on Section 1 on the first reading, perhaps supplemented with the results (but not derivations) of Sections 3 and 4.

2.1 The Nelson–Aalen and Kaplan–Meier estimators

2.1.1 Estimating the hazard

A major focus of the Cox model, and this book, is the hazard function. It turns out to be much easier to estimate the cumulative or integrated hazard, $\Lambda(t) = \int_0^t \lambda(s)ds$, than the hazard function. For the no-covariate case, the most common estimate of the cumulative hazard is the Nelson–Aalen estimate, which makes it a logical place to begin. The first data application for this chapter is a sample of right-censored failure times taken from the

4.5	4.6+	11.5	11.5	15.6+	16.0	16.6+	18.5+	18.5+	18.5+
18.5+	18.5+	20.3+	20.3+	20.3+	20.7	20.7	20.8	22.0+	30.0+
30.0+	30.0+	30.0+	31.0	32.0+	34.5	37.5+	37.5+	41.5+	41.5+
41.5+	41.5+	43.0+	43.0+	43.0+	43.0+	46.0	48.5+	48.5+	48.5+
48.5+	50.0+	50.0+	50.0+	61.0+	61.0	61.0+	61.0+	63.0+	64.5+
64.5+	67.0+	74.5+	78.0+	78.0+	81.0+	81.0+	82.0+	85.0+	85.0+
85.0+	87.5+	87.5	87.5+	94.0+	99.0+	101.0+	101.0+	101.0+	115.0+

TABLE 2.1: *Generator fan failure data in thousands of hours of running time; + indicates censoring*

paper in which the Nelson–Aalen estimator was introduced [111]. The data come from a field engineering study of the time to failure of diesel generator fans. The ultimate goal was to decide whether to replace the working fans with higher quality fans to prevent future failures. The engineering problem was to determine whether the failure rate was decreasing over time. It was possible that the initial failures removed the weaker fans (an early application of the idea of *frailty*), and the failure rate on the remaining fans would be tolerably low. Seventy generators were studied. For each one, the number of hours of running time from its first being put into service until fan failure or until the end of the study(whichever came first) was recorded. Table 2.1 shows the 70 observations conveniently ordered by followup time.

Let T_i^* denote the running time until fan failure for the ith generator, $i = 1, \ldots, 70$. We assume that the T_i^*s are iid with pdf $f(t)$, survivor function $S(t)$, and failure rate given by the hazard function $\lambda(t)$ which we want to estimate. The assumption of independent failure times seems reasonable, but the alert reader may question the assumption of identical failure time distributions — we said just above that the fans might be heterogeneous, with the weaker fans tending to fail first. However, we have no fan-specific information and thus must work with the marginal distribution of failure time. $S(t)$ is thus a mixture of survivor distributions for the different qualities of fan and the T_i^*s are iid from this distribution. We observe $T_i = \min(T_i^*, C_i^*)$, where C_i^* is the censoring time.

To put this into counting process notation, $Y_i(t) = I\{T_i \geq t\}$ is the indicator function that fan i is still under observation at time t; it is 1 from time $t = 0$ (when the fan is put on test) until failure or censoring and 0 thereafter. $N_i(t)$, the number of observed failures for fan i, is 0 until the moment of failure (if observed) and 1 thereafter. For the first fan, $Y_1(t) = 1$ for all $t \leq 4.5$ and is 0 thereafter, and $N_1(t) = 0$ for all $t < 4.5$ and is 1 thereafter. Note the difference between the use of $<$ and $\leq$ in the definitions.

The cumulative hazard estimator is based on the aggregated processes $\overline{Y}(t) = \sum_i Y_i(t)$ and $\overline{N}(t) = \sum_i N_i(t)$. $\overline{Y}(t)$ is the number of fans "at risk for failure" at time t. More formally, it is the number at risk during an interval of time $(t-\epsilon, t]$ for some small ϵ, since any fan that fails at precisely

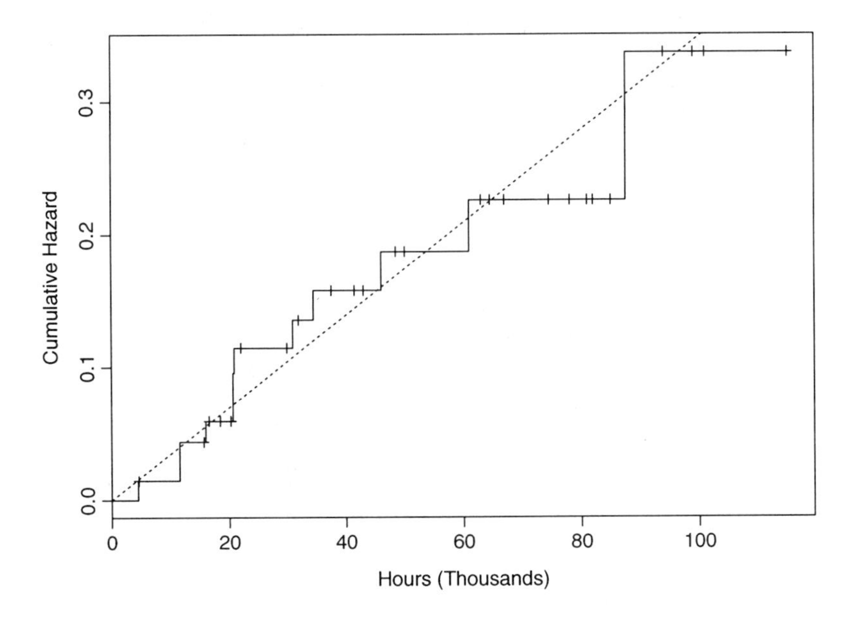

FIGURE 2.1: *Nelson–Aalen estimate for the generator fan failure data*

t must be both in the risk set at the failure time and known to be at risk before the failure occurred. (The gambling analogy provides justification — you can't win a lottery if you are not in it, and you must join before the drawing.) $\overline{N}(t)$ is the total number of fan failures up to and including t. To motivate the Nelson–Aalen estimator [50, p.4], consider a brief interval of time:

$$\begin{aligned} \Lambda(s+h) - \Lambda(s) &\approx \lambda(s)h \\ &= \Pr(\text{event in}(s, s+h] \,|\, \text{at risk at s}). \end{aligned}$$

It is natural to estimate this by $[\overline{N}(s+h) - \overline{N}(s)]/\overline{Y}(s)$. Summing these quantities over subintervals of $(0, t]$ and letting the subintervals get small enough that they contain at most one event time gives the Nelson–Aalen estimator:

$$\hat{\Lambda}(t) = \int_0^t \frac{d\overline{N}(s)}{\overline{Y}(s)}. \tag{2.1}$$

Counting process/integral notation can be a bit intimidating at first. The element $d\overline{N}$ is a shorthand that allows mixed continuous and discrete processes to be handled by a single notation. It can be heuristically decomposed as $d\overline{N}(t) = \Delta\overline{N}(t) + n(t)dt$ where the discrete part $\Delta\overline{N}(t) = \overline{N}(t) - \overline{N}(t-)$ is the number of of events occurring precisely at t and $n(t)dt$ is the change in the continuous portion, the familiar differential from elementary calculus. Counting processes are purely jump processes, so $d\overline{N}(t) = \Delta\overline{N}(t)$. Let t_1

Failure No.	Hours $\times 10^3$	Hazard	$\hat{\Lambda}(t)$	$\text{var}(\hat{\Lambda}(t))$
1	04.5	1/70	.0143	.0143
2–3	11.5	2/68	.0437	.0252
4	16.0	1/65	.0591	.0296
5–6	20.7	2/55	.0954	.0392
7	20.8	1/53	.1143	.0435
8	31.0	1/47	.1356	.0484
9	34.5	1/45	.1578	.0533
10	46.0	1/34	.1872	.0608
11	61.0	1/25	.2257	.0720
12	87.5	1/8	.3368	.1324

TABLE 2.2: *Computation of the Nelson–Aalen estimator for the generator fan data*

denote the first failure time, t_2 denote the second, and so on. An equivalent representation of the Nelson-Aalen estimate is a sum:

$$\hat{\Lambda}(t) = \sum_{i:t_i \leq t} \frac{\Delta \overline{N}(t_i)}{\overline{Y}(t_i)}. \tag{2.2}$$

Computations for the Nelson–Aalen integrated hazard estimate are summarized in Table 2.2. For example, $\hat{\Lambda}(2) = 0$ as there were no fan failures in $(0, 2]$ (the first is at time 4.5). At $t_1 = 4.5$ the curve increases by (# failures at 4.5)/(# fans at risk at 4.5) $= 1/70$, at $t_2 = 11.4$ it has a further increase of $2/68$, and so on. The last failure occurred at $t_{12} = 87.5$. So for any $t \geq 87.5$, we have:

$$\begin{aligned} \hat{\Lambda}(t) &= \frac{\text{\# failures at 4.5}}{\text{\# fans at risk at 4.5}} + \ldots + \frac{\text{\# failures at 87.5}}{\text{\# fans at risk at 87.5}} \\ &= \frac{1}{70} + \frac{2}{68} + \ldots + \frac{1}{8} \\ &= 0.3368. \end{aligned}$$

The estimate is plotted in Figure 2.1. The "+" marks on the curve show the followup time for censored observations.

There are two ways of interpreting the Nelson–Aalen estimate.

1. $\hat{\Lambda}(t)$ estimates the average number of failures in $(0, t]$ for a unit "perpetually at risk." For the fan data, this means the number of fan failures expected in t thousand hours of running if a generator were put into service at $t = 0$ and each time a fan failed, the generator were to be replaced by a working one of the same risk level (i.e., with the same cumulative thousand hours of running). In the reliability literature, this is called minimal repair [18]. Table 2.2 shows that a minimal repair policy would yield only .337 failures on average for 87,500 hours of running time.

2. The slope of the plot estimates $\lambda(t)$. There are numerous formal smoothing techniques that could be applied to the displayed step function; informally, one can smooth the plot visually and thus "see" the slope. Figure 2.1 shows little change in slope with time. A constant slope (i.e., constant hazard) corresponds to an exponential failure time distribution. As is well known, the MLE of the hazard λ for right-censored data from an exponential distribution is the total number of failures divided by the total time on trial, $\hat{\lambda} = \sum \delta_i / \sum T_i$. For these data $\hat{\lambda} = 12/3443 = 0.0035$. A line through 0 with slope 0.0035 is superimposed on the plot and fits reasonably well, and Nelson concluded that these data were compatible with a constant hazard. A strategy of replacing fans before they failed would not pay off.

The Nelson–Aalen estimator is essentially a *method of moments* estimator. Its variance is estimated consistently by

$$\text{var}[\hat{\Lambda}(t)] = \int_0^t \frac{d\overline{N}(s)}{\left[\overline{Y}(s)\right]^2} \tag{2.3}$$

$$= \sum_{i:t_i \le t} \frac{\Delta \overline{N}(t_i)}{\overline{Y}^2(t_i)}. \tag{2.4}$$

These properties can be justified informally by exploiting the Poisson connection: virtually any counting process can be modeled as a Poisson process, at least locally over short time periods. The increment $\Delta_h \overline{N}(t) = \overline{N}(t+h) - \overline{N}(t)$, the number of events in a small interval from t to $t+h$, is approximately a Poisson count for small h. Recall that for a Poisson random variable, the expected number of events is the product of the event rate, the time period, and the number of units available to have an event. Conditional on the past, $\Delta_h \overline{N}(t)$ is Poisson with mean $\int_t^{t+h} \overline{Y}(s)\lambda(s)ds \approx \overline{Y}(t)\lambda(t)h$, so

$$\mathcal{E}[\Delta_h \overline{N}(t)/\overline{Y}(t)] \approx \lambda(t)h. \tag{2.5}$$

The Nelson–Aalen estimator is essentially the sum of the scaled increments $\Delta_h \overline{N}(s)/\overline{Y}(s)$. Since the variance of a Poisson random count equals its mean, conditional on the past, $\text{var}[\Delta_h \overline{N}(s)/\overline{Y}(s)] \approx \lambda(s)h/\overline{Y}(s)$ which can be estimated by $\Delta_h \overline{N}(s)/\overline{Y}^2(s)$. Poisson increments are independent, so we sum these variance estimators and equation (2.4) results. The final column of Table 2.2 gives the variance estimate for the generator fan data. (Of course, truly Poisson data has continuous interevent intervals and would not have any tied event times, which occur at 11.5 and 20.7 in the fan data. This is expanded upon later.)

One might then suspect that confidence intervals for the Nelson–Aalen would be more accurate if they were done on the log scale, since this transformation improves the accuracy of confidence limits in parametric Poisson

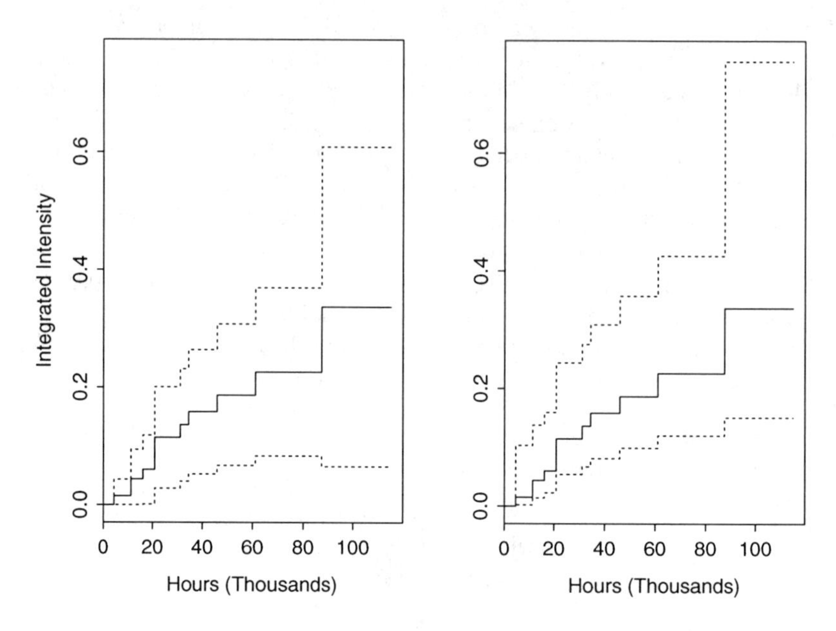

FIGURE 2.2: *95% confidence intervals for Nelson–Aalen estimator for fan failure data. Those in the right panel are based on a log transform*

models. The delta method gives $\text{var}[\log(\hat{\Lambda}(t))] \approx \text{var}[\hat{\Lambda}(t)]/\hat{\Lambda}^2(t)$ as the estimated variance for the log transform, and thus $\hat{\Lambda}(t)\exp\{\pm c_{\alpha/2}\hat{\sigma}(t)/\hat{\Lambda}(t)\}$ as the $100 \times (1-\alpha)\%$ confidence interval, where $\hat{\sigma}^2$ is the variance of $\hat{\Lambda}$ and $c_{\alpha/2}$ is the appropriate quantile of a normal distribution. This transformation was suggested by Kalbfleisch and Prentice [73, p. 15] and systematically examined by Bie et al. [15], whose simulations showed that the log-based confidence intervals had coverage probabilities much closer to the nominal values than the untransformed for a variety of failure distributions and censoring intensities. The authors concluded that for 90 or 95% confidence intervals, "about 10 deaths, and a similar number still at risk, are sufficient for the transformed intervals to perform reasonably well, and even with five individuals in these categories, the intervals will be accurate for many purposes." They found that the untransformed intervals required substantially larger sample sizes, by a factor of eight or so. Also, intervals with larger confidence coefficients (e.g., 99%) required larger sample sizes.

The right-hand panel of Figure 2.2 shows these confidence intervals for the fan data. They are obviously asymmetric, with greater spread above $\hat{\Lambda}(t)$ than below, appropriately reflecting the long right-hand tail of the distribution of $\hat{\Lambda}(t)$.

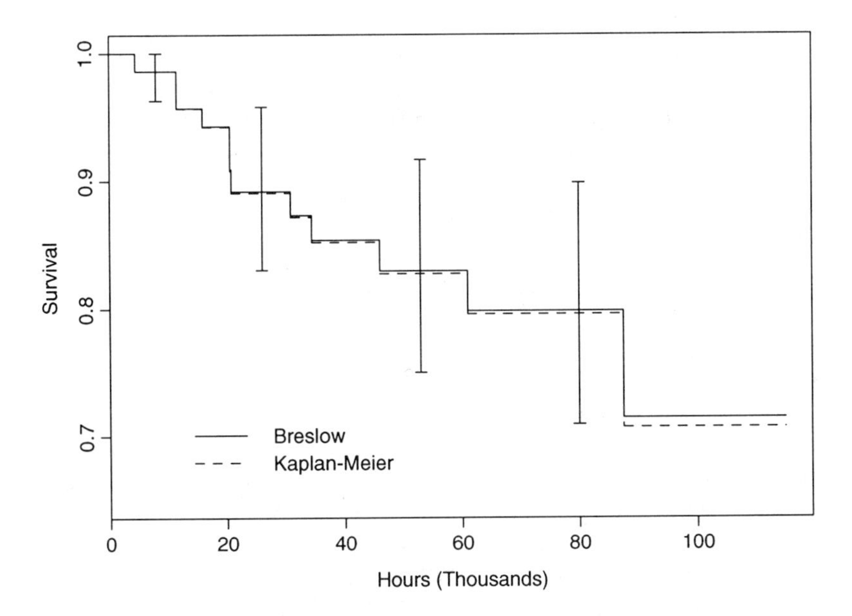

FIGURE 2.3: *Breslow and Kaplan–Meier estimates of survival for the generator fan data, with confidence bars for the Breslow estimate*

The Nelson–Aalen estimate satisfies a constraint on the total hazard:

$$\sum_{i=1}^{n} \hat{\Lambda}(T_i) = \sum_{i=1}^{n} N_i(T_i), \tag{2.6}$$

where, recall, T_i is the observed followup time for individual i. In words, "the total estimated hazard, summed over subjects equals the total number of observed events." Because $\hat{\Lambda}(T_i) = \int_0^\infty Y_i(s)d\hat{\Lambda}(s)$ and $N_i(T_i) = N_i(\infty)$, the constraint can also be written:

$$\sum_i \left[N_i(\infty) - \int_0^\infty Y_i(s)d\hat{\Lambda}(s) \right] = 0. \tag{2.7}$$

We will see that $N_i(\infty) - \int_0^\infty Y_i(s)d\hat{\Lambda}(s)$ is a useful residual derived from a martingale; the constraint means that these martingale residuals sum to 0.

2.1.2 *Estimating the survival function*

For any continuous distribution, the survival function and the hazard are connected by the simple relation $S(t) = \exp[-\Lambda(t)]$. Breslow [21] suggested $S_B(t) = \exp[-\hat{\Lambda}(t)]$ as a nonparametric estimator of the survival function. Fleming and Harrington [49] showed the close relationship between the

Breslow and Kaplan–Meier estimators, and compared them numerically for several sample sizes and censoring percentages. As above, let t_1, t_2, $\ldots$ be the unique failure times. Let $d\hat{\Lambda}(t_i) = d\overline{N}(t_i)/\overline{Y}(t_i)$, the increment in the Nelson–Aalen estimator at the ith failure (e.g., 1/65 for $t = 4$ in the fan data). Then the Breslow estimator can be written as

$$\hat{S}_B(t) = \prod_{j:t_j \le t} e^{-d\hat{\Lambda}(t_j)}$$

and the Kaplan–Meier estimate is

$$\hat{S}_{KM}(t) = \prod_{j:t_j \le t} [1 - d\hat{\Lambda}(t_j)].$$

Since $e^{-x} \approx 1 - x$ for small x, the two estimators are quite similar when the increments $d\hat{\Lambda}$ are small, that is, when there are many subjects still at risk. The two estimates are in fact asymptotically equivalent, since as $n \to \infty$ the individual increments get arbitrarily small. Since $e^{-x} \ge 1 - x$, $\hat{S}_B(t) \ge \hat{S}_{KM}(t)$ in finite samples; most notably, if the largest time T in a data set is a death, $\hat{S}_{KM} = 0$, but $\hat{S}_B$ is positive. Figure 2.3 compares the two estimators on the fan failure data. The difference between them is scarcely noticeable until the last failure when only eight fans are at risk. The plot also shows 90% confidence intervals at selected points; the difference in estimators is miniscule compared to their precision. Figure 2.4 presents the two estimates along with a 95% confidence interval about the Kaplan–Meier for the advanced lung cancer data set, 228 patients from a study of prognostic variables in advanced lung cancer [95], showing that the difference becomes truly negligible for moderate n. Here is the S-Plus code to create Figure 2.4.

```
> afit <- survfit(Surv(time, status) ~1, data=lung,
                        type='fleming-harrington')
> kfit <- survfit(Surv(time, status) ~1, data=lung,
                        type='kaplan-meier')
> plot(kfit, mark.time=F, xscale=365.25,
          xlab="Years", ylab="Survival")
> lines(afit, lty=2, mark.time=F, xscale=365.25)
> print(kfit)

   n events mean se(mean) median 0.95LCL 0.95UCL
 228    165  376     19.7    310     285     363
```

The left-hand side of the formula declares the response variable to be a survival object; the right-hand side `~1` is a "null" model, treating all subjects as a single group. The `type` argument could have been abbreviated to any unique string: `type='fl'`, for example, and could have been omitted for the Kaplan–Meier estimate since that is the default type. The `plot` command

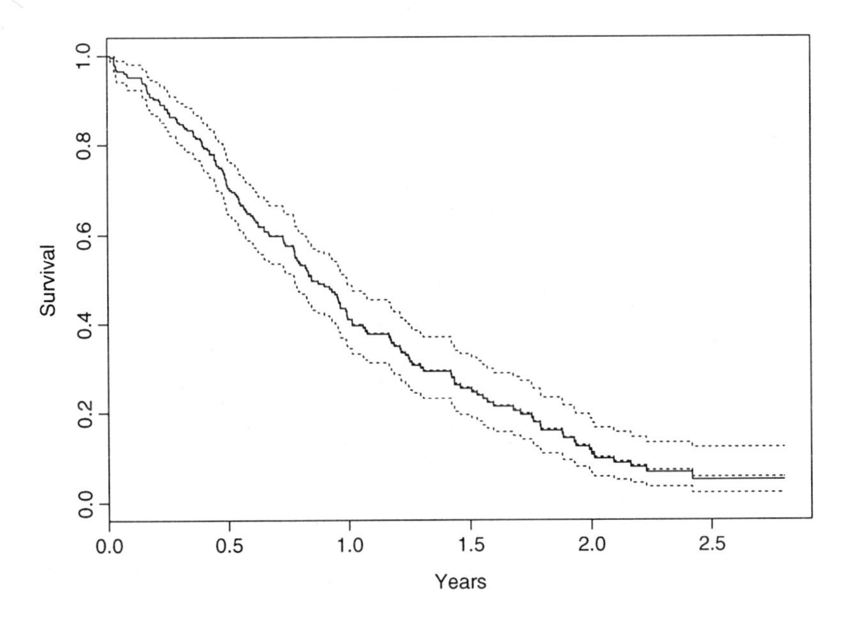

FIGURE 2.4: *Kaplan–Meier (solid) and Nelson–Aalen estimates for the lung cancer data set, along with pointwise 95% confidence intervals for the Kaplan–Meier*

draws the Kaplan–Meier curve, along with its 95% confidence intervals, the axes and their labels. The `lines` command adds the Nelson–Aalen line to the current plot. In the plot command, `mark.time=F` prevents "+" marks from being added at the censoring times (a purely artistic choice — we felt that they made this particular plot too "busy"). The `xscale` argument is used to plot the horizontal axis in years instead of days; alternatively, one could have fit the model as `survfit(Surv(time/365.25, status) ...)` to get a curve in years.

Since the step sizes of the Breslow estimate are always smaller than those of the Kaplan–Meier, it has a uniformly lower variance. It is biased upward, however, especially when the estimate(s) are close to zero. In comparing mean square error these aspects trade off. Fleming and Harrington [49] compared the estimates for sample sizes of n =10, 20, 50, and 100. Using theoretical calculations for uncensored data and simulations for censored data, they found that the Breslow estimate has smaller mean square error than the Kaplan–Meier for t such that $S(t) \geq .20$, and larger MSE for smaller $S(t)$. For instance, for $n = 20$ and uncensored data, MSE ratios for Breslow/Kaplan–Meier at $S(t) = .9$ and .1 were $4.3/4.5 = 0.96$ and $4.7/4.5 = 1.04$.

When there are ties in the data, the difference in the estimators can be substantially larger, and an alternative to the Breslow estimate is appealing. Assume that the "true" data are not tied, but that ties arise due to a lack of precision in our measurements. For the fan data, for instance, it is unlikely that both the third and fourth entries failed after exactly 11,500.00 hours of service. If the true failure times were 11.48 and 11.52, the increments to the Nelson–Aalen estimate would be $1/68 + 1/67$ instead of the value of $2/68$ obtained for the grouped data. A pleasing feature of the Kaplan–Meier is that it is invariant to such coarsening: the K–M at time 12 is $(69/70)(66/68)$. If the 11.5 tied data are replaced with 11.48 and 11.52, the new calculation has one more term but the same outcome: $(69/70)(67/68)(66/67) = (69/70)(66/68)$.

Nelson suggested replacing each tied failure time by failures equally spaced throughout a small interval. Other authors add a small amount of uniformly distributed random "jitter" to each event time thus breaking any ties. Fleming and Harrington [49] proposed a similar tie breaking to compute a modified Breslow estimate of survival. For the fan data, $\hat{S}_{FH}(12) = \exp(-[1/70 + 1/68 + 1/67]) = 0.9570$, very slightly smaller than the Breslow estimate of $\hat{S}_B(12) = \exp(-[1/70 + 2/68]) = 0.9572$ and closer to the K–M value of 0.9567. Of course, with only two tied and 68 at risk, the differences are small. However, consider a five-way tie with 15 at risk. It would contribute $\exp(-5/15) = 0.717$ to the Breslow estimate, $\exp(-[1/15 + 1/14 + 1/13 + 1/12 + 1/11]) = 0.678$ to the modified Breslow estimate, and $10/15 = 0.667$ to the Kaplan–Meier. Fleming and Harrington's proposal gives an estimator nearer to the Kaplan–Meier and smaller than the Breslow for tied data. We show later that their method generalizes directly to Efron's suggestion for tied failure times in fitting the Cox model. In S-Plus, it can be obtained using the option `type='fh2'` in the `survfit` function.

Confidence intervals for the survival curve can be calculated using either of two different variance formulae and on any of several scales. Based on a binomial argument, Greenwood's formula for the variance of the cumulative hazard is

$$\text{var}_g \hat{\Lambda}(t) = \int_0^t \frac{d\overline{N}(s)}{\overline{Y}(s)\left[\overline{Y}(s) - d\overline{N}(s)\right]},$$

which is larger than the Aalen estimate of variance (2.4). Confidence intervals can be computed on the scale of $S(t)$ as $\hat{S}(t) \pm 1.96\sqrt{\text{var}[\hat{S}(t)]}$ where $\text{var}[\hat{S}(t)] \approx \hat{S}^2(t)\text{var}[\hat{\Lambda}(t)]$. (We call this the *plain* scale.) They have also been suggested on the log–survival (cumulative hazard), log–log, and logit scales. Several authors have examined the choices with somewhat different conclusions. The one certain and common thread in the reports is the marked inferiority of the plain scale: it results in intervals that may extend below 0 or above 1, and has poor coverage properties. Anderson et al. [6] prefer the logit over the log–log transform; they do not consider using a log transform, however. Link [90, 91] considers confidence intervals for the baseline survival function after a Cox model, and finds the log transform to be superior to either the logit or log–log, with the latter giving conservative estimates. These are for the Breslow estimate only, however. Klein [75] shows that for estimating the cumulative hazard the Aalen variance is superior, but for estimating the survival the Greenwood variance is preferred. He does not consider any transformations. We would suggest the Kaplan–Meier, Greenwood variance, and either a log or logit transform for survival, and the Nelson–Aalen, Aalen variance, and log transform for cumulative hazard. Actually, as long as one avoids the "plain" intervals, all of the options work well.

The following SAS code generates Kaplan–Meier curves for the two treatment arms of the PBC data set, first using the `lifetest` procedure and then the `%surv` macro; the macro contains several extra options that we find useful. Neither of these supports the Breslow estimator, but this is no great deficiency. The `cl=7` option of `%surv` specifies a logit scale for computation of the confidence intervals; `lifetest` supports only the plain scale.

```
proc lifetest data=pbc plots=(s);
    time  hours * status(0);
    strata group;

%surv(time=hours, event=status, class=group, plottype=4, cl=7);
```

In summary, it is worth remembering that the differences among the survival estimators are small, except for very small n or a large number of ties. Small n usually occurs at the tail of a survival curve, where the confidence bands are huge anyway. As to ties, the Kaplan–Meier estimator is invariant to ties created by grouping the data, but the Breslow estimate may be improved by using the jittered calculation of Fleming and Harrington if the number of ties is large. There really is no reason not to use the Kaplan–Meier for ordinary data analysis. Hazard-based methods such as the Breslow estimate, however, can be easily extended to more complicated situations, for example, baseline survival curves after a Cox model, and play an important role later in the book.

2.2 Counting processes and martingales

This section provides a gentle introduction to counting processes and the martingale theory used to analyze them. To keep things simple, we focus on failure time data from a single sample. We introduce the reader to *martingales, submartingales, histories, compensators, the Doob–Meyer decomposition, predictable* and *quadratic variation processes, martingale transforms,* and the *martingale central limit theorem.* We emphasize concepts, not proofs or regularity conditions.

We are particularly interested in those parts of the theory that are useful for the analysis of data. The centerpiece of this chapter is the Nelson–Aalen nonparametric estimator of the cumulative hazard function. It is a beautiful example of martingale theory in action. Simple martingale concepts will allow a more careful look at some ideas presented above: justification for variance estimators and confidence limits, handling of ties, and comparison to parametric models.

2.2.1 Modeling the counting process

In order to develop a statistical model, we need to specify the information on which it is based. For counting process data this is done by specifying the *history*, often called the *filtration*, denoted $\{\mathcal{F}_t; t \geq 0\}$. A natural choice is to let $\mathcal{F}_t$ denote the history of the experiment up to and including time t. This time is not necessarily calendar or "wall clock" time. Instead, we realign the counting and risk processes to have a common origin, using a time scale appropriate to the data at hand.

In the data of our example the most natural scale is "running time since installation": all fans start at t = 0 and accumulate runtime (when turned on) from that point forward, Thus two fans, one put in service at noon on February 3, 1965 and failing at 3 PM, February 10, 1967 after running for 10,000 hours and the other put in service at noon on February 3, 1961 and failing at noon on February 3, 1964 after running 10,000 hours have simultaneous failures in the failure time scale. $\mathcal{F}_t$ contains all the information available to an observer who has been watching each fan from the time it was put in service until it has run for t hours. This would include any fan failures or censorings in $[0, t]$. Generally, $\mathcal{F}_t$ denotes the history of the N_is and any auxiliary processes, such as at risk processes Y_i and, when available, covariate processes X_i. The covariates may be vector-valued and must be predictable on the failure time scale.

Using the notation of σ-algebras, this is often written

$$\mathcal{F}_t = \sigma(N_i(s), Y_i(s+), X_i(s);\ i = 1, \ldots, n;\ 0 \leq s \leq t).$$

For $s \leq t$, $\mathcal{F}_s \subseteq \mathcal{F}_t$, reflecting the increase in information with the passage of time.

To specify the model for our example in terms of this history, let $dN_i(t)$ denote the increment in N_i over the infinitesimal time interval $[t, t + dt)$. Note that $\mathcal{F}_{t-}$ contains all the information on $[0, t)$. Then, we have:

$$\mathcal{E}(dN_i(t)|\mathcal{F}_{t-}) = Y_i(t)\lambda(t)dt. \tag{2.8}$$

To justify this equation, note that $dN_i(t)$ can be only 1 or 0, so

$$\mathcal{E}(dN_i(t)|\mathcal{F}_{t-}) = \Pr(dN_i(t) = 1|\mathcal{F}_{t-}).$$

Because the generators are independent, the only component of the history relevant to $dN_i(t)$ is the history of fan i. In turn, the only relevant part of its history is its status at $t-$, $Y_i(t)$. Therefore, $\Pr(dN_i(t) = 1|\mathcal{F}_{t-}) =$

$\Pr(dN_i(t) = 1|Y_i(t))$. If $Y_i(t) = 0$, then either the fan has already failed or is no longer under observation, and $dN_i(t) = 0$ with probability 1. If $Y_i(t) = 1$, the fan is at risk to fail, and

$$\Pr(dN_i(t) = 1|Y_i(t) = 1) = \Pr(t \le T_i^* < t + dt | t \le T_i^*, t \le C_i^*). \tag{2.9}$$

The independence of T_i^* and C_i^* means that

$$\begin{aligned} \Pr(t \le T_i^* < t + dt | t \le T_i^*, t \le C_i^*) &= \Pr(t \le T_i^* < t + dt | t \le T_i^*) \\ &= \lambda(t)dt \end{aligned}$$

by the definition of hazard. We can easily combine these two possibilities into one equation:

$$\Pr(dN_i(t) = 1|Y_i(t)) = Y_i(t)\lambda(t)dt,$$

thus obtaining equation (2.8).

2.2.2 *Martingale basics*

The statistical properties of the Nelson–Aalen estimator can be derived immediately from elementary martingale theory, which we now present. Consider the process

$$M_i(t) = N_i(t) - \int_0^t Y_i(s)\lambda(s)ds, \tag{2.10}$$

which is a counting process martingale wrt the history given above. A martingale wrt a filtration $\{\mathcal{F}_t\}$ is a stochastic process that, in addition to some technical conditions, including right-continuous sample paths with left-hand limits, possesses the key martingale property: for any $t > 0$,

$$\mathcal{E}(dM(t)|\mathcal{F}_{t-}) = 0. \tag{2.11}$$

Equivalently, for any $0 \le s < t$,

$$\mathcal{E}(M(t)|\mathcal{F}_s) = M(s) \tag{2.12}$$

which implies,

$$\mathcal{E}(M(t)|M(u); 0 \le u \le s) = M(s).$$

Thus, a martingale is a process *without drift.* Conditional on its past, the best prediction of any future value is its current value. The simplest martingale is the discrete-time symmetric random walk, the cumulative sum of mean zero iid random variables. General martingales retain two of its properties.

1. Martingale increments have mean 0 (cf. equations (2.11) and (2.12)) and thus any martingale has a constant mean. A counting process martingale is 0 at time 0 (there are no observed events until one is at risk) and therefore is a mean 0 martingale.

2. Martingale increments are uncorrelated, although not necessarily independent. For $t, u, s > 0$,

$$\begin{aligned} \text{Cov}[M(t), M(t+u) - M(t)] &= 0 \\ \text{Cov}[M(t) - M(t-s), M(t+u) - M(t)] &= 0. \end{aligned}$$

According to the *Doob–Meyer decomposition* theorem, any counting process may be uniquely decomposed as the sum of a martingale and a predictable, right-continuous process, 0 at time 0, called the *compensator* (assuming certain mathematical conditions, of course, which are true of the counting processes we consider). As an example, equation (2.10) shows that $\int_0^t Y_i(s)\lambda(s)ds$ is a compensator. This process is predictable because the integrand is the product of two predictable processes and right-continuous, in fact continuous, by properties of integrals. The fan data are a very simple situation. With more complex data, unit-specific covariates are available and they may change over time. A unit may experience multiple events. However, the compensator frequently retains the form suggested by equation (2.8) and one can write

$$N_i(t) = M_i(t) + \int_0^t Y_i(s)\lambda_i(s)ds,$$

where $\lambda_i(s)$ may be a complicated function of time and covariates. In actual applications, λ_i will encode the model that we are currently entertaining for the data.

The decomposition: counting process = compensator + martingale is analogous to the statistical decomposition: data = model + noise or, more to the point since we are dealing with counts, observed count = expected count + error. If we denote the process $\int_0^t Y_i(s)\lambda_i(s)ds$ by $E_i(t)$ for "expected," the counting process Doob–Meyer decomposition becomes simply:

$$N_i(t) = E_i(t) + M_i(t). \tag{2.13}$$

This analogy has been very fruitful, as we show, particularly in motivating residuals and related diagnostics. But one must use care: the analogy is not as strict as one might like. The compensator is predictable, but unlike the usual model, need not be deterministic. In the statistical decomposition, we have $\mathcal{E}(\text{data})$ = model, but with the Doob–Meyer decomposition, we have only $\mathcal{E}(\text{counting process}) = \mathcal{E}(\text{compensator})$. Like noise, the martingale has mean zero, but a noise process has zero autocorrelation and constant variance, whereas a martingale has positive autocorrelation

$\text{Cov}[M(t+s), M(t)] = \text{Var}[M(t)]$ and increasing variance. The decomposition of counting process differentials

$$dN_i(t) = dE_i(t) + dM_i(t)$$

gives a better analogy to the statistical decomposition. Given $\mathcal{F}_{t-}$, the differential $dE_i(t) = Y_i(t)\lambda_i(t)dt$ is deterministic and therefore independent of $dM_i(t)$, and the $dM_i(t)$ are mean 0 and uncorrelated, but not necessarily of equal variance. Unfortunately, differentials are more difficult to work with in practice.

If we replace "=" in equations (2.11) and (2.12) with"$\geq$", the resulting process is a *submartingale*, e.g., a gambling process in which the winnings generally *increase* over time. (Perhaps *sub*martingale would refer to a casino's view of the process.) Of course, a counting process is a submartingale. It is strictly monotone, but a general submartingale need not be; even in a biased game the gambler does not always win. Since M has mean 0, the variance of M is $\mathcal{E}(M^2)$. By Jensen's inequality, M^2 is a submartingale; it has the same history $\mathcal{F}_t$ as M. The Doob–Meyer decomposition applies to submartingales: M^2 can be uniquely decomposed into a compensator and a martingale. The martingale portion must be 0 at time 0 (winnings are identically 0 just before the game starts, and thus of variance 0), and so is a mean 0 martingale. The compensator is called the *predictable variation* process and is usually written with angle brackets $\langle M, M\rangle(t)$ or, more compactly, $\langle M\rangle(t)$. It is the limit in probability of $\sum_i \mathcal{E}[\{M(t_{i+1}) - M(t_i)]^2\}|\mathcal{F}_{t_i}] = \sum_i \text{Var}[\{M(t_{i+1}) - M(t_i)\}|\mathcal{F}_{t_i}]$ over increasingly fine partitions of the interval $[0,t]$, $0 = t_0 < t_1 < \cdots < t_n = t$. In differential notation, we get:

$$d\langle M\rangle(t) = \text{var}(dM(t)|\mathcal{F}_{t-}).$$

For a counting process martingale,

$$d\langle M\rangle(t) = \text{var}(dN(t) - Y(t)\lambda(t)dt|\mathcal{F}_{t-}).$$

Given $\mathcal{F}_{t-}$, $dN(t)$ is a Poisson random variable with mean and variance $Y(t)\lambda(t)dt$ so

$$\langle M\rangle(t) = \int_0^t Y(s)\lambda(s)ds = E(t);$$

that is, the predictable variation for a counting process martingale equals the compensator for the counting process. Counting processes behave locally, and often globally, like Poisson processes with time-varying rate functions.

The *quadratic variation* (also called *optional variation*) process, a related but simpler process, is the limit in probability of $\sum\{M(t_{i+1})-M(t_i)\}^2$ over increasingly fine partitions of the interval $[0,t]$. It is denoted $[M](t)$ and often called the square brackets process. Like $\langle M\rangle$, it is right-continuous, and has the property that $M^2-[M]$ is a martingale, so that it is an unbiased estimator of the variance of a mean 0 martingale. When M has continuous sample paths, $[M] = \langle M \rangle$. When M is not continuous, the usual case in this book except for Brownian motion [4, p. 69],

$$[M](t) = \sum_{s \le t} \Delta M(s)^2$$

where $\Delta M(s) = M(s) - M(s-)$, so [M](t) is the sum of squares of jump heights. Therefore, a counting process martingale with an absolutely continuous compensator has $[M] = N$, since it jumps only when the counting process jumps, and by definition, the jumps are size 1 [4, p. 74]. In this case, $[M]$ is a submartingale with $\langle M \rangle$ as its compensator. It is, essentially, the observed information while $\langle M \rangle$ is the expected information. For a counting process (or any mean 0) martingale

$$\text{Var}\{M(t)\} = \mathcal{E}\{\langle M \rangle(t)\} = \mathcal{E}\{[M](t)\} = \mathcal{E}\{E(t)\}.$$

Because martingale increments are uncorrelated,

$$\text{cov}(\text{M}(\text{t}), \text{M}(\text{s})) = \text{Var}\{\text{M}(\text{t} \wedge \text{s})\}.$$

There are two other useful ways of creating martingales, in addition to the submartingale minus compensator that produces counting process martingales.

1. Consider a collection of n martingales with respect to a common filtration $\{\mathcal{F}_t, t \ge 0\}$. Then, $\overline{M}(t) = \sum_i M_i(t)$ is a martingale wrt $\{\mathcal{F}_t, t \ge 0\}$. The variance process for $\overline{M}$ depends on the covariation among these martingales. The product $M_i M_j$ is the difference of two submartingales:

$$M_i M_j = (1/4)[(M_i + M_j)^2 - (M_i - M_j)^2].$$

   Therefore, it has a compensator $\langle M_i, M_j \rangle$, the *predictable covariation* process, the limit over increasingly finer partitions of $[0, t]$ of $\sum \text{cov}[\{\text{M}_\text{i}(\text{t}_{\text{i}+1}) - \text{M}_\text{i}(\text{t}_\text{i})\}, \{\text{M}_\text{j}(\text{t}_{\text{i}+1}) - \text{M}_\text{j}(\text{t}_\text{i})\} | \mathcal{F}_{\text{t}_\text{i}}]$. If $\langle M_i, M_j \rangle = 0 \; \forall t$, then M_i and M_j are called *orthogonal* martingales. This means that the product $M_i M_j$ is a martingale. For counting process martingales, $\mathcal{E}\{\langle M_i, M_j \rangle\} = \text{cov}(\text{M}_\text{i}, \text{M}_\text{j})$ so orthogonal counting process martingales are uncorrelated. There is also the *optional covariation* process $[M_i, M_j]$, the limit of $\sum[\{M_i(t_{i+1}) - M_i(t_i)\}\{M_j(t_{i+1}) - M_j(t_i)\}]$. If the martingales are continuous, $[M_i, M_j] = \langle M_i, M_j \rangle$; otherwise

$$[M_i, M_j](t) = \sum_{s \le t} \Delta M_i(s) \Delta M_j(s).$$

   $\langle M_i, M_j \rangle$ is the compensator of $[M_i, M_j]$. This leads to the useful result that if two counting process martingales on a common filtration have no simultaneous jumps, they are orthogonal. No simultaneous jumps means $[M_i, M_j] = 0$ which forces $\langle M_i, M_j \rangle = 0$. This can lead to some rather surprising situations: strongly dependent counting processes can have uncorrelated martingales. Consider two machine components where A has a failure time distribution with hazard $\lambda(t)$ and component B keeps working as long as A is operative, but fails precisely 10 minutes after A fails. Assume no censoring. Although counting process B is a deterministic function of counting process A, the components cannot fail simultaneously, so the two martingales are orthogonal. This example is purposely extreme; the compensator of A is the usual $\int_0^t Y_A(s)\lambda(s)ds$ but the compensator for B is $N_A(t+10) = N_B(t)$! So the martingale for B is identically 0 and thus orthogonal to anything. As one would expect, independent counting processes have orthogonal counting process martingales.

The predictable and quadratic variation processes for $\overline{M}$ depend on the predictable and optional covariation processes of the summand martingales:

$$
\begin{aligned}
\langle \overline{M} \rangle (t) &= \sum_i \sum_j \int_0^t d\langle M_i, M_j \rangle (s) \\
[\overline{M}](t) &= \sum_i \sum_j \int_0^t d[M_i, M_j](s)
\end{aligned}
$$

[50, Theorem 2.4.5, p. 73]. $\text{Var}\overline{M}(t) = \mathcal{E}\{\langle \overline{M} \rangle (t)\} = \mathcal{E}\{[\overline{M}](t)\}$. The above formulae are just martingale versions of the familiar fact that the variance of a sum is the sum of the covariances of all possible pairs of summands. If the M_is are orthogonal counting process martingales, then $\langle M_i, M_j \rangle = [M_i, M_j] = 0$ and

$$
\begin{aligned}
\langle \overline{M} \rangle (t) &= \sum_i \langle M_i \rangle (t) \\
[\overline{M}](t) &= \sum_i [M_i](t).
\end{aligned}
$$

These are martingale versions of an even more familiar result: the variance of a sum of uncorrelated random variables is the sum of the variances. Independent martingales will of course be uncorrelated.

2. If M is a mean 0 martingale wrt a filtration and H is a predictable process wrt to the same filtration and is sufficiently well behaved (being bounded is sufficient), then the martingale transform $U(t) = \int_0^t H(s)dM(s)$ is also a mean zero martingale. It is easy to prove using equation (2.11):

$$
E[dU(t)|\mathcal{F}_{t-}] = E[H(t)dM(t)|\mathcal{F}_{t-}]
$$

$$
\begin{aligned}
&= H(t)E[dM(t)|\mathcal{F}_{t-}] \\
&= H(t)\,0 = 0\,.
\end{aligned}
$$

Since H is predictable it is contained in the σ-algebra defined by $\mathcal{F}_{t-}$, and can be factored out of the expectation. This famous theorem is sometimes called the *gambler's ruin*: any betting strategy that does not look into the future (a predictable process) will not change the expected value of the game. Of course in the casino's case the gambler is facing a martingale M describing a fair random variation process plus a compensator T (for *tax*) representing the house's advantage. (T is how much the casino would have to refund you, for each chip purchased, to make it a fair game.) The gambler's losses will be $\int H(t)[dM(t)+dT]$: the first part has expectation 0 no matter how he or she bets.

One can show that the predictable and quadratic variation processes for U are simple transforms of those for M:

$$
\begin{aligned}
\langle U\rangle(t) &= \int_0^t H^2(s)\,d\langle M\rangle(s) \\
[U](t) &= \int_0^t H^2(s)\,d[M](s).
\end{aligned}
$$

If M is a counting process martingale, these can be written in terms of the compensator and counting process for M, respectively: $M(t) = N(t) - \int_0^t Y(s)\lambda(s)ds$; then

$$
\begin{aligned}
\langle U\rangle(t) &= \int_0^t H^2(s)Y(s)\lambda(s)ds \\
[U](t) &= \int_0^t H^2(s)dN(s).
\end{aligned}
$$

One can combine addition and transformation. If M_i, $i = 1,\ldots,n$ is a collection of martingales with respect to a common filtration $\{\mathcal{F}_t, t \geq 0\}$ and $H_i, i = 1,\ldots,n$ is a collection of bounded processes wrt to $\{\mathcal{F}_t, t \geq 0\}$, then $\sum_i \int H_i dM_i$ is a martingale wrt to that filtration. The utility of this simple result can not be overstated. Almost all of the estimators and test statistics used in the study of censored data can be written as some (suitably transformed) predictable process H, with respect to the martingale formed by the observed event data $dN(t)$ and compensator based on the fitted model for λ. Since

$$
\begin{aligned}
\left\langle \int_0^t H_i(s)dM_i(s), \int_0^t H_j(s)dM_j(s) \right\rangle &= \int_0^t H_i(s)H_j(s)d\langle M_i, M_j\rangle \\
\left[\int_0^t H_i(s)dM_i(s), \int_0^t H_j(s)dM_j(s) \right] &= \int_0^t H_i(s)H_j(s)d[M_i, M_j]
\end{aligned}
$$

[4, p.71–72], martingale transforms of orthogonal martingales are orthogonal. Using the martingale central limit theorem for orthogonal martingales below, statistical properties of the estimators are immediate.

Under regularity conditions, suitably normalized sums of orthogonal martingales converge weakly to time-transformed Brownian motion $W^*(t)$ as the number of summand martingales increases, where

1. $W^*(t)$ has continuous sample paths;
2. $W^*(0) = 0$
3. $\mathcal{E}\{W^*(t)\} = 0 \; \forall t$;
4. independent increments: $W^*(t) - W^*(u)$ is independent of $W^*(u)$ for any $0 \leq u \leq t$; and
5. Gaussian process: for any positive integer n and time points $t_1, \ldots, t_n$, the joint distribution of $\{W^*(t_1), W^*(t_2), \ldots, W^*(t_n)\}$ is multivariate normal.

See Fleming and Harrington [50, p. 203]. For standard Brownian motion, $\text{Var}[W(t)] = t$. Time–transformed Brownian motion generalizes the variance function: $\text{Var}[W^*(t)] = \alpha(t)$, where $\alpha(t)$ is an absolutely continuous, nonnegative, nondecreasing function, 0 at $t = 0$. Because of independent increments, for $t_1, t_2 > 0$,

$$\text{Cov}[W^*(t_1), W^*(t_2)] = \alpha(t_1 \wedge t_2),$$

where $x \wedge y = \min(x, y)$. In fact, $W^*(t)$ is often written $W(\alpha(t))$. In the transformed time scale where time is measured in $\alpha(t)$ units, $W(\alpha)$ is standard Brownian motion, hence the name "time–transformed Brownian motion." It is a martingale. Unlike counting process martingales, its predictable and quadratic variation processes are identical and deterministic, $\alpha(t)$.

Let $U^{(n)}(t) = \sum_{i=1}^{n} \int_0^t H_i^{(n)}(s) dM_i^{(n)}(s)$, a sum of n orthogonal martingale transforms, where as in Fleming and Harrington [50, p. 201], the notation indicates the dependence on sample size n. Then under regularity conditions which essentially entail that

1. the jumps of $U^{(n)}$ become negligible as n increases, so that the sample paths become continuous and
2. the variation processes become deterministic. Mathematically, this translates as either

   (a)

$$\langle U^{(n)} \rangle(t) = \sum_i \int_0^t \{H_i^{(n)}\}^2(s) d\langle M_i^{(n)} \rangle(s) \xrightarrow{P} \alpha(t),$$

or (b)

$$[U^{(n)}](t) = \sum_i \int_0^t \{H_i^{(n)}\}^2(s) d[M_i^{(n)}](s) \xrightarrow{P} \alpha(t);$$

then, both 2(a) and 2(b) hold and $U^{(n)}$ converges weakly to $W(\alpha)$.

Weak convergence has a highly technical definition (see Appendix B in Fleming and Harrington [50]), but, for practical purposes, it means the following.

1. Any finite-dimensional distribution of the U^n process converges to a multivariate mean 0 normal distribution with variance matrix given by the appropriate values of $\alpha(t)$. For example, for any time point $t > 0$, $U^n(t)$ converges in distribution to $N(0, \alpha(t))$ and for any two points $t_1, t_2 > 0$, the vector $\{U^n(t_1), U^n(t_2)\}$ converges in distribution to a bivariate normal with mean $\{0, 0\}$ and variance matrix

$$\begin{bmatrix} \alpha(t_1) & \alpha(t_1 \wedge t_2) \\ \alpha(t_1 \wedge t_2) & \alpha(t_2) \end{bmatrix}.$$

2. Sample path properties converge; that is, the path of U^n on $[0, \tau]$ has approximately the same distribution as the path of a particle undergoing time-transformed Brownian motion, as in Billingsley [16, pp.4–5]. The continuous mapping theorem [50, p. 332] says that for bounded, continuous functionals f, $f\{U^n(s) : 0 \le s \le \tau\}$ converges in distribution to $f\{W^*(s) : 0 \le s \le \tau\}$. For example, $\sup_{0 \le s \le \tau} U^n(s) \xrightarrow{\mathcal{D}} \sup_{0 \le s \le \tau} W^*(s)$ and $\int_0^t U^n(s) ds \xrightarrow{\mathcal{D}} \int_0^t W^*(s) ds$ for $t \in (0, \tau)$.

2.3 Properties of the Nelson–Aalen estimator

2.3.1 Counting process results

The properties of the Nelson–Aalen estimator follow from the fact that $\hat{\Lambda}(t) - \Lambda(t)$ is very nearly a martingale. The "very nearly" comes from its nonparametric nature; the estimator at t is not defined if one runs out of data (no subjects left in the study) before the prespecified time t. This motivates the two usual regularity conditions for asymptotic results.

1. Over the chosen time interval $[0, \tau)$ for which results are desired, there will be subjects available. More formally, as n goes to infinity the proportion at risk converges uniformly to a strictly positive function of time denoted $\pi(s)$:

$$\sup_{s \in [0,\tau]} |\overline{Y}(s)/n - \pi(s)| \xrightarrow{P} 0, \qquad \inf_{s \in [0,t)} \pi(s) > 0.$$

2. The integrated hazard is finite, $\int_0^\tau \lambda(s)ds < \infty$.

For finite sample results, we use a truncated estimate, up to the point of losing our last subject. Let $J(s) = I\{\overline{Y}(s) > 0\}$, the indicator process for at least one observation still at risk. Let $\Lambda^*(t) = \int_0^t J(s)\lambda(s)ds$ and define $J(s)/\overline{Y}(s)$ as 0 whenever $J(s) = \overline{Y}(s) = 0$. Then,

$$\hat{\Lambda}(t) - \Lambda(t) = \hat{\Lambda}(t) - \Lambda^*(t) + \Lambda^*(t) - \Lambda(t). \tag{2.14}$$

With this notation, $\hat{\Lambda}(t) = \int_0^t J(s)d\overline{N}(s)/\overline{Y}(s)$ and is really estimating $\Lambda^*(t)$ rather than $\Lambda(t)$. In fact it is easy to show that $\hat{\Lambda}(t) - \Lambda^*(t)$ is a mean 0 martingale.

$$\begin{aligned}\hat{\Lambda}(t) - \Lambda^*(t) &= \int_0^t \frac{J(s)}{\overline{Y}(s)}(d\overline{N}(s) - \overline{Y}(s)\lambda(s)ds) \\ &= \int_0^t H(s)dM(s),\end{aligned}$$

where $H(s) = J(s)/\overline{Y}(s)$, a bounded predictable process, and $M(s) = \overline{N}(s) - \int_0^s \overline{Y}(u)\lambda(u)du$, a counting process martingale. So, $\hat{\Lambda}(t) - \Lambda^*(t)$ is a mean 0 martingale transform and thus a mean 0 martingale.

As an estimate of $\Lambda(t)$, $\hat{\Lambda}(t)$ will of course be slightly biased in the right tail: if the data run out before time t then $\hat{\Lambda}(t)$ remains constant at the value it had achieved when the last subject "left" observation, whereas $\Lambda(t)$ in the true population is presumably still increasing. This bias is asymptotically negligible for $t < \tau$, and practically negligible for any part of the curve where the confidence bands are less than outrageously wide. From equation (2.14) and the martigale results

$$\begin{aligned}E[\hat{\Lambda}(t) - \Lambda(t)] &= E[\Lambda^*(t) - \Lambda(t)] \\ &= -\int_0^t \Pr(\overline{Y}(s) = 0)\lambda(s)ds \\ &\rightarrow 0.\end{aligned}$$

The convergence is usually exponential because typically, $\Pr(\overline{Y}(s) = 0) = O(e^{-n})$.

The variance $E[\hat{\Lambda}(t) - E\{\hat{\Lambda}(t)\}]^2$ is asymptotically equivalent to that of the martingale $\hat{\Lambda}(t) - \Lambda^*(t)$, which has predictable variation process

$$\begin{aligned}\langle \hat{\Lambda} - \Lambda^* \rangle(t) &= \int_0^t H^2(s)d\langle M \rangle(ns) \\ &= \int_0^t \lambda(s)/\overline{Y}(s)ds,\end{aligned}$$

so the variance is asymptotically $E[\int_0^t \lambda(s)/\overline{Y}(s)ds]$, which requires knowledge of the censoring process for its computation. It can be consistently estimated, however, by the quadratic variation process:

$$[\hat{\Lambda} - \Lambda^*](t) = \int_0^t H^2(s) d[M](s) = \int_0^t d\overline{N}(s)/\overline{Y}^2(s) ds \,, \tag{2.15}$$

which is the Nelson–Aalen variance estimate given earlier (2.4), and justified at that point by an ad hoc Poisson argument.

One could also estimate the integrated hazard by $-\log[\hat{S}_{KM}(t)]$, which, as we have seen, is asymptotically equivalent to the Nelson–Aalen estimator and slightly larger in finite samples. It has a consistent variance estimator given by the well-known Greenwood formula [36, pp. 50–51],

$$\widehat{\text{Var}}\{-\log[\hat{S}_{KM}(t)]\} = \int_0^t \frac{d\overline{N}(s)}{\overline{Y}(s)[\overline{Y}(s) - \Delta\overline{N}(s)]}. \tag{2.16}$$

This is slightly larger than the Nelson–Aalen variance estimator in keeping with the larger size of the cumulative hazard estimator. In finite samples, however, the logarithm of the Kaplan–Meier is not a good estimate of the hazard in the tails. In particular, if the last subject in the study dies, the estimator is infinite.

The properties of the estimate then follow directly from the general martingale results. The Nelson–Aalen estimator is uniformly consistent [4, Theorem IV.1.1]; for any $t < \tau$:

$$\sup_{s \in [0,t]} |\hat{\Lambda}(s) - \Lambda(s)| \xrightarrow{P} 0.$$

The variance estimator is also uniformly consistent:

$$\sup_{s \in [0,t]} \left| \int_0^s n d\overline{N}(s)/\overline{Y}^2(s) - \int_0^s \lambda(s)/\pi(s) ds \right| \xrightarrow{P} 0.$$

Under an additional regularity condition that assures that the jumps are becoming negligible [4, Condition B, Theorem IV.1.2], the martingale central limit theorem applies and

$$\sqrt{n}\{\hat{\Lambda}(s) - \Lambda(s)\} \overset{n \to \infty}{\Longrightarrow} W(\alpha(s)) \quad \text{on } [0, \tau], \tag{2.17}$$

where

$$\alpha(t) = \int_0^t \lambda(s)/\pi(s) ds. \tag{2.18}$$

2.3.2 *Efficiency*

Nonparametric methods are less efficient than parametric methods, sometimes substantially so. For purposes of comparison, Figure 2.5 shows the

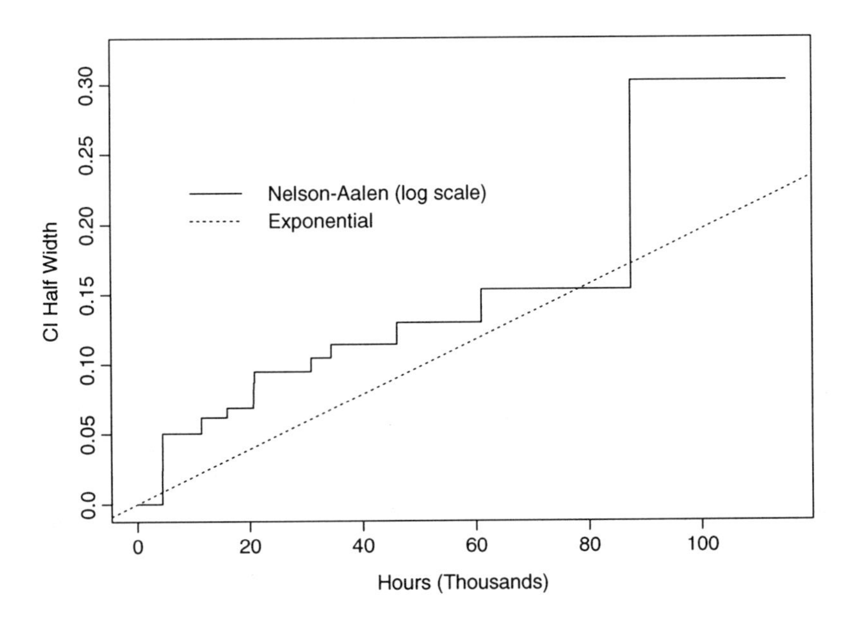

FIGURE 2.5: *Comparison of confidence interval widths*

half-widths of the Nelson–Aalen confidence intervals along with that for the simplest parametric model, exponential failure time. The confidence interval for the parametric estimate is based on the likelihood ratio test using the approximation suggested in Cox and Oakes [36, p. 38]: let $d = \sum_i \delta_i$, the number of failures. Then, $2d\lambda/(\hat{\lambda})$ is distributed approximately as chi-squared on $2d$ degrees of freedom and a $100 \times (1 - \alpha)$ confidence interval for the integrated hazard λt is

$$\frac{\hat{\lambda} t c^*_{2d,1-\alpha/2}}{2d} < \lambda t < \frac{\hat{\lambda} t c^*_{2d,\alpha/2}}{2d},$$

where $c^*_{p,\alpha}$ is the upper α point of the chi-squared distribution with p degrees of freedom. Over much of the range, the confidence intervals for the Nelson–Aalen are about 1.8 times as wide.

We can compute the asymptotic relative efficiency (ARE) in closed form for a simple case. Suppose T^* and C^*, the true survival and censoring times, are distributed exponentially with parameters λ and γ, respectively. Then the observed time $T = T^* \wedge C^*$ is exponential with parameter $\lambda + \gamma$, and $\pi(t) = e^{-(\lambda+\gamma)t}$ is the expected proportion of subjects still at risk at time t. Applying equations (2.17) and (2.18), the scaled Aalen estimate $\sqrt{n}[\hat{\Lambda}_a(t) - \Lambda(t)]$ has asymptotic variance

$$\alpha(t) = \frac{\lambda\{\exp[(\lambda + \gamma)t] - 1\}}{\lambda + \gamma}.$$

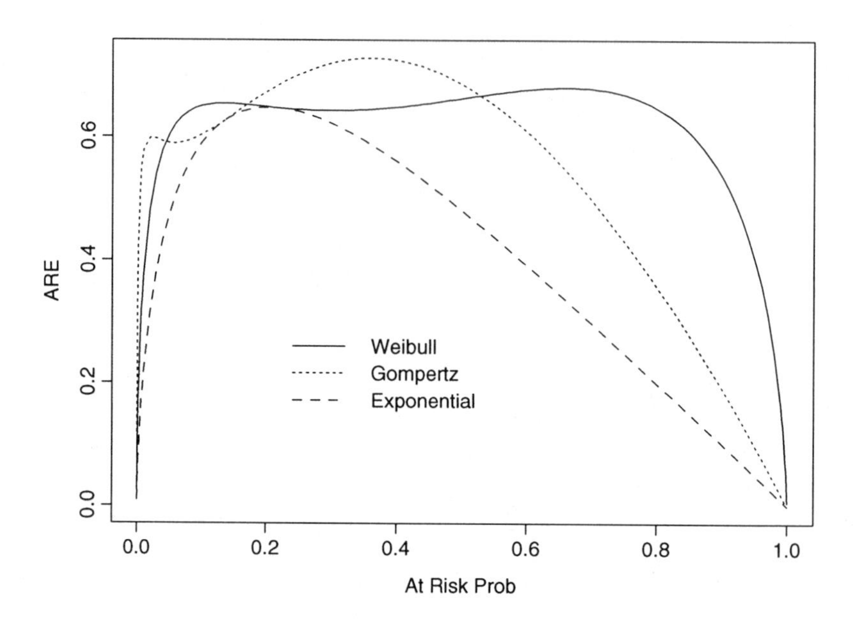

FIGURE 2.6: *Asymptotic relative efficiency when both failure and censoring are exponential*

The scaled parametric estimate $\sqrt{n}(\hat{\Lambda}_p - \Lambda) = \sqrt{n}(\hat{\lambda} - \lambda)t$ has asymptotic variance $t^2/E[-\ddot{\ell}] = t^2\lambda(\lambda + \gamma)$, where $\ell(\lambda) = \delta_i \log(\lambda) - \lambda T_i$ the loglikelihood for a single observation, $\dot{\ell}$ and $\ddot{\ell}$ are the first and second derivatives wrt λ, and $E[-\ddot{\ell}]$ is the Fisher (expected) information. The ARE is the ratio of the asymptotic variances:

$$\text{ARE} = \frac{(\lambda + \gamma)^2 t^2}{\exp[(\lambda + \gamma)t] - 1}.$$

This is identical to the ARE derived by Miller in his paper "What price Kaplan–Meier", for comparing the exponential and non-parametric estimates [104, equation (7)]. Considered as a function of the probability of being at risk, $\pi = \pi(t) = \exp[-(\lambda + \gamma)t]$, the ARE becomes

$$\text{ARE} = \frac{\pi(\log \pi)^2}{1 - \pi},$$

a concave function attaining its maximum of 0.648 at $\pi = 0.203$; see Figure (2.6).

The efficiency is not very impressive; but the poor showing of the non-parametric estimator should not be a surprise. The asymptotic efficiency relative to the exponential model effectively compares the variability in fitted values between a one-parameter and a (# deaths)-parameter model. The Nelson–Aalen estimator does better when compared to the fit from a model with more parameters. We consider two different two parameter distributions: the Weibull, $\lambda(t) = \alpha\lambda^\alpha t^{\alpha-1}$ and the Gompertz, $\lambda(t) = \lambda\exp(\alpha t)$; each reduces to the exponential for particular values of α. Using the same likelihood expansion method

$$\begin{aligned} \text{ARE(Gompertz)} &= \text{ARE(exp)}\{1 + \frac{[(\lambda+\gamma)t - 2]^2}{4}\} \\ \text{ARE(Weibull)} &= \text{ARE(exp)}\{1 + \frac{6\,[1 - c - \log((\lambda+\gamma)t)]^2}{\pi^2}\}, \end{aligned}$$

where c denotes Euler's constant 0.577215.... As with the exponential model, these AREs are functions of the probability of being at risk and so can be superimposed on Figure 2.6. The range over which efficiency $< .5$ has been substantially decreased, but still the ARE barely exceeds 60% over the range of likely values. These efficiencies are comparable to those of some other widely used nonparametric estimators; for (noncensored) Gaussian data, the median has ARE $2/\pi = 0.637$ relative to the sample mean [65], and the MAD and interquartile range both have ARE 0.735, relative to the sample standard deviation [68, Chap. 5, Exhibit 5.7.3].

2.4 Tied data

So far, we have assumed that each event time corresponds to exactly one event, an assumption required by an absolutely continuous integrated hazard function. However, tied event times are the rule rather than the exception; they exist in nearly every data set used in this book.

There are two conceptually different approaches to dealing with ties. The first, which we call the grouped approach, views the presence of tied data as an artifact of the imprecision of real world measurement. Ties happen because of intermittent observation and/or rounded event times. The AML study had both; clinical assessment for remission occurred only at certain times and remission and censoring times are recorded to the nearest week. The failure and censoring times of the generator data were rounded to the nearest hundred hours.

If ties result from imprecision, then the obvious approach is to break the ties randomly, reconstucting, in some sense, what the data "would have been" without the imprecision. If the rounding is small this recovery is essentially perfect. For instance, if followup time is recorded in days and data accuracy is such that an event recorded as day 44 really preceded an event at day 45, then the only issue is breaking ties within a day. The computed result for $\hat\Lambda(t)$ (i.e., cumulative hazard through the end of day t) is invariant to the order in which the ties are broken, and can be written as

$$\hat{\Lambda}_G(t) = \int_0^t \left[\sum_{j=0}^{d\overline{N}(s)-1} \frac{1}{\overline{Y}(s) - j} \right]. \tag{2.19}$$

This is a simple variant on equation (2.1), replacing the term $dN(s)/\overline{Y}(s)$ with a sum of estimated hazards over the broken tie; for example, if there were three events and 10 at risk we have $(1/10 + 1/9 + 1/8)$ instead of $3/10$. This is the estimate described earlier when discussing a modified Breslow estimate of survival; it is implemented in S-Plus using the option `fh2` to `survfit`. The variance formula found in equation (2.4) is similarly modified to use a sum of squared terms:

$$\widehat{\text{Var}}\hat{\Lambda}_G(t) = \int_0^t \sum_{j=0}^{d\overline{N}(s)-1} \frac{1}{[\overline{Y}(s) - j]^2}. \tag{2.20}$$

For three deaths out of 10 at risk, the variance increment will be $(1/100 + 1/81 + 1/64)$ instead of $3/100$. Because we are just "recreating" the results that would have been obtained with the uncoarsened data, the counting process results of Section 2.2 apply directly (e.g., justification for the variance estimate and asymptotic normality).

If the grouping is quite wide (e.g., all deaths in 0–1 year are recorded as "1", 1–2 as "2", etc.) then we may want to make some adjustment to the plotted form of the estimate. The usual plot will have a horizontal line from 1 to 2 years at the 1-year level, a jump to the 2-year estimate, a horizontal line to 3 years, and so on. If we assume that deaths actually occurred throughout the interval, then the horizontal segments, especially near their right-hand ends, are almost surely an *underestimate* of the hazard. (A printed listing, showing only the computed values at 0, 1, ..., doesn't have this problem.)

The second approach to ties is to treat the data as genuinely discrete. Ties are real, not spurious, and we should extend the mathematical model to accomodate them. This extension does introduce changes in the counting process notation and formulae. Discreteness means that, like the estimator $\hat{\Lambda}$, the true cumulative hazard function Λ has jumps. Let $\Delta\Lambda(t) = \Lambda(t) - \Lambda(t-)$ be the jump at the time points with positive probability of an event. Not surprisingly, $\Delta\Lambda(t)$ is the event probability

$$\mathcal{E}(dN_i(t)|\mathcal{F}_{t-}) = Y_i(t)\Delta\Lambda(t); \tag{2.21}$$

cf. equation (2.8). For a purely discrete distribution, Λ is a step function.

Mixtures of discrete and continuous are also possible. Such a distribution could arise, for example, if generator fans were replaced according to a protocol: replace at failure or after 150,000 hours of running time, whichever occurs first. This would produce a discrete atom at 150,000 hours. $\Lambda(t)$

would be strictly increasing with a jump at 150,000 hours, and $\Delta\Lambda(t)$ would be zero at all time points except $t = 150,000$, while $d\Lambda(t)$ (the underlying failure *rate*) would be > 0 at all t. We do not pursue an estimate for the mixed grouped/discrete case, although presumably one could break the "false" ties while keeping the real ones (assuming one knew which was which).

For a discrete or mixed continuous/discrete situation, each counting process $N_i, i = 1, \ldots, n$ has compensator $\int_0^t Y_i(s)d\Lambda(s)$. The counting process martingales $M_i(t) = N_i(t) - \int_0^t Y_i(s)d\Lambda(s)$ have predictable variation processes

$$\langle M_i \rangle(t) = \int_0^t Y_i(s)(1 - \Delta\Lambda(s))d\Lambda(s)$$

[4, p. 74] and [50, p. 80] and quadratic variation processes

$$[M_i](t) = N_i(t) - 2\int_0^t Y_i(s)\Delta\Lambda(s)dN_i(s) + \int_0^t Y_i(s)\Delta\Lambda(s)d\Lambda(s)$$

[4, p. 75]. In this setting $\overline{N}(t)$ is not formally a counting process since jumps can exceed 1, but it is a submartingale. It follows from the Doob–Meyer decomposition or from the summation of independent counting process martingales, that

$$\overline{N}(\cdot) - \int_0^t \overline{Y}(s)d\Lambda(s)$$

is a martingale. A moments argument gives the Nelson–Aalen estimator

$$\hat{\Lambda}_D(t) = \int_0^t d\overline{N}(s)/\overline{Y}(s). \tag{2.22}$$

Andersen et al. point out that for the model with discrete components the Nelson–Aalen estimate is a nonparametric maximum likelihood estimator (see the technical discussion in [4, Section IV.1.5]) rather than merely a method of moments estimator.

As before,

$$\hat{\Lambda}(t) - \Lambda^*(t) = \int_0^t \frac{J(s)}{\overline{Y}(s)}[d\overline{N}(s) - \overline{Y}(s)]d\Lambda(s)$$

so $\hat{\Lambda}_D(t) - \Lambda^*(t)$ is a martingale with

$$\langle \hat{\Lambda}_D - \Lambda^* \rangle(t) = \int_0^t \frac{J(s)}{\overline{Y}(s)}(1 - \Delta\Lambda(s))d\Lambda(s)$$

and

$$[\hat{\Lambda}_D - \Lambda^*](t) = \sum \{\Delta\overline{N}(s)/\overline{Y}(s) - \Delta\Lambda(s)\}^2,$$

where the sum is over time points $s \le t$ such that $\Delta\Lambda(s) > 0$. Note that if $\Delta\Lambda(t)$ is zero for all t (i.e., if there are no discrete data points), then these formulae all reduce to the untied case discussed earlier.

Three consistent and asymptotically equivalent variance estimators have been proposed.

1. The simple "Poisson" variance estimate

$$\hat{\sigma}_s^2 = \int_0^t \frac{d\overline{N}(s)}{\overline{Y}^2(s)}.$$

This comes from the moments argument we have seen before: if one assumes a Poisson model with conditional mean $\overline{Y}(s)\Delta\Lambda(s)$, then each summand $\Delta\overline{N}(s)/\overline{Y}(s)$ has conditional variance $\Delta\Lambda(s)/\overline{Y}(s)$. Estimating $\Delta\Lambda(s)$ by $\Delta\overline{N}(s)/\overline{Y}(s)$ gives $\hat{\sigma}_s^2$ [4, p. 223–225]. Note that this is formally the same as equation (2.15) but has a different derivation in the discrete setting, where it can not be justified as the quadratic variation process.

2. The "plug-in" estimator

$$\hat{\sigma}_p^2 = \int_0^t \frac{\{\overline{Y}(s) - \Delta\overline{N}(s)\}d\overline{N}(s)}{\overline{Y}^3(s)}.$$

This is formed by substituting $d\overline{N}(s)/\overline{Y}(s)$ for $d\Lambda(s)$ and $\Delta\overline{N}(s)/\overline{Y}(s)$ for $\Delta\Lambda(s)$ in the predictable variation formula [4, equation (4.1.7), p. 181].

3. The binomial estimator

$$\hat{\sigma}_b^2 = \int_0^t \frac{\{\overline{Y}(s) - \Delta\overline{N}(s)\}d\overline{N}(s)}{\overline{Y}^2(s)(\overline{Y}(s) - 1)}.$$

In a purely discrete model, conditional on the past, the number of events has a binomial distribution $B(\overline{Y}(s), \overline{Y}(s)\Delta\Lambda(s))$ at any time point. As noted by Fleming and Harrington [50, p. 94], an estimator of the binomial variance, which is *unbiased* for $\overline{Y}(s) > 1$, is

$$\overline{Y}(s)\frac{\sum_i(\Delta N_i(s) - \overline{N}(s)/\overline{Y}(s))^2}{\overline{Y}(s) - 1} = \frac{\Delta\overline{N}(s)(\overline{Y}(s) - \Delta\overline{N}(s))}{(\overline{Y}(s) - 1)}. \quad (2.23)$$

So each summand $\Delta\overline{N}(s)/\overline{Y}(s)$ in $\hat{\Lambda}_D$, except possibly the last, has an unbiased conditional variance estimator which is equation (2.23) divided by $\overline{Y}^2(s)$. Because the summands are asymptotically uncorrelated, $\hat{\sigma}_b^2$ results [50, Theorem 3.2.2].

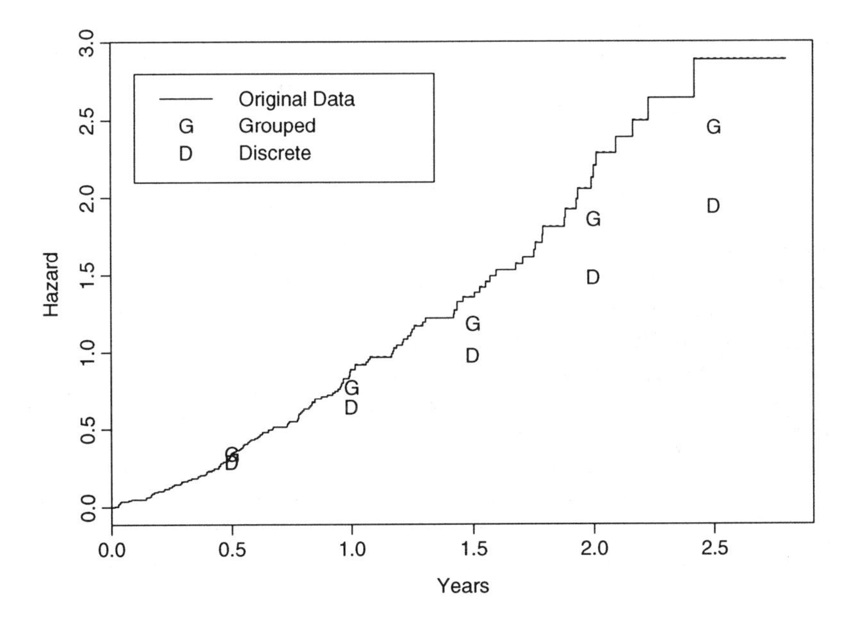

FIGURE 2.7: *Comparison of the cumulative hazards for the lung cancer data, and for grouped versus discrete computations on a coarsened version*

The variance estimators are ordered:

$$\hat{\sigma}^2_p < \hat{\sigma}^2_b \leq \hat{\sigma}^2_s.$$

(If there are no ties, $\hat{\sigma}^2_s$ and $\hat{\sigma}^2_b$ are the same.) All are smaller than Greenwood's estimator, equation (2.16). We are aware of no systematic comparison of these estimators in the presence of ties, but there have been some evaluations of special cases: Klein compared $\hat{\sigma}^2_s$ and $\hat{\sigma}^2_p$ analytically and by simulation for continuous failure time data. He found that for time points such that $\mathrm{E}\overline{Y}(t) \geq 10$, differences between the estimators were negligible:5 $\hat{\sigma}^2_s$ tended to overestimate the true variance, whereas $\hat{\sigma}^2_p$ tended to underestimate it. Andersen et al. [4, p. 182–183] suggested that the issue of the best choice to optimize confidence interval coverage was still open, but that the larger size of σ^2_s meant conservative confidence intervals, an advantage under many circumstances.

In practice, the discrete and grouped estimators of cumulative hazard hardly differ on data sets with modest amounts of ties. Figure 2.7 shows the Nelson–Aalen hazard estimator for the lung cancer data set. For this data set the grouped and discrete estimates are identical almost to the resolution of the figure, even though there are 22 ties and 1 triple in the set of 165 event times. The figure also shows the results of equations (2.22) (discrete) and (2.19) (grouped) when applied to a derived data set where time was recorded only to the nearest half year; that is, all deaths and/or censorings in days 0–182 are relabeled as 182, all those in days 182–365 are relabeled as 365, and so on. By the end of the study a substantial difference has accumulated between the two estimates. (The grouping is coarse enough that a correction for the censored observations is also needed; this is why the grouped estimate falls below the curve in Figure 2.7. In actual data gathered at this granularity, an actuarial estimate of survival would usually be computed; see, for instance, Miller [103, Chapter 3].)

Although they frequently give very similar numerical values, the difference between these two estimators is more fundamental than the difference between the Breslow and Kaplan–Meier estimators of the survival function for untied data. They are *not* two ways of estimating the same thing. If the data truly arise by grouping a set of continuous event times, the discrete approach yields a biased, inconsistent estimate and vice versa.

Suppose the data actually arise from a grouping mechanism and that the grouping intervals of $(0, \tau]$ are $(t_0, t_1], (t_1, t_2], \ldots, (t_{n-1}, t_n]$ with $t_n = \tau$ and $t_0 = 0$. Let t_k be a point of interest, and for simplicity assume no censoring. In this case we can write out the bias for both the discrete and grouped estimators. For the grouped estimate the prior counting process results show that

$$\begin{aligned}
\mathcal{E}\{\hat{\Lambda}_G(t_k)\} &= \mathcal{E}\Lambda^*(t_k) \\
&= \int_0^{t_k} \Pr(\overline{Y}(s) > 0)\lambda(s)ds \\
&= \Lambda(t_k) - \int_0^{t_k} \Pr(\overline{Y}(s) = 0)\lambda(s)ds,
\end{aligned}$$

with

$$\Pr(\overline{Y}(s) = 0) = [1 - \exp(-\Lambda(s))]^n.$$

There is a small negative bias, but only because we may have "run out" of data before time t_k, and the estimator is being extended as a horizontal line from the last datapoint. This probability decreases exponentially with increasing sample size.

For the discrete estimate,

$$\mathcal{E}\hat{\Lambda}_D(t_k) = \sum_{i=1}^{k} \mathcal{E}\left\{\frac{\Delta\overline{N}(t_i)}{\overline{Y}(t_i)}\right\}.$$

Let $\Delta_i = \Lambda(t_i) - \Lambda(t_{i-1})$, the true change in the cumulative hazard between t_i and the prior time point. Given $\overline{Y}(t_i)$, $\Delta\overline{N}(t_i) \sim \text{Bin}(\overline{Y}(t_i), 1 - \exp(-\Delta\Lambda_i))$. So the bias is

$$\mathcal{E}\{\hat{\Lambda}_D(t_k) - \Lambda(t_k)\} = \sum_{i=1}^{k}\{1 - \exp(-\Delta_i) - \Delta_i\}.$$

This is a function only of the grouping, *not* a function of the sample size, and so does not converge to zero. Using the lung cancer data in Figure 2.7 as an example, assume six intervals with each $\Delta_i = .5$ (the ungrouped data have a cumulative hazard of approximately 1 unit/year). Then the expected bias at interval six is $6(1 - \exp(.5) - .5) \approx -.64$. The bias becomes negligible if the grouping of the time axis is sufficiently fine: for 60 steps of size $\Delta_i = .05$ the expected bias is $-.074$; for 600 steps of size .005 it is $-.0075$.

When estimating the integrated hazard for a data set with ties, the analyst should give some thought to the mechanism generating the ties. In our experience, grouping of continuous data is far more common than genuinely discrete data.

3

The Cox Model

3.1 Introduction and notation

The Cox proportional hazards model [35] has become by a wide margin the most used procedure for modeling the relationship of covariates to a survival or other censored outcome.

Let $X_{ij}(t)$ be the jth covariate of the ith person, where $i = 1, \ldots, n$ and $j = 1, \ldots, p$. It is natural to think of the set of covariates as forming an $n \times p$ matrix, and we use X_i to denote the covariate vector for subject i, that is, the ith row of the matrix. When all covariates are *fixed* over time X_i is just a vector of covariate values, familiar from multiple linear regression. For other data sets one or more covariates may vary over time, for example a repeated laboratory test. We use X_i for both time-fixed and time-varying covariate processes, employing $X_i(t)$ when we wish to emphasize the time-varying structure.

The Cox model specifies the hazard for individual i as

$$\lambda_i(t) = \lambda_0(t) e^{X_i(t)\beta}, \tag{3.1}$$

where λ_0 is an unspecified nonnegative function of time called the *baseline hazard*, and β is a $p \times 1$ column vector of coefficients. Event rates cannot be negative (observed deaths can not unhappen), and the exponential thus plays an important role in ensuring that the final estimates are a physical possibility.

Because the hazard ratio for two subjects with fixed covariate vectors X_i and X_j,

$$\frac{\lambda_i(t)}{\lambda_j(t)} = \frac{\lambda_0(t) e^{X_i\beta}}{\lambda_0(t) e^{X_j\beta}} = \frac{e^{X_i\beta}}{e^{X_j\beta}},$$

is constant over time, the model is also known as the *proportional hazards* model.

Estimation of β is based on the partial likelihood function introduced by Cox [35]. For untied failure time data it has the form

$$PL(\beta) = \prod_{i=1}^{n} \prod_{t \geq 0} \left\{ \frac{Y_i(t) r_i(\beta, t)}{\sum_j Y_j(t) r_j(\beta, t)} \right\}^{dN_i(t)}, \tag{3.2}$$

where $r_i(\beta, t)$ is the *risk score* for subject i, $r_i(\beta, t) = \exp[X_i(t)\beta] \equiv r_i(t)$. The log partial likelihood can be written as a sum

$$l(\beta) = \sum_{i=1}^{n} \int_0^{\infty} \left[Y_i(t) r_i(t) - \log\left(\sum_j Y_j(t) r_j(t) \right) \right] dN_i(t), \tag{3.3}$$

from which we can already foresee the counting process structure.

Although the partial likelihood is not, in general, a likelihood in the sense of being proportional to the probability of an observed dataset, nonetheless it can be treated as a likelihood for purposes of asymptotic inference. Differentiating the log partial likelihood with respect to β gives the $p \times 1$ score vector, $U(\beta)$:

$$U(\beta) = \sum_{i=1}^{n} \int_0^{\infty} [X_i(s) - \bar{x}(\beta, s)]\, dN_i(s), \tag{3.4}$$

where $\bar{x}(\beta, s)$ is simply a weighted mean of X, over those observations still at risk at time s,

$$\bar{x}(\beta, s) = \frac{\sum Y_i(s) r_i(s) X_i(s)}{\sum Y_i(s) r_i(s)}, \tag{3.5}$$

with $Y_i(s) r_i(s)$ as the weights.

The negative second derivative is the $p \times p$ information matrix

$$\mathcal{I}(\beta) = \sum_{i=1}^{n} \int_0^{\infty} V(\beta, s) dN_i(s), \tag{3.6}$$

where $V(\beta, s)$ is the weighted variance of X at time s:

$$V(\beta, s) = \frac{\sum_i Y_i(s) r_i(t) [X_i(s) - \bar{x}(\beta, s)]' [X_i(s) - \bar{x}(\beta, s)]}{\sum_i Y_i(s) r_i(s)}. \tag{3.7}$$

The maximum partial likelihood estimator is found by solving the partial likelihood equation:

$$U(\hat{\beta}) = 0.$$

The solution $\hat{\beta}$ is consistent and asymptotically normally distributed with mean β, the true parameter vector, and variance $\{\mathcal{E}\mathcal{I}(\beta)\}^{-1}$, the inverse of the expected information matrix. The expectation requires knowledge of the censoring distribution even for those observations with observed failures; that information is typically nonexistent. The inverse of the observed information matrix $\mathcal{I}^{-1}(\hat\beta)$ is available, has better finite sample properties than the inverse of the expected information, and is used as the variance of $\hat\beta$.

Both SAS and S-Plus use the Newton–Raphson algorithm to solve the partial likelihood equation. Starting with an initial guess $\hat\beta^{(0)}$, the algorithm iteratively computes

$$\hat\beta^{(n+1)} = \hat\beta^{(n)} + \mathcal{I}^{-1}(\hat\beta^{(n)})U(\hat\beta^{(n)}) \tag{3.8}$$

until convergence, as assessed by stability in the log partial likelihood, $l(\hat\beta^{(n+1)}) \approx l(\hat\beta^{(n)})$. This algorithm is incredibly robust for the Cox partial likelihood. Convergence problems are very rare using the default initial value of $\hat\beta^{(0)} = 0$ and easily addressed by simple methods such as step-halving. As a result many packages (e.g., SAS) do not even have an option to choose alternate starting values.

Fitting the Cox model is very easy for the end user with either S-Plus or SAS. The example below is based on the PBC data set, which is used multiple times in the book. The data come from a Mayo Clinic trial in primary biliary cirrhosis of the liver conducted between 1974 and 1984. PBC is a progressive disease thought to be of an autoimmune origin; the subsequent inflammatory process eventually leads to cirrhosis and destruction of the liver's bile ducts and death of the patient. A description of the study along with a listing of the data set can be found in Fleming and Harrington [50]. A more extended discussion can be found in Dickson et al. [40]. The agents in the trial were found not to be effective in prolonging survival. The data were used to develop a model for survival for PBC patients in a "natural history setting." The model has been used for patient counseling, medical decision making (e.g., timing of liver transplantation), and stratification in subsequent clinical trials. Here are the commands from each package to fit a five-variable Cox model to the PBC data.

```
> fit.pbc <- coxph(Surv(futime, status==2) ~ age + edema +
                   log(bili) + log(protime) + log(albumin),
                     data=pbc)
> print(fit.pbc)

                  coef exp(coef) se(coef)      z       p
          age   0.0396    1.0404  0.00767   5.16 2.4e-07
        edema   0.8963    2.4505  0.27141   3.30 9.6e-04
    log(bili)   0.8636    2.3716  0.08294  10.41 0.0e+00
 log(protime)   2.3868   10.8791  0.76851   3.11 1.9e-03
 log(albumin)  -2.5069    0.0815  0.65292  -3.84 1.2e-04

Likelihood ratio test=231  on 5 df, p=0  n=416
    (2 observations deleted due to missing)
```

```
data temp; set pbc;
    lbili = log(bili);
    lpro  = log(protime);
    lalb  = log(albumin);

proc phreg data=temp;
    model futime * status(0 1) = age edema lbili lpro lalb
                                          /ties = efron;
```

(This generates two full pages of SAS output).

The `status` variable records each patient's status at his/her last followup (`futime`), and is coded as 0 = censored, 1 = liver transplant, and 2 = death. The S-Plus code via use of `Surv(futime, status==2)` and the SAS code by use of `status(0 1)` both specify that this is a model of time to death, treating liver transplantation as censoring. (S-Plus expects one to specify the *event* codes, and SAS the *nonevent* codes.) If instead one wished to treat both death and transplantation as a single composite event, "liver death," one would use `Surv(futime, status > 0)` and `futime *status(0)` respectively, in the two packages.

The estimated βs are labeled `coef` in the S-Plus output. Interpretation is clearest for the exponentiated coefficients, provided by the column `exp(coef)`, as this represents the multiplicative change in risk due to each covariate.

- Bilirubin is the most important variable, as evidenced by the large z-statistic, and has been entered using a log transformation due to its skewness (range 0.3–28, median of 1.4). Each 1 point change in log(bilirubin) is associated with a 2.4-fold increase in a patient's risk. The first and third quartiles of bilirubin are 0.8 and 3.4, respectively, which translates into an $\exp[0.864 * (\log(3.4) - \log(0.8))] \sim 3.5$-fold risk ratio for an "average" subject in the top half versus one in the bottom half of the bilirubin distribution.

- Each additional year of age is associated with an estimated 4% increase in risk; an additional decade corresponds to a nearly 50% increase, $\exp(10 * 0.0396) = 1.486$. Ages in the study range from 26 to 78 years, with quartiles at 43 and 58 years of age, so there is an 81% difference in risk between the quartiles. Age is of course strongly confounded with the duration of disease, which is usually not precisely known because of the slow and insidious onset.

- Edema is coded 0 for no edema, 0.5 for moderate, and 1 for severe edema. The estimated risk of death in patients with severe edema is 2.45 times that of patients with no edema, holding other covariates constant, since `exp(coef)` for edema is 2.4505. Patients with moderate edema have an estimated $\exp(.8963 * .5) = 1.57$-fold increase in risk compared to patients without edema. Although the numerical size of the effect is larger than that for age, only 44/418 and 20/418 subjects have moderate and severe edema, respectively.

- The risk accruing for each unit change in log(prothrombin time) is the greatest, 10.9, but the overall impact on study patients is much less than bilirubin or age; the first and third quartiles of `protime` are 10 and 11.1, respectively, corrresponding to a 28% difference in risk.

- Albumin, also fit in the log scale, has a negative estimated coefficient. This necessary substance is manufactured at least in part by the liver and a decrease in blood levels is a marker of dysfunction.

A strength and a weakness of the Cox model, or any model, is its succinct summarization of each covariate's effect with a single number. To the extent that the model is correct, this will be a good thing. To the extent that the model is wrong, the summary will be misleading. As a simple example, consider a fit to the PBC data using only bilirubin.

```
> coxph(Surv(futime, status==2) ~ log(bili), pbc)

              coef exp(coef) se(coef)    z p
log(bili) 0.989        2.69   0.0784 12.6 0

Likelihood ratio test=153  on 1 df, p=0  n= 418
```

The fit states that each unit increase in log(bilirubin) will give a 2.7-fold increase in risk. If this is true, then the survival curves $S_j(t)$ for three hypothetical cohorts of subjects with bilirubin values of 1, 1.6, and 2.7 = $\exp(0, .5, 1)$ (equally spaced on the log scale) should be such that

$$\log\{-\log[S_j(t)]\} = \log(\Lambda_0) + \beta x$$

are parallel curves spaced $.989/2 = .49$ units apart. The actual data set does not contain enough subjects with these precise values of bilirubin to check this directly, but we can look at a grouped approximation. Split the PBC subjects into three cohorts based on bilirubin levels of < 1.1, 1.1–3.3, and > 3.3, corresponding to 1 and 3 times the upper limit of bilirubin for normal subjects. The total count of subjects is 177, 133, and 108, respectively, with median bilirubin values within groups of 0.7, 1.8, and 6.6. A plot of the log–log survival curves is given in Figure 3.1, along with three visual reference lines that are .989∗log(1.8/0.7) and .989∗log(6.6/1.8) units apart, respectively. (The slope of the line was chosen by eye to roughly match the center curve.)

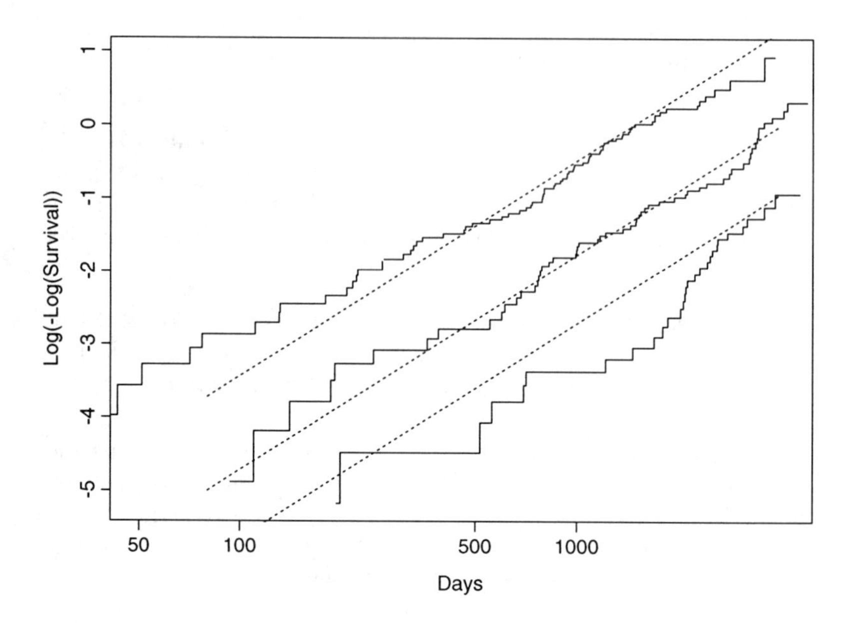

FIGURE 3.1: *Testing the fit of a model with bilirubin only*

```
> group <- 1*(pbc$bili > 1.1) + 1*(pbc$bili > 3.3)
> cfit <- survfit(Surv(futime, status==2) ~ group, data=pbc)
> plot(cfit, mark.time=F, fun='cloglog', xlab='Days',
        ylab='Log(-Log(Survival))')
> lines(c(80, 4000), c(-5, 0), lty=2)
> lines(c(80, 4000), c(-5, 0)- log(1.8/0.7) * .989, lty=2)
> lines(c(80, 4000), c(-5, 0)+ log(6.6/1.8) * .989, lty=2)
```

In this particular case the data appear to match the assumptions quite well. More complete methods to examine the assumptions and the fit of the model are the subject of Chapters 5 through 7.

3.2 Stratified Cox models

An extension of the proportional hazards model allows for multiple strata. The strata divide the subjects into disjoint groups, each of which has a distinct baseline hazard function but common values for the coefficient vector β. Assume that subjects $i = 1, \ldots, n_1$ are in stratum 1, subjects $n_1+1, \ldots, n_1+n_2$ are in stratum 2, and so on. The hazard for an individual i, who belongs to stratum k is

$$\lambda_k(t)e^{X_i\beta}.$$

Analysis of multicenter clinical trials frequently uses stratification. Because of varying patient populations and referral patterns, the different clinical centers in the trial are likely to have different *baseline* survival curves, ones that do not have the simple parallel relationship shown in Figure 3.1. Strata play a role similar to blocks in randomized block designs analyzed by two-way analysis of variance.

Computationally, the overall loglikelihood becomes a sum

$$l(\beta) = \sum_{k=1}^{K} l_k(\beta),$$

where $l_k(\beta)$ is precisely equation (3.3), but summed over only the subjects in stratum k. The score vector and information matrix are similar sums $U(\beta) = \sum U_k(\beta)$ and $\mathcal{I}(\beta) = \sum \mathcal{I}_k(\beta)$. These make use of $\bar{x}_k(t)$, the weighted mean of all subjects *in stratum* k who are still alive and at risk at time t, and $V_k(t)$, the weighted variance matrix of those subjects. To fit a model to the PBC data, but stratified on the presence/absence of ascites, we use

```
> coxph(Surv(futime, status==2) ~ age + edema + log(bili) +
            log(protime) + log(albumin) + strata(ascites),
                      data=pbc)

------------

data temp; set pbc;
    lbili = log(bili);
    lpro  = log(protime);
    lalb  = log(albumin);

proc phreg data=temp;
    model futime * status(0 1) = age edema lbili lpro lalb
                                    /  ties=efron;
    strata ascites;
```

Because they are used to divide the subjects or observations into a disjoint set of groups, stratification variables are effectively treated as categorical. If multiple stratification variables are given, the result is a separate baseline hazard for each unique combination of categories. For example, stratifying the PBC analysis on both sex and edema results in 6 different strata, one of which (males with severe edema) has only 3 subjects in it. That particular baseline hazard is, of course, quite poorly estimated. The S-Plus code would have `+ strata(edema, sex)` in the model specification and SAS would have the statement `strata edema sex;`.

The major advantage of stratification is that it gives the most general adjustment for a confounding variable. Disadvantages are that no direct estimate of the importance of the strata effect is produced (no p-value), and that the precision of estimated coefficients and the power of hypothesis tests may be diminished if there are a large number of strata [83].

The standard approach in stratified Cox models does not consider strata by covariate interactions. However, it is not always reasonable to assume that the effect of every covariate is constant across strata; for example, an analysis of a placebo-controlled drug trial, stratified by institution, yields a coefficient for treatment of -0.22, showing a 20% overall improvement in death rate for the new therapy ($\exp(-.22) = .8$). Are we willing to assume that although the baseline (placebo) survival differs between centers, that treatment is giving a uniform 20% improvement to each? An example where inclusion of such an interaction might be mandatory would be a cancer study involving tumor grade in which one of the institutions employed significantly different methods in the pathology department. The variable `grade` at this institution is not the same variable as at the others, and requires its own coefficient.

Strata by covariate interactions are simple to specify. Here is an example of testing an age by strata interaction for the PBC model stratified on edema.

```
data temp; set pbc;
    age1 = age * (edema=0);
    age2 = age * (edema=.5);
    age3 = age * (edema=1);
    lbili= log(bili);

proc phreg data=temp;
    model futime * status(0 1) = age1 age2 age3 lbili/ ties=efron;
    strata edema;
    Interact: test age1 = age2, age1 = age3;
```

```
        Summary of the Number of Event and Censored Values

                                                         Percent
Stratum   EDEMA        Total      Event    Censored    Censored

      1   0              354        116         238       67.23
      2   0.5             44         26          18       40.91
      3   1               20         19           1        5.00
-------------------------------------------------------------------
  Total                  418        161         257       61.48


              Testing Global Null Hypothesis: BETA=0

              Without     With
Criterion Covariates Covariates Model Chi-Square

-2 LOG L    1459.002   1311.224   147.777 with 4 DF (p=0.0001)
Score                             158.451 with 4 DF (p=0.0001)
Wald                              147.927 with 4 DF (p=0.0001)
```

```
            Analysis of Maximum Likelihood Estimates

                   Parameter     Standard       Wald          Pr >
Variable   DF       Estimate        Error   Chi-Square   Chi-Square

AGE1        1       0.035518      0.00880     16.30800       0.0001
AGE2        1       0.057035      0.02175      6.87596       0.0087
AGE3        1       0.108171      0.03085     12.29665       0.0005
LBILI       1       0.963203      0.08490    128.72036       0.0001

                     Linear Hypotheses Testing

                      Wald                                Pr >
     Label         Chi-Square                DF      Chi-Square
     INTERACT          5.4838                 2          0.0644
```

And in S-Plus the example is as follows.

```
> fit <- coxph(Surv(futime, status==2) ~ log(bili) +
                     age * strata(edema),  data=pbc)
>fit

                                coef exp(coef) se(coef)      z       p
                  log(bili) 0.9631      2.62   0.0849 11.345 0.0e+00
                        age 0.0355      1.04   0.0088  4.038 5.4e-05
agestrata(edema)edema=0.5 0.0215      1.02   0.0235  0.919 3.6e-01
  agestrata(edema)edema=1 0.0727      1.08   0.0321  2.265 2.4e-02

Likelihood ratio test=148  on 4 df, p=0  n= 418

> waldtest(fit, 3:4)
  chisq  df     p
   5.49   2 0.064
```

As always, there are many ways to code the dummy variables for an interaction. In SAS, we have created a separate age coefficient per stratum. In the S-Plus code, we have allowed the package to generate the dummy variables, and it has created contrasts. The first contrast of .0215 is equal to the difference of the SAS coefficients `AGE2 - AGE1` and the second is the contrast `AGE3 - AGE1`. (Because of different convergence criteria, the SAS code executed four iterations and S-Plus three iterations for these data, giving trivial coefficient differences.) The automatically generated S-Plus labels do leave something to be desired.

If all of the covariate by strata interaction terms are added to a model, then the result is identical to doing separate fits for each stratum. The combined fit allows one to test for the significance of strata by covariate differences, however.

3.3 Handling ties

The partial likelihood for the Cox model is developed under the assumption of continuous data, but real data sets often contain tied event times. Four variants of the computing algorithm are commonly used to address this. If there are no ties all four are precisely equivalent, and if there are very few tied death times they will be nearly so.

- Breslow approximation. This is the simplest formula to write down and the easiest to program. Consequently it was the only method available in the earliest Cox model routines, and is still the default method in *almost* all packages. The solution is the least accurate, but the method is fast.
- Efron approximation. The formula for this method looks much more difficult than the Breslow method on the surface, but in actuality it is nearly as easy to program. It is quite accurate unless the proportion of ties and/or the number of tied events relative to the size of the risk set is extremely large, and it is as fast as the Breslow method. It is the default in S-Plus.
- Exact partial likelihood. This method involves an exhaustive enumeration of the possible risk sets at each tied death time, and can require a prohibitive amount of computation time if any of the individual death times has a large number of events (>10 say). Interestingly, the evaluation is equivalent to the likelihood for a matched case-control study. SAS calls this the `discrete` option, S-Plus the `exact` option.
- Averaged likelihood. This is often very close to the Efron approximation. It also involves an exhaustive enumeration, but a substitution allows this to be replaced by numerical evaluation of an integral. This is not implemented in S-Plus; in SAS it is called the `exact` option.

As discussed previously, ties may occur because the event time scale is discrete or because continuous event times are grouped into intervals. The two possibilities imply different probability structures, which are reflected in the approximation that is chosen.

As we have seen in equation (3.2), the partial likelihood for untied data is a product over event times. If observation i is an event at time t_i, it will contribute a term

$$\frac{r_i(t_i)}{\sum_j Y_j(t_i) r_j(t_i)}. \tag{3.9}$$

This term is the conditional probability that individual i with risk score $r_i(t_i)$ had an event, given that an event occurred at t and given the set of risk scores available to have an event. Now assume that ties have been introduced into the data because of grouping. For a simple example, assume five subjects in time order, with the first two both dying at the same recorded time. If the time data had been more precise, then the first two terms in the likelihood would be either

$$\left(\frac{r_1}{r_1 + r_2 + r_3 + r_4 + r_5}\right)\left(\frac{r_2}{r_2 + r_3 + r_4 + r_5}\right) \tag{3.10}$$

or

$$\left(\frac{r_2}{r_1 + r_2 + r_3 + r_4 + r_5}\right)\left(\frac{r_1}{r_1 + r_3 + r_4 + r_5}\right) \tag{3.11}$$

but we don't know which. (Notice that the product of the numerators remains constant, but that of the denominators does not.) One may use either the average of the terms or some approximation to the average.

The simplest approximation, proposed independently by Breslow [21] and by Peto [118] uses the complete sum $r_1 + r_2 + \ldots + r_5$ for both denominators. However, it is the least accurate approximation. In particular, it counts failed individuals more than once in the denominator, producing a conservative bias and estimated β coefficients too close to 0 in absolute value [36, p. 103].

A much better approximation, due to Efron, uses the average denominator $.5r_1 + .5r_2 + r_3 + r_4 + r_5$ in the second term, giving a likelihood contribution of

$$\left(\frac{r_1}{r_1 + r_2 + r_3 + r_4 + r_5}\right)\left(\frac{r_2}{.5r_1 + .5r_2 + r_3 + r_4 + r_5}\right).$$

If there were three tied deaths out of n subjects, the three Efron denominators would have a weight of 1, 2/3, and 1/3 for the deaths in denominators 1, 2, and 3, respectively. One way to think of this is that each of the subjects who perished is certain to be in the first denominator, has 2/3 chance of being in the second (was not the first of the three to have an event), and 1/3 chance of being in the third denominator. If the tied deaths all happen to have an identical risk score r, the Efron solution will be exact. This approximation is only slightly more difficult to program than the Breslow version. In particular, since the downweighting is independent of β it does not change the form of the first or second derivatives; the extra computation throughout the code is essentially the same as that introduced by adding case weights.

A more ambitious approach is to use the average of the terms. The average likelihood calculation is nearly untractable computationally when the number of tied events at any time is even moderately large. Assume there were d tied events; then there will be $d!$ possible denominator patterns, one for each ordering of the events, and each pattern is itself a product of d terms. DeLong et al. [38] have shown that the averaged partial likelihood has an equivalent representation in terms of integrals. The sum of (3.10) and (3.11) can also be written

$$\int_0^\infty \left[1 - \exp\left(-\frac{r_1 t}{r_3 + r_4 + r_5}\right)\right]\left[1 - \exp\left(-\frac{r_2 t}{r_3 + r_4 + r_5}\right)\right] e^{-t}\, dt$$

and the general term for a d-way tie with n at risk is

$$\int_0^\infty \prod_{l=1}^{d} \left[1 - \exp\left(-\frac{r_l t}{r_{d+1} + r_{d+2} + \ldots + r_n}\right)\right] e^{-t}\, dt.$$

(Use integration by parts to repeatedly decompose the integral into $d!$ evaluable pieces; those pieces turn out to be exactly the terms in our sum.) The first and second derivatives involve integrals that are essentially the same type. Because these integrals are well-conditioned numerically, with positive smooth integrands, they can be efficiently evaluated by numerical approximation methods. The resulting algorithm is $O(d^2)$, far faster than the nominal $O(d!)$. It has been implemented in SAS where it is called the "exact" option, but it is not currently part of S-Plus.

For data considered to be discrete, there is a single term in the partial likelihood at a tied event time. If there were d tied events out of n individuals at risk, it compares the selection of the d individuals who actually had the event to all possible ways of choosing d items from a pool of n. That probability is

$$\frac{r_1 r_2 \cdots r_d}{\sum_{S(d,n)} r_{k_1} r_{k_2} \cdots r_{k_d}}, \tag{3.12}$$

where $S(d,n)$ denotes the set of all possible selections. There are, of course, a huge number of selections. For the above example of 2 events with 5 at risk there are 10 unique pairs and the likelihood term is

$$\frac{r_1 r_2}{r_1r_2 + r_1r_3 + r_1r_4 + r_1r_5 + r_2r_3 + r_2r_4 + r_2r_5 + r_3r_4 + r_3r_5 + r_4r_5}.$$

The computational burden grows very quickly — for 10 tied events in 1,000 at risk the denominator has $2.6 * 10^{23}$ terms. Gail et al. [52] develop a recursive algorithm for this computation that is much faster than the naive approach of separately counting all subsets, an order of magnitude or more when there are tied events with $d > 3$. SAS implements this as the "discrete" option for ties; S-Plus labels this as the "exact" option and uses the brute force approach.

The model corresponding to equation (3.12) is *not* the familiar form

$$\lambda_i(t) = \lambda_0(t) \exp(X_i(t)\beta),$$

but a logistic model [35, p. 192]

$$\frac{\lambda_i(t)}{1 + \lambda_i(t)} = \frac{\lambda_0(t)}{1 + \lambda_0(t)} \exp(X_i\beta), \tag{3.13}$$

with the risk score multiplying the odds ratio rather than the hazard. Compared to an individual with covariate vector X_1, an individual with X_2 has an $\exp[(X_2 - X_1)\beta]$-fold increase in the odds of an event. Not surprisingly, this model is formally equivalent to the logistic regression model for matched (stratified) case-control studies. Each tied event is analogous to a stratum with d cases, $n - d$ controls, and exposure vectors $X_1, X_2, \ldots, X_n$ with the first d belonging to the cases and $X_{d+1}, \ldots, X_n$ belonging to the controls.

Cox model programs are an efficient and simple tool for fitting matched case-control data. The data setup to do so is minimal.

1. Set the observation time to a dummy value `time=1` (or any positive number).
2. Set the status variable to 1 = case, 0 = control.
3. Create a stratum variable, not necessarily numeric, that uniquely identifies each case-control group (e.g., 1 = cases and controls in the first matched set, 2= cases and controls in the second matched set, etc.).
4. Fit a proportional hazards model with the `discrete`(SAS) or `exact`(S-Plus) option for ties. (If there is only one case per case-control set, all four methods for handling ties are identical.)
5. No special preprocessing of the predictor covariates is needed.

A concrete example comparing the four approaches is shown in Table 3.1. We first use the standard PBC data set. This has very few tied death times, only 5 tied pairs. Then the test is repeated on a coarsened PBC data set with time recorded quarterly instead of in days. The number of ties becomes

Multiplicity	1	2	3	4	5	6	7	8	9	10	11
Count	8	8	9	6	1	1	3	3	1	1	1

so there are only 8 quarters with a single event, 8 that have 2 events, ..., and one with 11 events.

```
data test; set pbc;
    futime2 = round(futime/91.25);
    age = age/10;              *rescale the age coef for the table;
    lbili = log(bili);
    lalb  = -1* log(albumin);   *make all signs positive in table;


proc phreg data=test;
    model futime * status(0 1)= age edema lbili lalb/ties=efron;
proc phreg data=test;
    model futime * status(0 1)= age edema lbili lalb/ties=breslow;
proc phreg data=test;
   model futime * status(0 1)= age edema lbili lalb/ties=discrete;
proc phreg data=test;
    model futime * status(0 1)= age edema lbili lalb/ties=exact;
```

		Coefficients		Compute	
Age	Edema	Log(bili)	Log(alb)	Time	
Original data					
Efron	0.395	1.040	0.895	2.595	126
Breslow	0.395	1.038	0.895	2.586	100
Discrete	0.396	1.040	0.896	2.591	156
Exact	0.395	1.040	0.895	2.596	153
Coarsened data					
Efron	0.393	1.058	0.895	2.521	106
Breslow	0.386	1.009	0.880	2.434	90
Discrete	0.403	1.116	0.925	2.580	362
Exact	0.393	1.063	0.896	2.528	345

TABLE 3.1: *Comparison of tied data methods for the raw and coarsened PBC data. The compute time is in arbitrary units*

```
proc phreg data=test;
   model futime2 * status(0 1)= age edema lbili lalb/ties=efron;
proc phreg data=test;
   model futime2 * status(0 1)= age edema lbili lalb/ties=breslow;
proc phreg data=test;
  model futime2 * status(0 1)= age edema lbili lalb/ties=discrete;
proc phreg data=test;
   model futime2 * status(0 1)= age edema lbili lalb/ties=exact;
```

The results are fairly typical. Viewing the data as genuinely discrete yields larger coefficients as the data is coarsened, the Efron and exact results are closest to the original data, and the Breslow approximation attenuates the coefficients. The impact of a fairly moderate number of ties on the compute time of the ambitious methods is substantial, while having essentially no effect on the two approximations.

Recommendations

We have applied the discrete data partial likelihood to grouped data for illustrative purposes. It is *not* a good idea. As discussed above, the discrete and grouped data partial likelihoods fit different models: a linear logistic hazard with β as a log–odds ratio parameter versus a log–linear hazard with β as a log–relative risk parameter.

If the data are genuinely discrete, the logistic model is appropriate. For very heavily tied data sets, however, the computation may become burdensome. An alternative in this case is the discrete relative risk model of Prentice and Gloeckler [121]. The data are recast in a way that allows the use of a standard binomial regression model with complementary log–log link function, such as the `glm` function in S-Plus or `genmod` in SAS. The fit includes parameters both for the covariates and for the baseline hazard, an estimated jump for each unique event time, so the model is not appropriate when the number of parameters approaches the total number of events (i.e., when the number of ties is modest or small).

For grouped continuous data with light or moderate ties, one has a choice between the averaged likelihood or an approximation. In our experience, the Efron approximation gives very similar results to the more complex computation, while remaining computationally feasible even with large tied data sets. It is unfortunate that backwards compatibility arguments continue to justify the less accurate Breslow approximation as the default in most packages.

3.4 Wald, score, and likelihood ratio tests

The standard asymptotic likelihood inference tests, the Wald, score, and likelihood ratio, are also available for the Cox partial likelihood to test hypotheses about β. Testing the global null hypothesis $H_0 : \beta = \beta^{(0)}$ is particularly easy because both S-Plus and SAS output provide all three test statistics. $\beta^{(0)}$, the initial value for $\hat\beta$, is always 0 in SAS and defaults to 0 in S-Plus unless overridden by the user.

- The likelihood ratio test is $2(l(\hat\beta) - l(\beta^{(0)}))$, twice the difference in the log partial likelihood at the initial and final estimates of $\hat\beta$.
- The Wald test is $(\hat\beta - \beta^{(0)})'\hat{\mathcal{I}}(\hat\beta - \beta^0)$, where $\hat{\mathcal{I}} = \mathcal{I}(\hat\beta)$ is the estimated information matrix at the solution, equation (3.6), or the stratified equivalent. For a single variable, this reduces to the usual z-statistic $\hat\beta/\text{se}(\hat\beta)$.
- The efficient score test statistic $U'(\beta^{(0)})\mathcal{I}(\beta^{(0)})^{-1}U(\beta^{(0)})$ can be computed using only the first iteration of the Newton–Raphson algorithm. Letting $\hat\beta^1$ be the first step of the solution algorithm we see from equation (3.8) that $\hat\beta^1 - \beta^{(0)} = -U'(\beta^{(0)})\mathcal{I}(\beta^{(0)})^{-1}$, showing that the score test is closely related to a Wald test based on the result of one iteration. (The single iteration estimate is an asymptotically consistent estimator of β under general regularity conditions, although it is less efficient than the fully iterated MLE.)

The null hypothesis distribution of each of these tests is a chi-square on p degrees of freedom. As usual, they are asymptotically equivalent, but in finite samples they may differ. If so, the likelihood ratio test is generally considered the most reliable and the Wald test is the least. These test statistics are approximately low-order Taylor series expansions of each other. For example, a second order Taylor expansion of the loglikelihood ratio statistic, $2(l(\hat\beta) - l(\beta^{(0)}))$ about the point $\beta^{(0)}$ gives the score test; the same expansion justifies Newton–Raphson iteration as a succession of quadratic approximations. The following table compares the three test statistics on five simulated data sets. Each is of size 100 with a single binary covariate, and differ only in the true value of β.

β	$\hat\beta$	LRT	Score	Wald	Max/Min
0.00	-0.23	0.79	0.79	0.78	1.004
0.25	0.26	1.24	1.25	1.25	1.009
0.50	0.79	8.52	8.52	8.12	1.049
1.00	1.14	20.87	21.93	19.88	1.103
2.00	2.79	83.44	89.19	60.85	1.466

For smaller values of $\hat\beta$ the tests are very similar, as might be expected since the Taylor series are "close" at $\hat\beta^{(0)} = 0$, with larger differences as $\hat\beta$ grows. Even at the largest value, however, there is no difference in the *statistical* conclusions: for a chi-square distribution on one degree of freedom any value over 20 means "tiny p-value." In this example, the score test statistic is largest and the Wald is smallest, but that pattern can vary.

When $p = 1$ and the single covariate is categorical, the score test is identical to the log–rank test. (If there are tied death times, the variance approximation used by Cox programs differs slightly from that used by log–rank programs, so the numerical results of the two will differ trivially.) For the PBC data both the log–rank test and the Cox model for edema give a test statistic of 131 on two degrees of freedom. For the coarsened PBC data, the log–rank test for edema gives a test statistic of 125, a Cox model with the Efron approximation a value of 132, and one with the Breslow approximation a value of 123. SAS code to generate these numbers, but not the output, is shown below. Note that edema is treated as a `class` variable via a `strata` statement in the `lifetest` procedure, and the use of explicit dummy variables in the `phreg` procedure.)

```
data temp; set pbc;
    edema0 = 1*(edema=0);
    edema1 = 1*(edema=1);
    futime2 = round(futime/91.25);
proc lifetest notable data=temp;
    time futime * status(0 1);
    strata edema;
proc lifetest notable data=temp;
    time futime2 * status(0 1);
    strata edema;
proc phreg data=temp;
    model futime * status(0 1) = edema0 edema1;
proc phreg data=temp;
    model futime2 * status(0 1) = edema0 edema1 / ties=breslow;
proc phreg data=temp;
    model futime2 * status(0 1) = edema0 edema1 / ties=efron;
```

Here is an example of the printout for the lung cancer data.

```
> lungfit <- coxph(Surv(time, status) ~ age + sex + meal.cal,
                      data=lung)
```

```
> summary(lungfit)

  n=181 (47 observations deleted due to missing)

                 coef exp(coef) se(coef)      z    p
     age  0.015292      1.015 0.010535  1.452 0.15
     sex -0.491266      0.612 0.190855 -2.574 0.01
meal.cal -0.000134      1.000 0.000238 -0.563 0.57

         exp(coef) exp(-coef) lower .95 upper .95
     age     1.015      0.985     0.995     1.037
     sex     0.612      1.635     0.421     0.889
meal.cal     1.000      1.000     0.999     1.000

Rsquare= 0.057   (max possible= 0.998 )
Likelihood ratio test= 10.7  on 3 df,   p=0.0138
Wald test            = 10.2  on 3 df,   p=0.0172
Score (logrank) test = 10.3  on 3 df,   p=0.0159
```

A portion of the SAS printout for the same model shows the same values.

```
            Without      With
Criterion  Covariates  Covariates  Model Chi-Square

-2 LOG L     1157.789    1147.136     10.653 with 3 DF (p=0.0138)
Score                                 10.335 with 3 DF (p=0.0159)
Wald                                  10.165 with 3 DF (p=0.0172)
```

We can also compare the three tests for an individual variable in the model. Because the Wald test is already printed for each coefficient it is the one most commonly quoted; e.g., the z-statistic of $-.0153/.0105 = 1.45$ for the age coefficient above. A likelihood ratio test for age requires that the data set be refit without age.

```
> lungfita <- coxph(Surv(time, status) ~ sex + meal.cal, lung)
> print(lungfita)

                 coef exp(coef) se(coef)      z      p
     sex -0.527473       0.59 0.189393 -2.785 0.0054
meal.cal -0.000216       1.00 0.000234 -0.924 0.3600

Likelihood ratio test=8.5  on 2 df, p=0.0143
  n=181 (47 observations deleted due to missing)
```

The LR test statistic is $(10.7 - 8.5) = 2.2$ on one degree of freedom, which differs only slightly from the Wald test for age of $1.452^2 = 2.11$. Missing values in the data set can also be a major nuisance when computing the LR test for a variable, however. If we naively compute the likelihood ratio test for meal calories

```
> coxph(Surv(time, status) ~ age + sex, lung)

      coef exp(coef) se(coef)     z      p
age  0.017     1.017  0.00922  1.85 0.0650
sex -0.513     0.599  0.16745 -3.06 0.0022

Likelihood ratio test=14.1  on 2 df, p=0.000857  n= 228
```

then the LR test statistic appears to be $(10.7 - 14.1) = -3.4$, an impossibility. The reason is that the second model includes 47 more patients than were in the first model `lungfit`; a proper computation requires that the second fit also exclude the patients with missing calories.

```
> coxph(Surv(time, status) ~ age + sex, data=lung,
                   subset=(!is.na(meal.cal)))
        coef exp(coef) se(coef)     z     p
age  0.0167     1.017   0.0103  1.63 0.100
sex -0.4745     0.622   0.1886 -2.52 0.012

Likelihood ratio test=10.3  on 2 df, p=0.00571  n= 181
```

The LR test of $(10.7 - 10.3) = 0.4$ now more closely matches the Wald value of $-.563^2 = .32$.

Computation of the score test for a single coefficient of the multivariate model requires two fits to the data as well. Since it is a test at $\beta = 0$, the first fit is to a model without the covariate of interest in order to get appropriate initial values, and the second uses all of the covariates.

```
> lungfitb <- coxph(Surv(time, status) ~ age + sex + meal.cal,
                   data=lung, init=c(0,coef(lungfita)), iter=0)
> lungfitb$score
[1] 2.11
```

The `phreg` procedure does not support initial values, so this test is not directly available in SAS. The test is rarely used in the "by hand" form shown above; if two models need to be run anyway, why not use the more trusted LR test? As well, the procedure has the same issue with missing values as the LR test. Because of its computational advantages with respect to the number of iterations required, however, the score test often *is* used in the forward selection stage of a stepwise Cox model program. In particular, note that the computation does not require the model to be iterated to a final solution. Subtracting the score statistics obtained from the full model `fit` and from the model without age `fita` is *not* a valid score test of `age`; that is, you should not subtract the test statistic for (`sex + meal.cal` vs. Null) from that for (`age + sex + meal.cal` vs. Null) and expect a useful result. If the coefficients common to the two fits are large, the subtraction can be subject to severe approximation error [84].

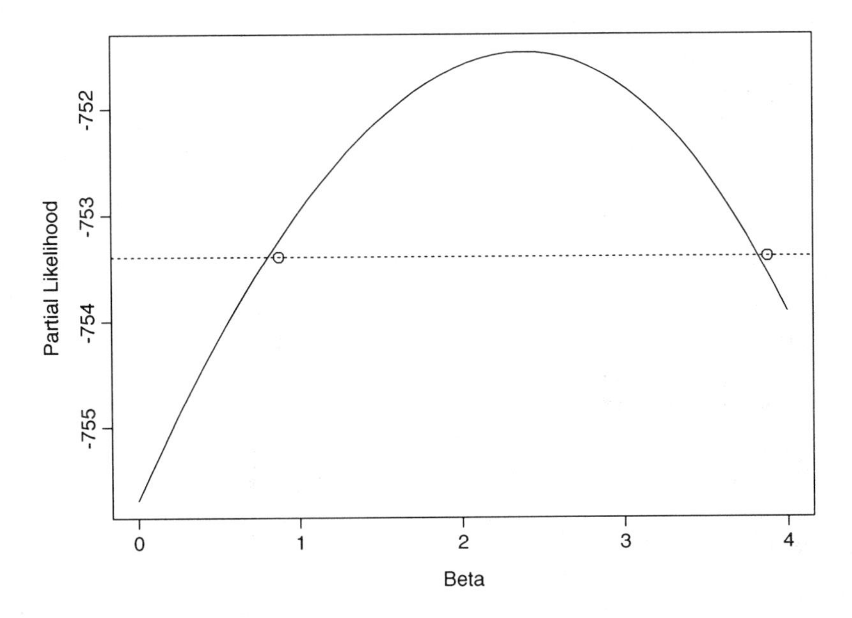

FIGURE 3.2: *Profile likelihood curve and 95% confidence interval cutoff for prothrombin time*

3.4.1 Confidence intervals

Confidence intervals are usually created based on the Wald statistics, as are printed above by the S-Plus `summary` function. The lower and upper CI values are $\exp(\hat\beta \pm 1.96\,\mathrm{se}(\hat\beta))$. More exact confidence limits can be created using a profile likelihood. The following code draws a profile likelihood for the variable `log(protime)` in a fit of the PBC data set; given the skewness of this variable and the width of its confidence interval, there might be some a priori concern about the adequacy of the standard calculation. The result is shown in Figure 3.2; the profile confidence limits are the intersection of the likelihood curve with a horizontal line 3.84/2 units below its maximum. (Twice the difference in the likelihood should be a chi-square on one degree of freedom.) The confidence interval based on a Wald approximation is shown by two circles; there is a slight but unimportant amount of asymmetric error in the approximate solution.

The computation was done in S-Plus as

```
> pbcfit <- coxph(Surv(futime, status==2) ~ age + edema +
                  log(bili) + log(albumin) + log(protime),
                  data=pbc)
```

```
> beta <- seq(0,4, length=50)
> llik <- double(50)
> for (i in 1:50) {
>     temp <- coxph(Surv(futime, status==2) ~ age + edema +
                    log(bili) + log(albumin) +
                    offset(beta[i] * log(protime)), data=pbc)
>     llik[i] <- temp$loglik[2]
>     }
> plot(beta, llik, type='l', ylab="Partial Likelihood")
>
> temp <-  pbcfit$loglik[2] - 3.84/2
> abline(h = temp, lty=2)
> sd <- sqrt(pbcfit$var[4,4])
> points(pbcfit$coef[4] + c(-1.96, 1.96)*sd, c(temp,temp), pch=1)
```

We first fit the overall model using all covariates. The second command creates a vector of trial values for the `log(protime)` coefficient, 50 evenly spaced values between 0 and 4. The range was chosen to include the Wald-based confidence interval. The third line creates a scratch vector of zeros. The loop then fits a sequence of Cox models. For each trial value of `beta`, an offset term is used to include `beta * log(protime)` in the model as a *fixed* covariate. This essentially fixes the coefficient at the chosen value, while allowing the other coefficients to be maximized, given `beta`. The result is saved in the `llik` vector. (The `loglik` component of the `coxph` fit is a vector of length 2, containing the partial likelihood at $\beta = 0$ and $\beta = \hat{\beta}$.) The curve is then plotted, and annotated with a horizontal line 3.84/2 units below the global maximum and two circles showing the Wald interval.

The profile likelihood will prove useful for frailty models in Chapter 9, but is not normally necessary for simpler cases such as this.

3.5 Infinite coefficients

Assume that a data set had the following structure at the time of analysis.

	Alive	Dead
Treatment	40	0
Control	30	10

Because the treatment group has no deaths its hazard rate is 0, and the hazard ratio of control/treatment is infinite. If a Cox model is fit to the data, the computer program will be attempting to converge to the true MLE of $\hat{\beta} = \infty$. A graph of the log partial likelihood function, although it is strictly increasing in $\hat{\beta}$, quickly approaches a horizontal asymptote. Since the `coxph` and `phreg` functions use the change in likelihood as their convergence criteria, rather than changes in $\hat{\beta}$, they will converge normally, ceasing to iterate once the change in loglikelihood becomes sufficiently small. Here is a simple example. We include the status variable as a predictor to force an infinite β.

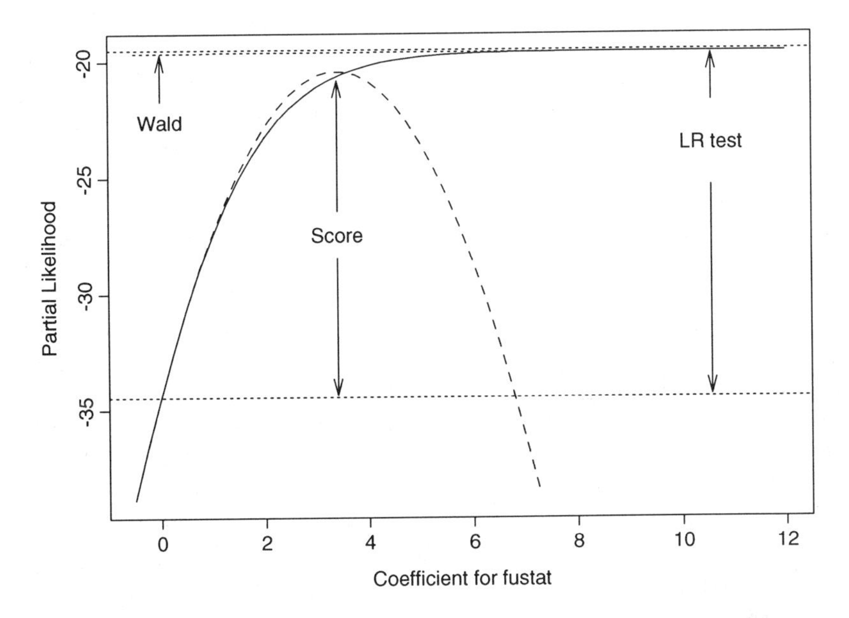

FIGURE 3.3: *Likelihood ratio, score, and Wald tests for an infinite coefficient*

```
>fit <-  coxph(Surv(futime, fustat) ~  rx + fustat, ovarian)
Warning messages:
  Loglik converged before variable  2 ; beta may be infinite.

>summary(fit)
  n= 26
          coef exp(coef) se(coef)      z    p
    rx  -0.557  5.73e-01     0.62 -0.898 0.37
fustat  10.582  3.94e+04    34.38  0.308 0.76

Likelihood ratio test= 30.8  on 2 df,   p=2.05e-07
Wald test             = 0.9  on 2 df,   p=0.637
Efficient score test = 29.1  on 2 df,   p=4.83e-07
```

The `coxph` function prints a warning message that one of the coefficients is approaching infinity, but this message is not totally reliable; that is, it can sometimes occur when there are collinear or skewed covariates that have converged to a finite (but large) value, and may miss infinite coefficients in some smaller data sets. Examination of the model output by the user, and thought, are the best guides for detecting when this problem has occurred.

Figure 3.3 shows the profile loglikelihood function along with the quadratic approximations used by the Wald and score tests. The actual LR statistic is the difference in the partial likelihood function at $\beta = 0$ and $\beta = \infty$. Clearly the difference printed by the program, based on the value at $\beta = 10.6$ (for S-Plus) or $\beta = 18.6$ (for SAS) is sufficiently close to the partial likelihood at infinity. And $\hat\beta$ is also close enough to ∞, at least from a medical point of view — a relative risk of death of exp(10.6) = 40,000-fold is essentially infinite.

The score test approximates the LR test using a quadratic Taylor expansion about $\beta = 0$, as shown by the dashed line on the figure; it reports the difference between the LR at $\beta = 0$ and the value that it believes the LR will have at $\hat{\beta}$. In this case the guessed value of -20.6 for the final value of the partial likelihood is a little small, but not bad. The maximum of the quadratic function, at $\beta = 3.4$, is the first iterate of the Newton–Raphson algorithm.

The Wald test creates a quadratic curve based on a Taylor series about $\hat{\beta}$, in this case either 10.6 or 18.6, depending on the number of iterations done by the routine. It is shown by the dotted line on the plot, nearly indistinguishable from the horizontal dotted line that is the asymptotic value of the likelihood curve. Its test is the difference between the LR at $\hat{\beta}$ and the value it extrapolates to be true at zero. Because it depends on an assumption that the log partial likelihood function is a quadratic near $\hat{\beta}$, the Wald test is worthless in this situation. (Normally the Wald test will be very small for infinite coefficients, since se($\hat{\beta}$) seems to iterate to infinity faster than $\hat{\beta}$ does.) The score and likelihood ratio tests are still valid, however.

Here is the same example in SAS. Because of a different convergence threshold the program has performed one more iteration than S-Plus. This hardly changes the overall loglikelihood or the values for the treatment covariate `rx`, but goes one step closer to infinity for the second covariate.

```
proc phreg data=ovarian;
    model futime * fustat(0) = rx  fustat /ties=efron;

                   Testing Global Null Hypothesis: BETA=0

                 Without        With
Criterion     Covariates    Covariates    Model Chi-Square

-2 LOG L          69.970        39.165     30.805 with 2 DF (p=0.0001)
Score                                      29.086 with 2 DF (p=0.0001)
Wald                                        0.806 with 2 DF (p=0.6682)

                   Analysis of Maximum Likelihood Estimates

                Parameter   Standard      Wald         Pr >          Risk
Variable DF      Estimate      Error  Chi-Square  Chi-Square        Ratio

RX        1     -0.556617    0.61994     0.80614      0.3693        0.573
FUSTAT    1     18.581741       1877   0.0000980      0.9921   1.1748E8
```

This situation is sometimes referred to in the literature under the title of “monotone likelihood” for the Cox model, and viewed as a problem.

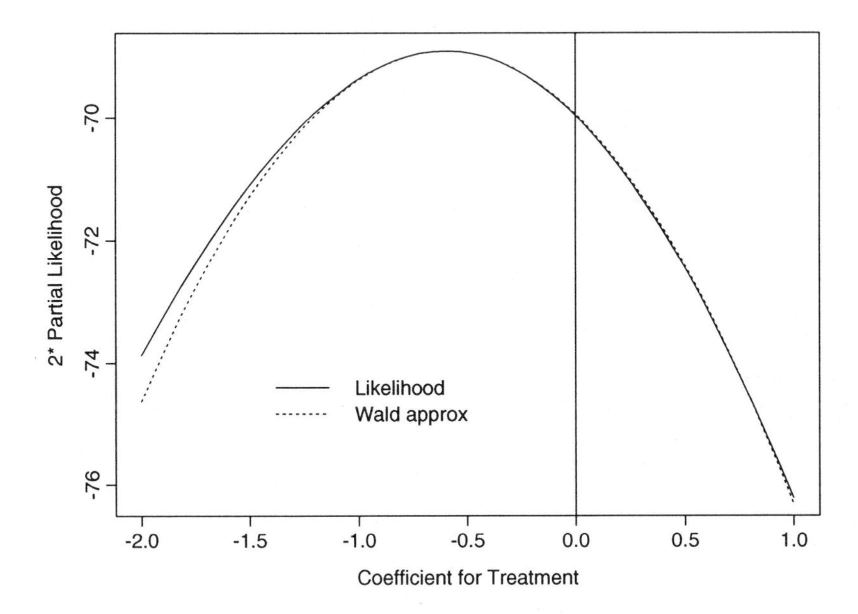

FIGURE 3.4: *The profile likelihood and Wald approximation for a finite β*

Bryson and Johnson [26], for instance, estimate the finite coefficients based on a stratified loglikelihood in which stratification is based on the distinct values of the covariates leading to infinity. Clarkson [33] demonstrates an efficient computer algorithm for this procedure.

We do not view this as a serious concern at all, other than an annoying numerical breakdown of the Wald approximation. One is merely forced to do the multiple fits necessary for a likelihood ratio or score test. A 95% confidence interval for the `fustat` variable can be based on the profile likelihood, and gives a value of $(2.75, \infty)$. Interestingly, similar concerns are rarely voiced about the use of the log–rank statistic in situations where one subset has no events.

Figure 3.4 shows the profile likelihood along with the Wald approximation in a more usual case. All three curves — profile, Wald, and score — are so close that only two could be distinctly shown.

3.6 Sample size determination

Consider an experiment comparing two groups, such as a clinical trial comparing a new treatment with a standard. For convenience, we refer to these as the experimental and control groups, although this terminology is not meant to preclude application to observational studies (e.g., comparing time from initial hiring to promotion in native vs. foreign-born employees in some job category). We want to detect a log–hazard ratio of β; that is, $\lambda_e(t) = e^{\beta}\lambda_c(t)$, where λ_e and λ_c denote the experimental and control group hazards, respectively. The total number of events required is

$$d = \frac{(c_\alpha + z_{power})^2}{pq\beta^2}, \tag{3.14}$$

where

- p is the proportion of study subjects in the experimental group,
- $q = 1 - p$,
- α is the type I error,
- c_α is the critical value for the test, and
- z_ν is the upper ν quantile of the standard normal distribution.

This is an asymptotic formula and can be derived from power calculations for the log–rank test [129], the Cox model score test for the treatment covariate whether or not other covariates are present [130], or for the score test under the parametric assumption of exponential failure time in both groups [14].

What value of β should you use? The answer is heavily dependent on the context, but the following are some considerations that we have found useful.

1. When dealing with rare events, e^β can be simply interpreted as the ratio of event probabilities. Let the survival functions in the two groups be $S_0(t)$ and $S_1(t)$, respectively, with corresponding distribution functions $F_0(t)$ and $F_1(t)$. By definition under proportional hazards,

   $$S_1(t) = S_0^{e^\beta}(t)$$

   so

   $$\begin{aligned} e^\beta &= \log(1 - F_1(t))/\log(1 - F_0(t)) \\ &\approx F_1(t)/F_0(t) \end{aligned}$$

   by a one-term Taylor expansion when $F_1(t)$ and $F_0(t)$ are small. Over intervals short enough that the event probability is small, a treatment that halves the hazard ratio will approximately halve the proportion of events.

2. In the case of exponential distributions, the reciprocal of the ratio of medians (or any other quantile) gives e^β. For example, if we want to detect a 50% increase in median survival time, we would set $e^\beta = 2/3$. For other distributions, relationships are not so simple, but the Weibull is only slightly more complicated. If S_0 and S_1 are Weibull distributions with shape parameter γ (i.e., $S_0(t) = \exp[-\lambda t^\gamma]$) then $e^\beta = (m_0/m_1)^\gamma$, where m_0 and m_1 denote the respective medians.

	e^β				
Power	1.15	1.25	1.50	1.75	2.00
.5	787	309	94	49	32
.7	1264	496	150	79	51
.8	1607	631	191	100	65
.9	2152	844	256	134	88

TABLE 3.2: *Number of events required under equal allocation with two-sided* $\alpha = 0.05$

3. In the specific context of medical studies with clinical event endpoints, such as heart attacks in studies of hypertension, values of $|\beta| \le 0.14$ (i.e., $0.87 \le e^\beta \le 1.15$) are regarded as small; in fact, hazard ratios closer to 1 are often regarded as pertaining to clinically equivalent treatments. At the other extreme, in cancer, AIDS, and chronic diseases, it is unusual to find a treatment that does better than halving the hazard rate. Therefore, clinical studies are often powered to detect hazard ratios of 1.25 or 1.50.

Example: suppose we wish to compare an experimental to a standard treatment. Five-year survival under standard treatment is approximately 30% and we anticipate that the new treatment will increase that to 45%, for $e^\beta = \log(.45)/\log(.3) = 0.663$. Assume that the study will use a two-sided test at $\alpha = .05$ and we want 90% power to detect the anticipated hazard ratio of 0.663. We have $c_\alpha = 1.96$ and $z_{power} = 1.28$. The study will allocate patients equally to the two treatments, so $p = q = .50$. The number of deaths required is $4 * (1.96 + 1.28)^2/(\log 0.663)^2 = 249$.

Table 3.2 gives the number of events required for selected values of power and e^β assuming a two-sided α level of 0.05 and equal allocation to the two groups. We have found this a handy reference. It is useful to keep in mind that e^β and its reciprocal require the same number of events. The line in the table for 50% power is a "hopelessness" lower bound; why conduct the study if you can do no better than flipping a coin? The greatest power and thus minimum number of events occur under equal allocation. For $p \ne 1/2$, divide the number in the table by $4p(1-p)$.

A one-tailed test of level α uses the same formula, equation (3.14), with a revised c_α value; for $\alpha = 0.05$, one would use 1.64 instead of 1.96. Table 3.3 is the one-sided analogue of Table 3.2. As expected, a smaller number of events are required.

The more challenging part of sample size computation is deciding how many subjects to enroll in the study in order to obtain the required number of events. Four factors are important for this second calculation: the length of the accrual (also called enrollment or recruitment) period a, the enrollment rate r, the additional followup time between the last enrollment and study closure f, and the survival curve for the control group S_c. Many computer programs exist to do this calculation, making various assumptions about the underlying survival curve. There is much room for complexity; our suggestion is to keep it simple.

	e^β				
Power	1.15	1.25	1.50	1.75	2.00
.5	554	217	66	35	23
.7	964	378	115	60	39
.8	1266	497	151	79	52
.9	1754	688	208	109	71

TABLE 3.3: *Number of events required under equal allocation with one-sided* $\alpha = 0.05$

Continuing with our numerical example: a prior study of this disease gave the following estimated survival curve for the control group.

t(yrs.)	2.0	2.5	3.0	3.5	4.0	4.5	5.0	5.5	6.0
$S_c(t)$	.86	.80	.65	.52	.43	.43	.30	.20	.12

Suppose we plan to recruit for $a = 3$ years and follow for $f = 2$. There are two approaches. For the first, consider each year of recruitment separately. Those recruited during the first year will have an average of 4.5 years of followup. Since $S_c(4.5) = .43$ and $S_e(4.5) = .43^{.663} = .57$, 100 patients randomized to control will provide 57 deaths, and 100 patients randomized to experimental treatment will provide 43 deaths. Those recruited during the second year will have an average 3.5 years of followup. $S_c(3.5) = .52$ and $S_e(3.5) = .65$, so they will provide 48 and 35 deaths, respectively, per 100 patients. Finally, those recruited during the third year will have 2.5 years of followup on average. $S_c(2.5) = .80$ and $S_e(2.5) = .86$, so they will provide 20 and 14 deaths, respectively, per 100 patients. The total number of deaths is 217, 125 from the controls and 92 from the experimental group.

The second approach is due to Schoenfeld [130]. He pointed out that the constant accrual rate means that the proportion surviving in each group is the average of the group's survival curve from time f to time $a + f$, which can be easily approximated by Simpson's rule, $(1/6)\{S(f) + 4S(f + .5a) + S(f + a)\}$. For our example, we get

$$\begin{aligned}\overline{S}_c &= (1/6)\{S_c(2) + 4S_c(3.5) + S_c(5)\}\\ &= (1/6)\{.80 + 4 * .52 + .30\}\\ &= 0.53.\end{aligned}$$

Similarly, for the experimental group, we get:

$$\begin{aligned}\overline{S}_e &= (1/6)\{S_e(2) + 4S_e(3.5) + S_e(5)\}\\ &= (1/6)\{.86 + 4 * .65 + .45\}\\ &= 0.652.\end{aligned}$$

The 300 controls would provide $(1 - .53) * 300 = 141$ deaths and the 300 experimentals would provide 105, for a total of 246. The two methods give different results, 246 versus 217, but they are "in the same ballpark."

There is an asymmetry between the two steps in the power computation. The first part involving the hazard rates, size, and power is fairly precise. The second, involving the expected accrual rate is usually based on, at best, an informed guess. Louis Lasagna was director of one of the research laboratories at Strong Memorial Hospital in the early 1980s, and one of his quotes (or at least attributed to him) was widely copied there as "Lasagna's law."

> At the commencement of a study the incidence of the condition under investigation will drop by one-half, and will not return to its former rate until the study is closed or the investigator retires, whichever comes first.

One suggestion is to word the statistical section of a protocol as "For a power of .80 to detect a 50% improvement in survival, using a two-sided test at $\alpha = .05$, the study needs 191 events. We *anticipate* that this will require the enrollment of $\ldots$," then allow accrual plans to be changed based on updated estimates of the total number of events. Investigators and especially accountants do not like this level of indeterminacy, but it is a truthful statement of how studies are actually run.

Complex designs

For more complex designs, a study-specific formula can be worked out fairly easily. A local example concerns a prospective study on risk factors for breast cancer, using women from a set of high-risk families and women who married into these families and thus were not selected for high familial breast cancer risk. One likely mechanism of risk for the high-risk group is a defect in DNA repair abilities, which might make the families particularly susceptible to certain risk factors; for example, factor x increases the risk of breast cancer by 25% in the population at large, but by 200% in the repair-compromised. Thus, we consider the possibility of a risk factor by risk group interaction. To be concrete, suppose our risk factor is smoking. Let γ_1 denote the log relative risk for breast cancer associated with smoking in the unselected population and γ_2 denote the log relative risk in the high-risk families. To assess the interaction, we test the null hypothesis of $\gamma_1 = \gamma_2$. Suppose that we want to detect a doubling of risk due to the gene-environment interaction; (that is $\gamma_2 - \gamma_1 = 0.693$. How many breast cancers will we need? We describe sample size calculations under two models. In the first, we stratify on unselected/familial status since the baseline survival curves for the two groups are known to be quite different, particularly with respect to early onset disease. We have two binary covariates, smoking and the gene-environment interaction. In the second, smoking status and family risk are two binary covariates in an (unstratified) Cox model and the interaction is a standard interaction covariate. It seems reasonable to assume that the proportion of smokers is the same in both groups and we let p_1 denote the proportion of smokers.

Consider the stratified model. It is convenient to code the two covariates, denoted x_1 and x_2, as follows: x_1 is a binary indicator of smoking status, 1 for smokers and 0 for nonsmokers, and x_2 is 1 for smokers in the high-risk family history group and 0 otherwise. The second coefficient in the fit, $\hat{\beta}_2$, is an estimate of $\gamma_1 - \gamma_2$ and the required test is the strata by covariate interaction test of $H_0 : \beta_2 = 0$. Sample size calculations require the variance of $\hat{\beta}_2$, which is a function of the information matrix $\mathcal{I}$, a sum over event times and over the two strata of weighted variance matrices of the covariates, see equation (3.7). We approximate this by computing the variance at $t = 0$ in each stratum.

Under H_0, $\beta' = (\beta_1, 0)$. In stratum 1, x_2 is identically 0 and $\bar{x}_1 = p_1 e^{\beta_1}/(p_1 e^{\beta_1} + 1 - p_1)$. Define

$$v = \frac{(1-\bar{x}_1)^2 p_1 e^{\beta_1} + \bar{x}_1^2(1-p_1)}{p_1 e^{\beta_1} + 1 - p_1}. \tag{3.15}$$

Then the variance matrix for (x_1, x_2) in stratum 1 is

$$V_1 = \begin{pmatrix} v_1 & 0 \\ 0 & 0 \end{pmatrix}.$$

In stratum 2, $x_1 = x_2$ and

$$V_2 = \begin{pmatrix} v_1 & v_1 \\ v_1 & v_1 \end{pmatrix}.$$

If we assume that the distribution of covariates stays roughly constant during the course of the study, then the total information will be

$$\mathcal{I} = d_1 V_1 + d_2 V_2 = \begin{pmatrix} (d_1 + d_2)v_1 & d_1 v_1 \\ d_1 v_1 & d_1 v_1 \end{pmatrix},$$

where d_1 and d_2 are the total number of events (breast cancers) in strata 1 and 2, respectively. The variance of $\hat{\beta}_2$ will be the 2,2 element of the inverse of $\mathcal{I}$, which is $(d_1 + d_2)/(d_1 d_2 v_1)$. The resultant power formula is very similar to equation (3.14):

$$\frac{d_1 d_2}{d_1 + d_2} = \frac{(z_{1-\alpha/2} + z_{power})^2}{v_1 .693^2}. \tag{3.16}$$

It is easy to see that the study has no power if d_1 or $d_2 = 0$, and in fact for any given total number of events $(d_1 + d_2)$ the power is maximized if half are in the high-risk families. In this best case, the required number of events is twice that for an ordinary test of treatment effect as found in equation (3.14), assuming $pq = v_1$.

As an alternate computation, assume that a covariate for family type were added to the Cox model, rather than stratifying on the variable. Now x_3 is family type, with an expected frequency of p_3, the proportion of familial subjects in the study. The covariate pattern at the start of the study is shown in Table 3.4. From this, the weighted variance matrix (3.6)

Pattern			Proportion	r
x_1	x_2	x_3	of Observations	
0	0	0	$(1-p_1)(1-p_3)$	1
1	0	0	$p_1(1-p_3)$	e^{β_1}
0	0	1	$(1-p_1)p_3$	e^{β_3}
1	1	1	p_1p_3	$e^{\beta_1+\beta_3}$

TABLE 3.4: *Patterns of covariates in a study of breast cancer risk, x_1 = smoking, 0 = no/1 = yes; x_3 = high-risk subject 0 = no/1 = yes; and $x_2 = x_1x_3$*

can be derived. The power formula is nearly identical to equation (3.14), with d as the total number of events in the study, but with the 2,2 element of the matrix's inverse in place of "pq".

The assumption that var(X) remains relatively constant throughout the course of a study is actually close to true in many if not most trials. Given the other unknowns, it is usually a benign assumption with respect to sample size computation. Violations can occur when the trial extends until nearly all of the subjects have had an event, in which case the sample size becomes very small for the last few deaths, but this affects only a handful of the $d = 100+$ risk sets in a study. The more serious possibility is aggressive censoring of the risk sets. Assume that a treatment is somewhat toxic, particularly for older patients, and thus a substantial fraction of the older subjects drop out in the first two months of a planned six-month treatment regimen. Sample size computations done in the manner above with respect to age as a covariate would be severely compromised. Algebraic solution based on an X matrix that varies over time would be quite difficult, and simulation becomes the more attractive solution for estimating the needed sample size.

3.6.1 The impact of strata on sample size

We said earlier that the use of many strata could have an impact on the sample size and power of a Cox model. How much impact does it have? The answer is "it depends."

To investigate this, we need to be somewhat more precise about the information matrix than we were in the sample size discussion above. For simplicity, we restrict ourselves to the case of $\hat\beta = 0$; technically then these comments only apply to the power of the score test, but the Wald and likelihood ratio results should be very similar. Assume, as we did earlier, that the weighted variance of $X(t)$ among those at risk remains constant as the study progresses. If the true variance of X is V, it is well known from any first-year statistics course that the expected value of the *computed* variance is $(n-1)/nV$.

Start with a very simple case: 10 subjects in the study, no tied death times, and no censoring. At the first death $n = 10$, at the second $n = 9$, and so on, so that the expected information matrix for the Cox model is

$$\mathcal{E}(\mathcal{I}) = V(\frac{9}{10} + \frac{8}{9} + \ldots + \frac{1}{2} + \frac{0}{1}).$$

For a rather standard-sized study with 200 events, again assuming no censoring, the result is $\mathcal{E}(\mathcal{I}) = V\sum_{i=1}^{200}(i-1)/i \simeq 194.1V$. Now say that the study were stratified into 4 strata of 50 events each. The overall information $\mathcal{I}$ of the model is the sum of the separate results for each stratum, or $\mathcal{E}(\mathcal{I}) = 4V\sum_{i=1}^{50}(i-1)/i \simeq 182.0$. The stratified study has a small loss of power of $(1 - 182/194.1) = 6\%$. Now suppose that it were 50 strata with 4 subjects per institution. The total information is now $\mathcal{E}(\mathcal{I}) = 50V\sum_{i=1}^{4}(i-1)/i \simeq 95.8V$; essentially half the power of the study is lost, and the sample size would need to be double that of an unstratified approach! This situation can be a real issue in some modern trials that utilize a very large number of enrolling centers; an alternate solution is discussed in Section 9.3.1.

The presence of censoring can greatly modify these calculations. In a study of adjuvant breast cancer, for instance, the fraction of subjects still alive at the end of followup may be quite high, over 85%. Sample size computations for 80% power to detect a 50% improvement, using a two-sided test at $\alpha = .05$ would still dictate a study of about 200 events, but in a total sample of over 1,200 patients. Assume for simplicity that all of the censored subjects have been followed for longer than the last observed event (nearly true in most studies); then the information in the unstratified study is $\mathcal{E}(\mathcal{I}) = V\sum_{i=1}^{200}(1200+i-1)/(1200+i) \simeq 199.86V$, and for one with 50 equal strata is $\mathcal{E}(\mathcal{I}) = 50V\sum_{i=1}^{4}(1200+i-1)/(1200+i) \simeq 199.83V$. In this case the stratified study has essentially no loss of power.

3.7 The counting process form of a Cox model

As discussed earlier the counting process approach has been extremely successful as a theoretical tool. Perhaps surprisingly, it has proven to be a very useful approach in the practical side of data analysis. The basic viewpoint is to think of each subject as the realization of a *very slow* Poisson process. Censoring is not "incomplete data," rather, "the geiger counter just hasn't clicked yet." The computing idea here is not completely new. Laird and Olivier [80] show how to use a Poisson regression program to fit a Cox model, and Whitehead [159] gave a GLIM macro to do the same.

To cast a data analysis in this framework has advantages as well. A Cox model program requires just one more variable. In the computer data file, we simply replace

```
time   status   strata   x1, x2, ...
```

with

```
(start, stop]   status   strata   x1, x2, ....
```

Each subject i is represented by a *set* of observations, each containing `start` and `stop` along with the usual status, strata, and covariate variables. Here `(start, stop]` is an interval of risk, open on the left and closed on the right; the status variable is 1 if the subject had an event *at* time `stop` and is 0 otherwise, and the strata and covariate values are the values that apply *over* the interval. Data sets like this are easy to construct with a package such as SAS or S-Plus (but easier with SAS). This simple extension allows

- time-dependent covariates,
- time-dependent strata,
- left truncation,
- multiple time scales,
- multiple events per subject,
- independent increment, marginal, and conditional models for correlated data, and
- various forms of case-cohort models.

The choice of an open bracket on the left end of the time interval and a closed bracket on the right is deliberate and important. First, it clarifies the issue of overlap. If a computer file contains two intervals `(0,35]` `(35,80]`, any internal computations at $t = 35$ will involve the former interval and not the latter. Secondly, it echoes the important mathematical constraints: computations done at $t = 35$ utilize covariate data known before time 35 (in this particular example the value for `x1` at 35 has held since time 0) so that covariates and at-risk intervals are predictable processes, and the event or death, if any, is at exactly $t = 35$, consistent with the counting process form of the outcome.

3.7.1 Time-dependent covariates

The most common type of time-dependent covariates is a repeated measurement on a subject or a change in the subject's treatment. Both of these are straightforward in the proposed formulation. As an example consider the well-known Stanford heart transplant study [37], where treatment is a time-dependent covariate. Patients 84 and 94 have times from enrollment to death of 102 and 343 days, respectively; the second patient had a transplant 21 days from enrollment; the first did not receive a transplant. The data file for these two would be

Id	Interval	Status	Transplant	Age	Prior Surgery
84	(0,102]	1	0	41	0
94	(0,21]	0	0	48	1
94	(21,343]	1	1	48	1

Note that static covariates such as "age at entry" are simply repeated for a patient with multiple lines of data.

One concern that often arises is that observations 2 and 3 above are "correlated," and would thus not be handled by standard methods. This is not actually an issue. The internal computations for a Cox model have a term for each unique death or event time; a given term involves sums over those observations that are available or "at risk" at the select event date. Since the intervals for a particular subject, "Jones" say, do not overlap (assuming of course that Jones does not have a time machine, and *could* meet himself on the street), any given internal sum will involve at most one of the observations that represent Mr. Jones; that is, the sum will still be over a set of independent observations. For time-dependent covariates, the use of (start, stop] intervals is just a mechanism, a trick almost, that allows the program to select the correct x values for Jones at a given time. (When there are multiple events per subject the situation does become more complicated, a subject for later chapters).

Multiple measurements over time are easily accommodated as well. For example, a patient with laboratory values of 0.30, 0.42, 0.39 measured on days 0, 60, and 120 who was followed to day 140 would be coded as three time intervals:

Interval	Status	Lab
(0,60]	0	0.30
(60,120]	0	0.42
(120,140]	0	0.39

This coding implicitly assumes that the time-dependent covariate is a step function with jumps at the measurement points. It might be more reasonable to break at the midpoints of the measurement times, or to use an interpolated value over many smaller intervals of time, but in practice these refinements appear to make little practical difference in the inference from the fitted model. If a lab test varies *markedly* from visit to visit, and the exact values are important to the risk model, then interpolation strategies may become important. But in this case adequacy of the study design would then also be in question, since the final result would depend critically on the way in which the interpolation was done.

The Stanford heart transplant data

Since the Stanford data set is so well known, it is worthwhile to show the data setup in complete detail. We use the data set as it is found in the paper by Crowley and Hu [37]; the first few lines of the raw data are shown in Table 3.5. A copy of the data can be obtained from `statlib` in the `jasa` section. Several issues arise in setting up the data.

1. The covariates in the data set are moderately collinear. Because of the presence of an interaction term, the coefficients found in Table 5.2 of Kalbfleisch and Prentice [73] will be recreated only if the covariates are defined in *exactly* the same way as was done there. (Conclusions

1	1 10 37	11 15 67	.	1 3 68	1	0
2	3 2 16	1 2 68	.	1 7 68	1	0
3	9 19 13	1 6 68	1 6 68	1 21 68	1	0
4	12 23 27	3 28 68	5 2 68	5 5 68	1	0
5	7 28 47	5 10 68	.	5 27 68	1	0
6	11 8 13	6 13 68	.	6 15 68	1	0
7	8 29 17	7 12 68	8 31 68	5 17 70	1	0
8	3 27 23	8 1 68	.	9 9 68	1	0
9	6 11 21	8 9 68	.	11 1 68	1	0

TABLE 3.5: *First nine lines of the Stanford heart transplant data file*

are not changed, however.) The appropriate definition for age is `(age in days)/365.25 - 40 years`, and that for year of enrollment is the number of years since the start of the study: `(entry date - Oct 1, 1967)/365.25`.

2. One subject died on the day of entry. However $(0, 0]$ is an illegal time interval for the programs. To avoid this, we treat this subject as dying on day 0.5.

3. A subject transplanted on day 10 is considered to be on medical treatment for days 1–10 and on surgical treatment for days 11–last contact. Thus if Smith died on day 10 and Jones was transplanted on day 10, we in effect treat the transplant as happening later in the day than the death; *except* for patient 38 who died during the procedure on day 5. This person should certainly be counted as a treatment death rather than a medical one. The problem is resolved by moving his transplant to day 4.9.

(Because all times are in days, subject 38 could have been labeled as a transplant on day $4.x$ for any $0 < x < 1$ without changing the result; the use of 4.9 as opposed to say, 4.5, is completely arbitrary.)

If there are ties between the time at which some time-dependent covariate changes value and an event or censoring time, two rules apply. Since time intervals are open on the left and closed on the right, changes in a covariate by default happen *after* the deaths and/or censoring at a given time point. For ties between death and censoring times SAS and S-Plus place deaths first, in accordance with common practice. (A subject who left the study on day 17 is considered to have been at risk for any death that occurred on day 17.)

Here is SAS code to create the analysis data set. The input data are assumed to be in the form shown in Table 3.5. Variables are the subject id, birth date, date of entry into the study, date of transplant (missing if not transplanted), last followup date and status on that date (0 = alive, 1 = dead), and whether the subject had had prior cardiac surgery.

```
data temp;
    infile 'data.jasa';
    input id  @6 birth_dt mmddyy8. @16 entry_dt mmddyy8.
              @26 tx_dt mmddyy8.   @37 fu_dt mmddyy8.
              fustat  prior_sx ;
    format birth_dt entry_dt tx_dt fu_dt date7.;

data stanford;
    set temp;
    drop fu_dt fustat birth_dt entry_dt tx_dt;

    age =  (entry_dt - birth_dt)/365.25  - 48;
    year = (entry_dt - mdy(10,1,67))/ 365.25;  *time since 1Oct67;
    wait =  tx_dt - entry_dt;                  *waiting time;
    if (id = 38) then wait = wait - .1;   *first special case;

    if (tx_dt =.) then do;
        rx = 0;                 * no transplant recieved;
        start = 0;
        stop  = fu_dt - entry_dt;
        if (id=15) then stop = 0.5;  *the other special case;
        status= fustat;
        output;
        end;

    else do;
        rx =0;           *first an interval on standard treatment;
        start = 0;
        stop  = wait;
        status= 0;
        output;

        rx =1;           *then an interval on surgical treatment;
        start = wait;
        stop  = fu_dt - entry_dt;
        status= fustat;
        output;
        end;

proc print;
    id id;
```

A line-by-line explanation of this particular code fragment, along with S-Plus code to create the same data set, can be found in Appendix A. However, note the last two lines of the code, which we consider critical. As easy as it is to create (start, stop] data sets, it is just as easy to mess up the creation. You must LOOK at the data you have created.

Here is S-Plus code to fit the six models found in Table 5.2 of Kalbfleisch and Prentice [73].

```
> sfit.1 <- coxph(Surv(start, stop, status) ~ (age + prior.sx)*rx,
                          data=stanford, method='breslow')
> print(sfit.1)
                coef exp(coef) se(coef)      z    p
        age  0.0139     1.014   0.0181  0.768 0.44
   prior.sx -0.5465     0.579   0.6109 -0.895 0.37
         rx  0.1195     1.127   0.3277  0.365 0.72
     age:rx  0.0346     1.035   0.0272  1.270 0.20
prior.sx:rx -0.2929     0.746   0.7582 -0.386 0.70

Likelihood ratio test=12.5  on 5 df, p=0.0288  n= 172

> sfit.2 <- coxph(Surv(start, stop, status)~ year* rx,
                          data=stanford, method='breslow')

> sfit.3 <- coxph(Surv(start, stop, status)~ (age + year)* rx,
                          data=stanford, method='breslow')

> sfit.4 <- coxph(Surv(start, stop, status)~ (year +prior.sx)*rx,
                          data=stanford, method='breslow')

> sfit.5 <- coxph(Surv(start, stop, status)~ (age + prior.sx)*rx
                   + year, data=stanford, method='breslow')

> sfit.6 <- coxph(Surv(start, stop, status)~ age* rx + prior.sx +
                   year, data=stanford, method='breslow')
```

Because of several tied death times in the data set, the solution differs slightly for different methods of handling ties. The Efron approximation is the default in S-Plus; the Breslow approximation matches the results in Table 5.2 of Kalbfleisch and Prentice.

At the time of writing, the SAS phreg procedure did not support either the class statement or interaction terms, as found in other SAS procedures such as reg. Thus the interactions with treatment found above have to be coded by hand, which is not particularly burdensome. The SAS code and a portion of the printout for the fifth model is as follows.

```
data temp2; set stanford;
    age_rx   = age * rx;
    prior_rx = prior_sx * rx;
proc phreg data=temp2;
    model start stop *status(0) = age prior_sx rx age_rx prior_rx;


-----------------

                    Event and Censored Values
                                                  Percent
           Total        Event     Censored       Censored
             172           75           97          56.40
```

```
             Testing Global Null Hypothesis: BETA=0

             Without      With
Criterion Covariates Covariates Model Chi-Square

-2 LOG L     596.651    584.199    12.452 with 5 DF (p=0.0291)
Score                              12.024 with 5 DF (p=0.0345)
Wald                               11.633 with 5 DF (p=0.0402)


             Analysis of Maximum Likelihood Estimates

                   Parameter   Standard     Wald        Pr >
 Variable  DF       Estimate      Error  Chi-Square  Chi-Square

 AGE        1       0.013823    0.01813     0.58165      0.4457
 PRIOR_SX   1      -0.545702    0.61091     0.79792      0.3717
 RX         1       0.118102    0.32769     0.12989      0.7185
 AGE_RX     1       0.034766    0.02725     1.62719      0.2021
 PRIOR_RX   1      -0.291631    0.75819     0.14795      0.7005
```

Discontinuous intervals of risk

Experimental units may have time periods when they are not "at risk" for various reasons. For example, they may be lost to observation. In a study of the relationship between tumor progression and the time course of a blood marker, the protocol called for measurement of the marker every three to six months; a sample of observations is shown in Table 3.6. One patient had a two-year hiatus in her visit record. See patient 2 in the table with the long interval $(96, 405]$ and the lab measurement given as "?". Rather than interpolate the values over that two-year period, the investigators chose to treat the measurements as missing data. One could either remove that row from the data file or simply use the missing data indicator (NA in S-Plus or "." in SAS) in place of "?", thus effectively removing the subject from the risk set over that interval, since the analysis programs first remove missing observations.

Another example occurs in clinical studies of multiple adverse events, such as injuries, where the treatment for an event temporarily protects the patient from further injury. In a study of falls in the elderly, hospitalization following a fall would protect the patient from additional falls. (For conditions with a low event rate, however, this refinement is likely to be insignificant.) An example where the refinement does matter, however, can be found in Therneau and Hamilton [144]. Patients with cystic fibrosis are at risk for recurrent lung infections, due in part to the lungs' inability to clear unnaturally thick mucus. In a study of rhDNase, an enzyme felt to help the condition, patients were by definition not at risk for a "new" infection during antibiotic treatment for the infection, nor for seven days after the end of antibiotic treatment. Thus, they contain gaps in their at risk

Subject	Interval	Status	Lab
1	(0, 90]	0	80
1	(90, 173]	0	75
1	(173,300]	0	91
2	(0, 96]	0	105
2	(96, 405]	0	?
2	(405, 487]	0	87
2	(487, 560]	0	80
⋮	⋮	⋮	⋮

TABLE 3.6: *A sample data set with discontinuous follow-up*

interval by protocol design. This example is discussed in more detail in the section on multiple events.

3.7.2 Alternate time scales

In most uses of the Cox model "time" is time since entry to the study. In some studies a more logical grouping might be based on another alignment, such as age or time since diagnosis. Andersen et al. [4] discuss this issue in several of their examples, and then in depth in Chapter 10 of their book. One example concerns nephropathy and mortality among insulin-dependent diabetics. Patients can be in one of three states: 0 = alive without diabetic nephropathy (DN), 1 = alive with DN, and 3 = dead. Relevant time scales for the 0–1 transition are age, calendar time, and duration of diabetes, and for the 1–2 transition the duration of DN.

As another example consider a study conducted at the Mayo Clinic on the effect of L-dopa for patients with Parkinson's disease. In a longe term condition such as this, the time interval between diagnosis and referral to Mayo might depend on driving distance, affluence, a relative's prior experience with the institution, or other non-disease factors. It was felt that time from diagnosis was the most appropriate time scale for analysis. However, Mayo is a major tertiary referral center, and many of the study's patients were not seen at Mayo until well after that date. For each patient we have the date of diagnosis, the date of referral to Mayo, and the date of last followup or death. The patient diagnosed on 2/8/82 with referral on 4/28/85 and last contact on 6/18/90 is represented as a single interval (1175, 3052]. It is not correct to enter them as (0, 3052] (which is equivalent to a standard noninterval Cox model with followup time of 3052) since the patient was not at risk for an *observable* death during the first 1,175 days of that interval. Such data, where the patient enters the risk set after time 0, is said to be *left truncated.*

3.7.3 Summary

Some of the other usages mentioned above, for example, time-dependent strata and multiple events are discussed in later sections. The flexibility afforded by the (start, stop] paradigm has proven to be truly surprising. It was first added to S code by the first author in 1984 as an ad hoc way to handle multiple events, without any inkling as to its eventual utility.

One problem that does arise with moderate frequency is zero length intervals such as (11,11]. S-Plus treats these as an error; SAS silently ignores them. (We prefer the S-Plus behavior, since we have found that such intervals often signal a programming mistake.) The intervals can arise legally in one situation, which is a death or covariate change on the first day of enrollment; the usual method of date subtraction will give an interval of (0,0]. We suggest moving the event to day 0.5 (or .1 or .8 or ...). The actual value chosen will not affect the model results, as long as the value is before the first actual death or censoring event. It will affect the plotted survival curve based on the Cox model (but requires good eyesight to see it), and can affect tests for proportional hazards.

One should avoid the temptation to create short intervals. For instance, in a study of PSA (prostate specific antigen) as a marker for recurrence of prostate cancer, we have a subject with visits at 0, 100, 200, and 300 days after enrollment, PSA values of 3.0, 3.1, 3.5, 5.1, and an event, detection of recurrence, at day 300. Using the argument that "it's the value of 5.1 that is relevant on day 300," one might create a data set with intervals of (0, 99.9], (99.9, 199.9], (199.9, 299.9], and (299.9, 300] containing the four PSA values. Beyond the fact that the mathematical bases for the fit (including p-values) have all been washed away by this stratagem, what exactly is the meaning of a model that can predict this afternoon's clinical findings only by use of this morning's laboratory value? In the case at hand, the high PSA value may also have promoted the search for other, definitive evidence of progression: PSA predicts progression because it makes us look. Any (start, stop] setup that forces "$-\epsilon$" intervals like this should be viewed with suspicion.

The key strength of the counting process approach is its flexibility: because the user creates the data, it is easy to code variants or situations not thought of by the Cox program's authors. No internal changes to the program are needed to fit these variants. This strength is also its weakness: because the user sets up the data, it is possible to mess up, and fit an absolutely idiotic model. As an example of the latter, we include a real example from our own institution, one which unfortunately made it all the way to the final manuscript before being caught.

The study in question was a placebo-controlled trial of a new drug whose main effect was expected to be on the symptoms of a chronic disease. A possible improvement in survival was a secondary endpoint. Some patients were expected to have, and did have, an early adverse reaction to the drug.

The total number was small (4%), and they were crossed over to placebo. To deal with these subjects in the analysis, a time-dependent treatment variable was created based on the variable `weeks on rx`, which was a part of the data form. (Since no placebo patient crossed over, the variable was only filled out for patients on the active arm.) Here is, essentially, the SAS code for analysis. (The actual code was much less succinct, being an ancillary part of a much larger endeavor.)

```
data anal; set main;
    futime = last_dt - entry_dt;
    if (rx=1 and futime > weeks*7) then do;
        start=0; stop = weeks*7; status=0; output;
        start=stop, stop=futime; status=death; rx=2; output;
        end;
    else do;
        start=0; stop=futime; status=death; output;
        end;
```

What could be wrong with 9 lines of code? Assume that subject "Smith," randomized to the active drug, died exactly one year after enrollment, without crossover. His covariates are `futime=365`, `weeks=52`, `weeks*7 = 364`. Due to roundoff, about 1/2 of the treatment patients are "crossed over" to placebo one to three days before death or last followup. The total number of deaths on treatment is dramatically lowered. Not surprisingly, a Cox model based on the above data set shows a 50% reduction in deaths due to treatment; the correct analysis gives $\hat{\beta} \approx 0$.

There are four steps to effective use of the counting process paradigm.

1. Think through the problem. As in the Stanford data set, decide upon the ordering of various events (death, transplant, enrollment) in the case of ties. Create appropriate dummy variables for interactions, choose the time scale, and so on.
2. Create the (start, stop] data set. This is usually tedious but straightforward.
3. Check the data set for sanity.
    - PRINT OUT some or all of the cases.
    - Read the printout carefully.
4. Fit the model (trivial), and think again about what the results appear to be saying.

4

Residuals

There are four major residuals of interest in the Cox model: the martingale, deviance, score, and Schoenfeld residuals, along with two others, the dfbeta and scaled Schoenfeld residuals, that are derived from these. This chapter gives an overview of the definitions and mathematical underpinnings of the residuals; later chapters take up their uses one by one in detail.

4.1 Mathematical definitions

Several ideas for residuals based on a Cox model have been proposed on an ad hoc basis, most with only limited success. The current, and most successful, methods are based on counting process arguments, and in particular on the individual-specific counting process martingale that arises from this formulation. Barlow and Prentice [10] provided the basic framework and further initial work was done by Therneau et al. [143]. The counting process martingale for the ith individual, $M_i(t) = N_i(t) - E_i(t)$, becomes

$$M_i(t) = N_i(t) - \int_0^t Y_i(s) e^{X_i(s)\beta} \lambda_0(s)\, ds. \tag{4.1}$$

It has associated predictable and optional variation processes

$$\begin{aligned} \langle M_i \rangle(t) &= \int_0^t Y_i(s)\lambda_i(s)\, ds, & (4.2) \\ [M_i](t) &= N_i(t), & (4.3) \end{aligned}$$

and $\text{Var}(M_i(t)) = \mathcal{E}\langle M_i \rangle(t) = \mathcal{E}[M_i](t) = \mathcal{E}E_i(t)$. The counting process martingales are uncorrelated under very general regularity conditions. Independence of the individuals in the study is sufficient, but not necessary; all that is needed is a common filtration and no simultaneous jumps.

Equation (4.1) generalizes the counting process martingale introduced in Chapter 2, equation(2.10). There we mentioned the (imperfect) analogy between the statistical decomposition of data = model + noise and the Doob decomposition of counting process = compensator + martingale. Having fit a model to data, one has another statistical decomposition, data = fit + residuals, with the counting process analogue, counting process = estimated compensator + martingale residual (process). The martingale residual process is

$$\begin{aligned}\widehat{M}_i(t) &= N_i(t) - \widehat{E}_i(t) \\ &= N_i(t) - \int_0^t Y_i(s) e^{X_i(s)\hat{\beta}} d\hat{\Lambda}_0(s).\end{aligned} \tag{4.4}$$

The vector $\hat{\beta}$ is the maximum partial likelihood estimate, discussed in the last chapter, and $\hat{\Lambda}_0$ estimates the baseline cumulative hazard. Estimation of $\hat{\Lambda}_0$ is discussed in detail in Chapter 10 on expected survival; for now, we need merely note that the simplest estimator is also the easiest from the standpoint of martingale theory:

$$\hat{\Lambda}_0(t) = \int_0^t \frac{d\overline{N}(s)}{\sum_{j=1}^n Y_j(s) e^{X_j(s)\hat{\beta}}}. \tag{4.5}$$

Notice that this reduces to the Nelson–Aalen estimator when $\hat{\beta} = 0$. An immediate consequence of equation (4.5) is that $\sum_i \widehat{M}_i(t) = 0$ for any t.

4.2 Martingale residuals

4.2.1 Properties

Define $M_i = N_i - E_i$ as the martingale residual process at the end of the study; formally $M_i = \widehat{M}_i(\infty) = N_i(\infty) - \widehat{E}_i(\infty)$. In the special situation of no time-dependent covariates and each subject under observation from 0 to t_i, the residual takes the simple nonintegral form $\widehat{M}_i = N_i - \hat{r}_i \hat{\Lambda}_0(\hat{\beta}, t_i)$.

The martingale residual is really a simple difference $O - E$ between the observed number of events for an individual and the conditionally expected number given the fitted model, followup time, and the observed course of any time-varying covariates. Four properties of martingale residuals parallel those familiar from an ordinary linear model.

1. $E(M_i) = 0$. The expected value of each residual is 0, when evaluated at the true (unknown) parameter vector β.

2. $\sum \widehat{M}_i = 0$. The observed residuals based on $\hat{\beta}$ must sum to 0.

Model	df	Martingale SS	Deviance SS
null	0	159	553
bili	1	169	502
log(bili)	1	165	462
5 variable	5	180	418

TABLE 4.1: *Martingale and deviance residuals for PBC data*

3. $\text{Cov}(M_i, M_j) = 0$. The residuals computed at the true parameter vector β are uncorrelated.
4. $\text{Cov}(\widehat{M_i}, \widehat{M_j}) < 0$. The actual residuals are negatively correlated, as a consequence of condition 2. The covariance is, however, very slight, $O(1/n)$ as with linear models.

4.2.2 Overall tests of goodness-of-fit

Despite these similarities, the martingale residuals can not play all the roles that linear model residuals do; in particular, the overall distribution of the residuals does not aid in the global assessment of fit. In linear models, the sum of squared residuals provides an overall summary measure of goodness-of-fit. Of several competing models with approximately the same number of parameters, the one with the smallest SS is preferred. With Cox regression however, the best model need not have the smallest sum of squared martingale residuals. For PBC, prior modeling along with multiple validations of the models on independent populations have verified that (a) bilirubin is a very important and predictive risk factor and that (b) it predicts better if it enters the model in the log scale. Furthermore, age, severity of edema, prothrombin level, and albumin are useful additional predictors. Table 4.1 shows the sums of squared martingale residuals for these four models. Surprisingly, the martingale residuals put the models in nearly the reverse order to that expected. The no-covariate model has the smallest sum of squared martingale residuals and the best model, the one with all five predictors, has the largest. The models based on bilirubin alone are intermediate.

4.2.3 Distribution

With linear models, the errors are assumed normally distributed, and if the model fit to the data is correct, the residuals should have approximately the normal distribution. There are numerous tests and diagnostic plots to assess normality; perhaps the most common is the normal QQ plot: the ordered residuals are plotted on the ordinate versus expected Gaussian order statistics on the abscissa. Residuals that are Gaussian in distribution give roughly a straight line, and nonlinearity indicates some departure from normality. The analogue for the Cox model is comparison of the martingale residuals to a unit exponential distribution. This would be a good idea if it worked.

The plot is motivated by the fact that if a random failure time T has a distribution with integrated hazard function Λ, then $\Lambda(T)$ has a unit exponential distribution. If the model fit is correct, then the set of values $\{\hat{\Lambda}_i(T_i)\}$ should behave as a(censored) iid sample from a unit exponential. For censored data recall that if $T \sim \exp(1)$, then $\mathrm{E}[T|T \geq c] = c+1$. Therefore, one could consider a plot with $\hat{\Lambda}_i(T_i)$ for the failure times and $\hat{\Lambda}_i(T_i)+1$ for the censored times. But this is just the set $\{1 - \widehat{M}_i\}$. Thus, it is tempting to assess the goodness-of-fit of a Cox model by assessing exponentiality of the martingale residuals, for example, by plotting against the expected values of exponential order statistics, the analogue of the normal QQ plot. However, this is a hopeless endeavor. The semiparametric estimator of the baseline cumulative hazard rescales the martingale residuals to be roughly exponential no matter how bad the model is. In fact, if there are no censored data points, the ordered set of values $\{1 - \widehat{M}_i\}$ from the null model will be, by the definition of $\hat{\Lambda}_0$, exactly the order statistics of a sample from the unit exponential, that is, $\{1/n, [1/n+1/(n-1)], [1/n+1/(n-1)+1/(n-2)], \ldots\}$. Thus, the residuals from the true model are a random sample from the exponential distribution, while those from the null model are a "perfect" sample: the null model is guaranteed to be the best fit, even if all the covariates have substantial impacts on the hazard. By contrast, for parametric models this approach has some merit.

Another common diagnostic tool for linear models is the plot of the residuals against the fitted values. If the model is correct, it will be a structureless, roughly horizontal band of points. This plot is useless for martingale residuals; the martingale residuals and the fitted values are negatively correlated, frequently strongly so. Consider the case of uncensored survival data, where each subject has exactly one event. Since $N_i(\infty) = 1 \; \forall i$, the plot is one of $1 - \widehat{E}_i$ versus $\widehat{E}_i$, a straight line of slope -1 for any model fit to the data.

4.2.4 Usage

At this point, one may wonder if the martingale residuals are good for anything. They are; two important uses are a direct assessment and for investigating functional form. By the former, we mean that examination of the residuals as a measure $O - E$ of "excess events" will reveal individuals that are poorly fit by the model — they either lived too long or died too soon. For the PBC data, for instance, the smallest residual from a null model is -1.03; the five variable model has two individuals with residuals < -3.5. These are persons with long survival times in spite of high-risk covariates, the cases may be worth further examination and thought.

Evaluation of the appropriate functional form for a covariate uses methods parallel to linear model plots of residuals versus a single or multiple predictor. It is discussed in Chapter 5.

4.3 Deviance residuals

The martingale residual is highly skewed, particularly for single-event (survival) data, with a long right-hand tail. The deviance residual is a normalizing transform [143], similar in form to the deviance residual for Poisson regression. If all covariates are time-fixed, the deviance residual is

$$d_i = \text{sign}(\widehat{M}_i) * \sqrt{-\widehat{M}_i - N_i \log((N_i - \widehat{M}_i)/N_i)}.$$

A one-term Taylor expansion shows that

$$d_i \approx \frac{N_i - \widehat{E}_i}{\sqrt{\widehat{E}_i}},$$

formally equivalent to the Pearson residual of generalized linear models. The deviance residual was designed to improve on the martingale residual for revealing individual outliers, particularly in plotting applications. In practice it has not been as useful as anticipated.

Table 4.1 would suggest that the sum of squared deviance residuals can be used to compare models. Although more often properly ordered than the sum of squared martingale residuals, this sum also is not guaranteed to decrease with improved model fit.

4.4 Martingale transforms

Barlow and Prentice [10] pointed out that a flexible family of residual processes arises from transformation of the individual counting process martingales:

$$R_i(h_i) = \int h_i(t)\, dM_i(t);\ i = 1, \ldots, n,$$

where h_i is a possibly vector-valued predictable process, that is, a process that depends only on information prior to time t. From results discussed in Section 2.2.2 on martingale basics, one can immediately conclude that these processes have mean 0, are orthogonal and therefore uncorrelated, and have predictable variation processes

$$\langle R_i \rangle = \int Y_i(s) h_i(s) h_i'(s) d\Lambda_i(s).$$

The corresponding observed residual process is

$$\widehat{R}_i(h_i) = \int h_i(t)\, d\widehat{M}_i(t),$$

with the "plug-in" variance estimator:

$$\widehat{\text{var}}(\widehat{R}_i) = \int Y_i(s) h_i(s) h_i'(s) d\hat{\Lambda}_i(s). \tag{4.6}$$

The martingale residual itself corresponds to $h_i(t) = 1$. Barlow and Prentice suggested three others: $h_i(t) = t$, $h_i(t) = \log(\hat{r}_i(t))$, and $h_i(t) = X_i(t) - \bar{x}(\hat{\beta}, t)$. The first two are suggested as residuals that would be sensitive to time trends and to incorrect specification of the covariate model, respectively, but have received little attention. The third gives rise to the score residual discussed below.

Assume that we have a counting process style of data set, where each subject may be represented by multiple (start, stop] intervals. One nice feature of the martingale and transformed martingale residuals is that the residual for a subject is the sum of the residuals for his or her observations. This is a natural consequence of the integral representation. For example, assume that subject "Smith" is represented in the data as four observations with intervals (0,10], (10,25], (25,27], and (27,50]. The martingale residuals for the individual observations are

$$\int_0^{10} Y_i(s)\hat{r}_i(s)\, d\hat{\Lambda}_0(s), \qquad \int_{10}^{25} Y_i(s)\hat{r}_i(s)\, d\hat{\Lambda}_0(s),$$
$$\int_{25}^{27} Y_i(s)\hat{r}_i(s)\, d\hat{\Lambda}_0(s), \quad \text{and} \quad \int_{27}^{50} Y_i(s)\hat{r}_i(s)\, d\hat{\Lambda}_0(s).$$

The martingale residual for the subject is the integral from 0 to 50, which is obviously the sum of these four quantities. The same argument holds for a martingale transform residual $R_i(h)$.

4.5 Score residuals

The score process for the ith individual is

$$U_i(\beta, t) = \int_0^t [X_i(s) - \bar{x}(\beta, s)]\, dM_i(s),$$

where $\bar{x}(\beta, s)$, defined in equation (3.5), is the weighted mean of the covariates over those at risk at time s. It is a row vector of length p, the number of covariates, with components $U_{ij}(\beta, t)$, $j = 1, \ldots, p$.

One can think of the set of score processes as a three-way array with dimensions of subject, covariate, and time. The time dimension is discrete when one considers only those time points with one or more events. Let t_k denote the kth event time. Then

$$U_{ijk}(\beta) = \int_{t_{k-1}}^{t_k} [X_{ij}(s) - \bar{x}_j(\beta, s)]\, dM_i(s). \tag{4.7}$$

Lin et al. [87] suggest a global test of the proportional hazards model based on the maximum of the array.

The *score residual* is defined as $U_{ij} = U_{ij}(\hat{\beta}, \infty)$. The set of score residuals forms an $n \times p$ matrix. It is easy to show using the definition of $\hat{\Lambda}_0$ in equation (4.5) that for all t,

$$\sum_i U_i(\hat{\beta}, t) = \sum_i \int_0^t [X_i(s) - \bar{x}(\hat{\beta}, s)]\, dN_i(s). \tag{4.8}$$

Also, $\sum_i U_{ij}(\hat{\beta}, \infty) = 0$. The right-hand side of equation (4.8) is recognizable as the estimating equation for the Cox model for $t = \infty$. Therefore, the score residuals form an additive decomposition of the Cox model estimating equation into subject-specific components that are *uncorrelated* because of their martingale structure. That is not true of the obvious decomposition of the right-hand side of (4.8) into single components $\int_0^t [X_i(s) - \bar{x}(\hat{\beta}, s)]\, dN_i(s)$ corresponding to each event. The score residuals are useful for assessing individual influence and for robust variance estimation, which is discussed in Chapter 7.

4.6 Schoenfeld residuals

Summing the score process array over individuals gives a process that varies over time. This yields a residual first proposed by Schoenfeld [128]. Because $\hat{\Lambda}_0$ is discrete, our estimated score process is also discrete, having jumps at each of the unique death times. The Schoenfeld residual at the kth event time is

$$\begin{aligned} s_k &= \int_{t_{k-1}}^{t_k} \sum_i [X_i - \bar{x}(\hat{\beta}, s)] d\widehat{M}_i(s) \\ &= \int_{t_{k-1}}^{t_k} \sum_i [X_i - \bar{x}(\hat{\beta}, s)] dN_i(s). \end{aligned} \tag{4.9}$$

The set of Schoenfeld residuals is a p column matrix with one row per event, the kth row as above. Since the residuals are defined at each unique death, their definition and computation is unchanged by a counting process formulation of the data set.

When there are no tied event times, then equation (4.9) above can be rewritten as

$$s_k = X_{(k)} - \bar{x}(\hat{\beta}, t_k), \tag{4.10}$$

where $X_{(k)}$ is the covariate vector of the individual experiencing the kth event, at the time of that event. When there are $k > 1$ tied events at a given time, the computer programs return k residuals, each one based on equation (4.10) applied to that event rather than an overall residual for that time point based on equation (4.9). (This choice is more useful for the residual plots discussed later.) Schoenfeld residuals are useful for assessing proportional hazards, and are discussed in Chapter 6.

5

Functional Form

In the Cox model, we assume that the hazard function satisfies

$$\lambda_i(t) = \lambda_0(t) \exp(X_i\beta)\,,$$

that is, a proportional hazards structure with a loglinear model for the covariates. For a continuous variable, age, for instance, this implicitly assumes the ratio of risks between a 45- and a 50-year-old is the same as that between an 80- and an 85-year-old. Yet experience with biological data shows that threshold effects, both upper and lower, are common. Perhaps the risk does not begin to rise until after age 65, or even rises and then falls again at a later age.

In this chapter we describe several methods useful for exploring the correct functional form for a covariate. Section 5.7 and Section 5.8 give theoretical development for methods based on martingale residuals and penalized likelihoods and may be omitted on a first reading.

5.1 Simple approach

The simplest approach is one examined by Therneau et al. [143] who suggested plotting the martingale residuals from a null model, that is, one with $\hat\beta = 0$, against each covariate separately and superimposing a scatterplot smooth. They show that if the correct model for covariate j is $\exp(f(X_j)\beta_j)$ for some smooth function f, then the smooth for the jth covariate will display the form of f, under certain assumptions. That is,

$$E(M_i|X_{ij} = x_j) \approx cf(x_j),$$

where c is roughly independent of x_j and depends on the amount of censoring. Since c simply scales the y axis, it has no effect on the visual appearance of the plot. In many ways, this plot is similar in spirit to the ordinary "y versus x" plots of the response variable against each predictor used for uncensored data in linear models.

5.1.1 *Stage D1 prostate cancer*

Winkler et al. [160] studied the utility of flow cytometry as a prognostic method for patients with stage D1 prostatic adenocarcinoma. There were 91 patients, all of whom received a radical prostatectomy as the surgical procedure. A clinical stage of D1 means that disease is present in local lymph nodes, but is not (yet) evident in distant sites such as the bone marrow. The available variables included demographics (age, date of surgery, ...), pathological staging, and flow cytometry. All patients had 5+ years of followup.

The flow cytometric analysis used archival tissue material from the excised tumor. The cell's DNA was stained with a fluorescent dye, and then 100,000 cells were individually passed through the beam of a low-power laser and the amount of DNA recorded. Each cell could then be individually classified. Diploid cells have the expected amount of DNA material (23 pairs). Tetraploid cells have double the expected amount of DNA; presumably these are cells that are midway through cell division (the DNA has replicated but the cytoplasm has not yet divided, known as G2 phase). Aneuploid cells are those with an abnormal number of chromosomes, which can be either greater or less than that of a diploid cell, perhaps due to the loss or duplication of a single chromosome or portion thereof.

Since aneuploidy is considered the most serious pattern, any tumor with a detectable fraction of aneuploid cells was classified as "aneuploid." Among the remainder, any tumor with $\geq 13\%$ cells in G2 phase was classified as "tetraploid," and the remainder of the tumors as diploid. We might expect tetraploid tumors to have a higher recurrence rate than diploid tumors, since they have a larger growth fraction of actively dividing cells. There were 38 diploid, 41 tetraploid, and 12 aneuploid tumors by these criteria.

The use of diploid/tetraploid as a variable in the model essentially enters the percentage of tetraploid cells as a step function: risk is considered to be constant below 13%, rise abruptly, and then remain constant for all growth fractions above this point. This model is not necessarily correct of course, and we would like to examine the data to see if they fulfill these assumptions. Perhaps the percentage in G2 phase should be entered as a linear term, or as linear up to some threshold, or some other form. The default cutoff value of 13% had been chosen as the mean + 3 standard deviations ($7.87 + 3 * 1.53$) of the g2 values from a sample of 60 specimens of noncancerous human prostate tissue (cases of benign prostatic hyperplasia). On the basis of these "normal" controls an upper limit of 13% was

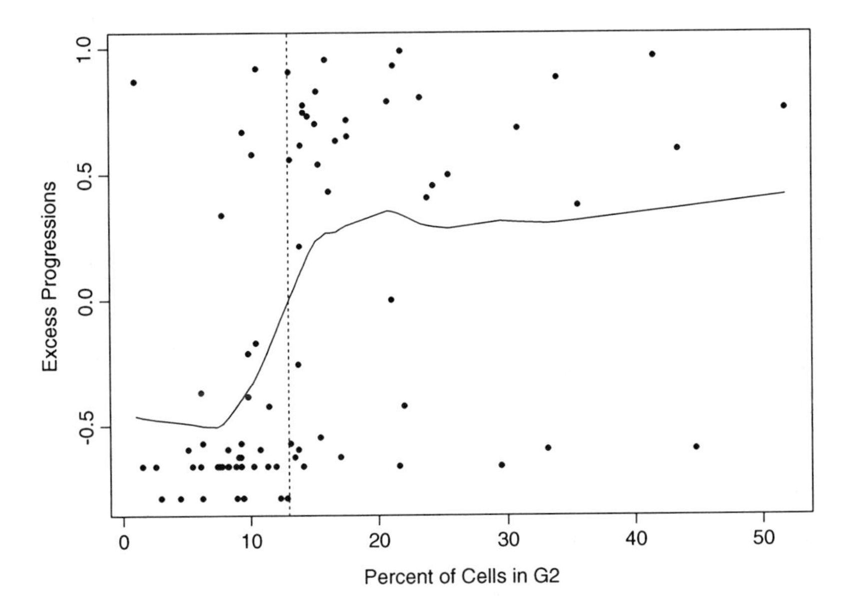

FIGURE 5.1: *Stage D1 prostate cancer*

defined. Although this cutoff might be expected to produce a relatively small number of false positives (indolent tumors labeled as "aggressive") there is no guarantee that it is the best overall cutoff. In particular, from a clinical point of view it is the other error, the labeling of an aggressive tumor as slow growing, that is the more serious mistake.

The following code uses the martingale residuals to explore the issue, with time to progression as the outcome.

```
> fit <- coxph(Surv(pgtime, pgstat) ~ 1, data=prostate)
> plot(prostate$g2, resid(fit),
                         xlab='Percent of Cells in G2',
                         ylab='Excess Progressions')
> smooth <- mlowess(prostate$g2, resid(fit), iter=0)
> lines(smooth)
> abline(v=13)
```

The result is shown in Figure 5.1. The y-axis of the figure, "Excess Progressions," was used in Winkler et al. [160] and seems to be a good choice for clinical audiences. In this case, the figure has validated the prior cutoff. The effect of G2% appears to have a threshold, and that threshold is quite close to 13%. A scatterplot smoother such as `lowess` will never give exactly a step function, of course.

The first line of the code fits an "intercept only" proportional hazards model by using $\sim$1 as the right-hand side of the model equation. Line 2 plots the `g2` values versus the martingale residuals. Line 3 computes a `lowess` smooth. This method has been shown, both in theory and long experience, to have good visual and practical smoothing properties. The `mlowess`

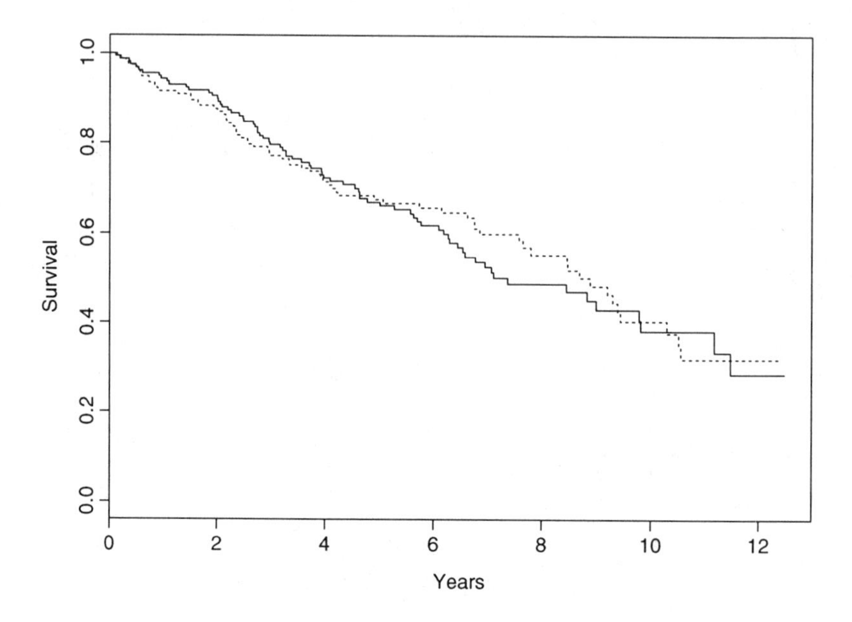

FIGURE 5.2: *Survival for the PBC study, by treatment arm*

function is a simple modification to the standard S-Plus `lowess` function which first removes missing values; that is, the 12 aneuploid patients that are missing `g2`. The smooth is then added to the plot, along with a vertical reference line at 13%. We are firm believers in the observation of Chambers et al. [28] that it is much easier for the human eye to see the pattern in a scatterplot when aided by a appropriate smoother (see their pages 101–104 "Why is smoothing scatterplots important?").

5.1.2 PBC data

A richer example is based on the PBC data set, introduced in Section 3.1, from a clinical trial comparing prednisone and placebo for patients suffering from primary biliary cirrhosis of the liver, a progressive, ultimately fatal disease. Liver transplantation is the only definitive treatment. Figure 5.2 shows the proportion alive without liver transplant for the two treatment arms of the study. Through previous work, the important variables and their proper transformation are already "known." Important covariates are the patient's age at first diagnosis, physical symptoms such as ascites or hepatomegaly, and blood values related to liver function such as bilirubin, albumin, and alkaline phosphotase.

The following code creates null residual plots for two covariates, age and bilirubin.

```
> fit.pbc0 <- coxph(Surv(futime, fustat) ~ 1,  data=pbc)
> rr <- resid(fit.pbc0)                          #martingale residuals
> plot(pbc$age, rr, xlab="Age", ylab='Residual')
```

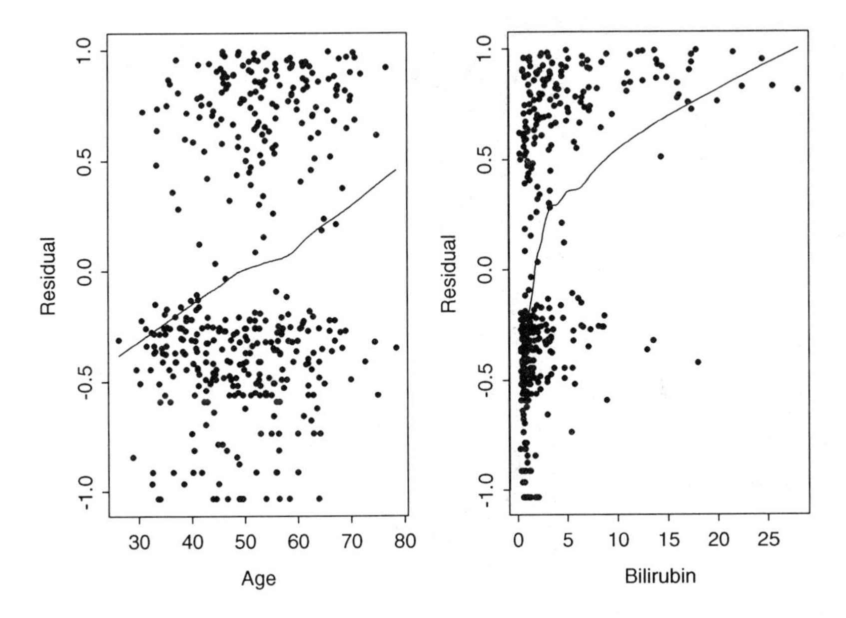

FIGURE 5.3: *PBC data, residual plots for age and bilirubin*

```
> lines(lowess(pbc$age, rr, iter=0), lty=2)
>
> plot(pbc$bili, rr, xlab="Bilirubin", ylab='Residual')
> lines(lowess(pbc$bili, rr, iter=0), lty=2)
```

Figure 5.3 shows that age is reasonably linear, but that bilirubin is certainly not so. A roughly logarithmic shape is suggested, and this can be easily checked by plotting on a log scale as shown in Figure 5.4.

```
> plot(pbc$bili, rr, log='x',
       xlab="Bilirubin", ylab='Residual')
> lines(lowess(pbc$bili, rr, iter=0), lty=2)
```

Creation of these plots in SAS is more subtle, as `phreg` has no option to directly fit a model without covariates. However, the procedure can be "fooled" by using a single dummy variable as follows. (Since it is not documented in the SAS manual, we can not be sure that this method for producing null residuals will work in future SAS releases.)

```
data temp; set pbc;
    dummy = 0;

proc phreg data=temp noprint;
    model futime*fustat(0)= dummy;
    output out=temp2 resmart=rr / order=data;

data temp3;
    merge temp temp2;
```

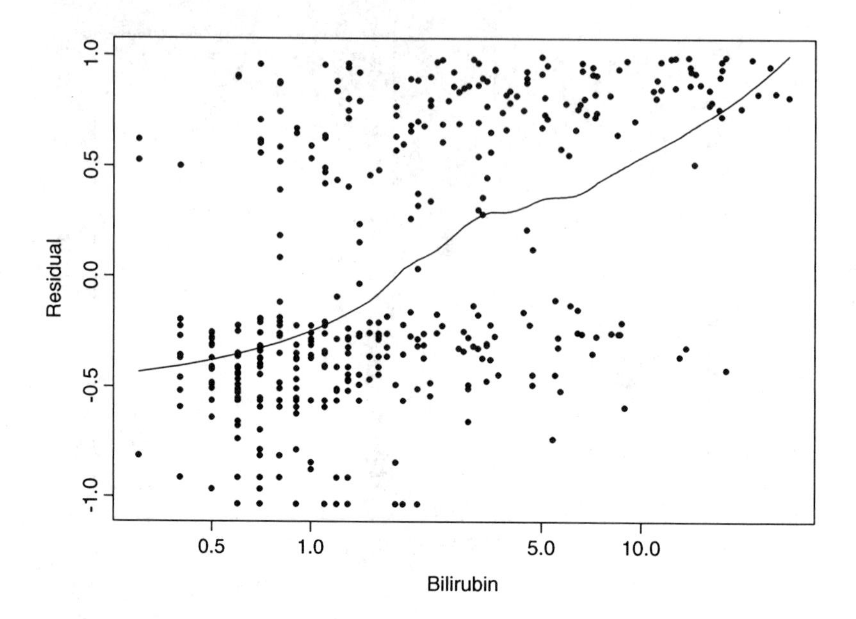

FIGURE 5.4: *PBC data, logarithmic plot for bilirubin*

```
proc gplot;
    plot rr * bili;
    symbol i=sm60s v=J font=special;
    label rr= 'Residual' bili= 'Bilirubin';
```

First a dummy variable is created such that $\hat{\beta}$ for this variable is guaranteed to be zero. The standard `phreg` printout is suppressed, and a model fit using only the dummy variable. The martingale residual is computed, and saved as variable `rr` in data set `temp2`. By default, the observations in the output data set are sorted in order of the time variable of the fitted data set; this is rarely useful, and we instead choose to have the output in the order of the input data set, which allows us to easily merge the residuals back into the original data set for further plotting. The scatterplot smoother that is used in this example is a smoothing spline built into the `gplot` procedure. The smoothing parameter ranges from 0 to 100; the value of 60 was chosen by inspection (plot not shown).

5.1.3 Heavy censoring

One feature of the above plot for residuals versus age is the horizontal "banding" of the points. There are a large number of residuals between -0.1 and -0.6, few between 0 and .3, and so on. This effect is particularly noticeable in data sets with a large amount of censoring. The PBC data

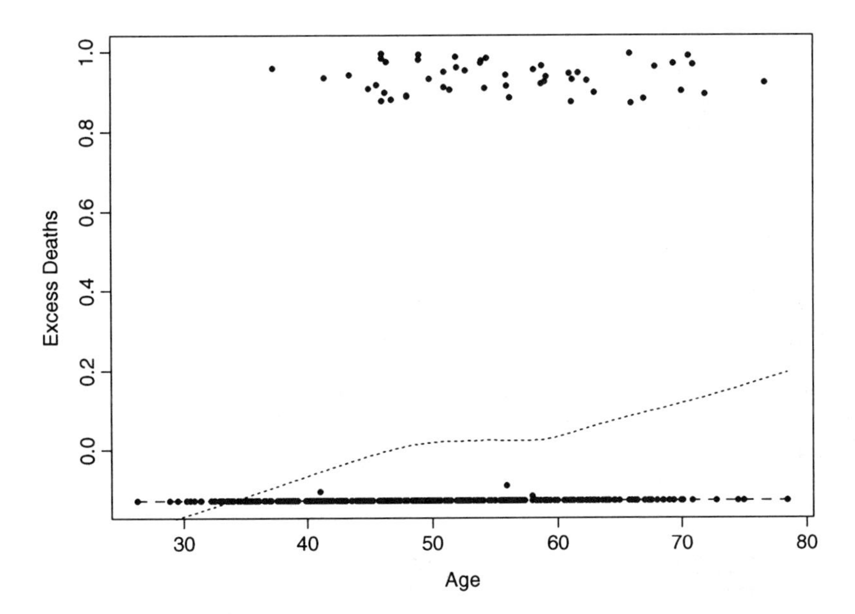

FIGURE 5.5: *Censored PBC data, functional form for age*

have followup times of between 0.1 and 13 years; we create a censored version by truncating followup for all subjects at 2 years.

Here is sample code in SAS to truncate the data and redraw the plot.

```
data pbc2; set pbc;
    dummy =0;
    if (fu_time < 730) then do;
        time2 = futime;
        stat2 = status;
        end;
    else do;
        time2 = 730;
        stat2 = 0;
        end;

proc phreg data=pbc2;
    model time2 * stat2(0) = dummy;
    output out=temp2 mresid=rr / order=data;

data temp3; merge pbc2 temp2;
proc plot;
    plot rr * age;
```

The S-Plus code is similar.

```
> time2 <- ifelse(pbc$futime <730, pbc$futime, 730)
> stat2 <- ifelse(pbc$futime <730, pbc$fustat, 0)
> fit0  <- coxph(Surv(time2, stat2) ~1)
> plot(pbc$age, resid(fit0))
```

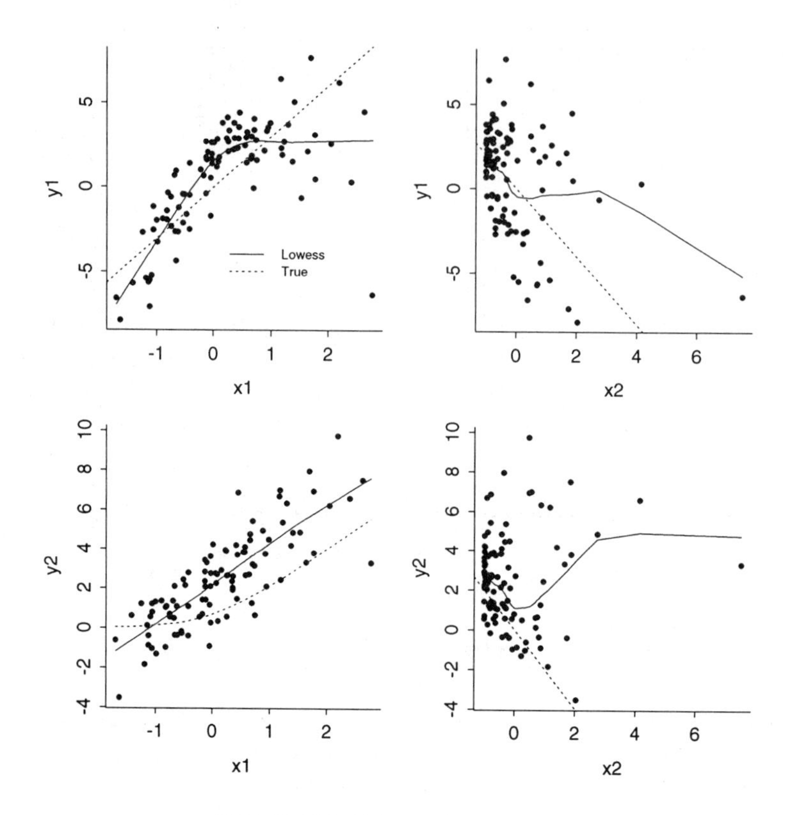

FIGURE 5.6: *Relationships for the simulated data*

```
> lines(lowess(pbc$age, resid(fit0), iter=0), lty=2)
> lines(lowess(pbc$age, resid(fit0)          ), lty=3)
```

As we can see from Figure 5.5, the results from heavily censored data look almost like a plot of binomial data. The martingale residual is $O - E$; in this case O, the observed number of events, is the 0/1 variable `stat2` and E, the expected number of events, ranges from 0.04 to 0.12.

The `iter` argument in the `lowess` function controls the number of iterations used for an outlier detection rule; setting the value to 0 effectively suppresses the outlier removal portion of the algorithm. The importance of the `iter=0` argument is apparent from the two lines drawn on the plot. In the second, the outlier rejection phase of `lowess` has decided that *all* of the deaths — residuals near 1 — are outliers, has eliminated them, and given as a result the boring and uninformative smooth of the remainder of the points, which is essentially a horizontal line near the bottom of the graph. (This second smooth is almost invisible on the plot.) The first smooth is much more useful.

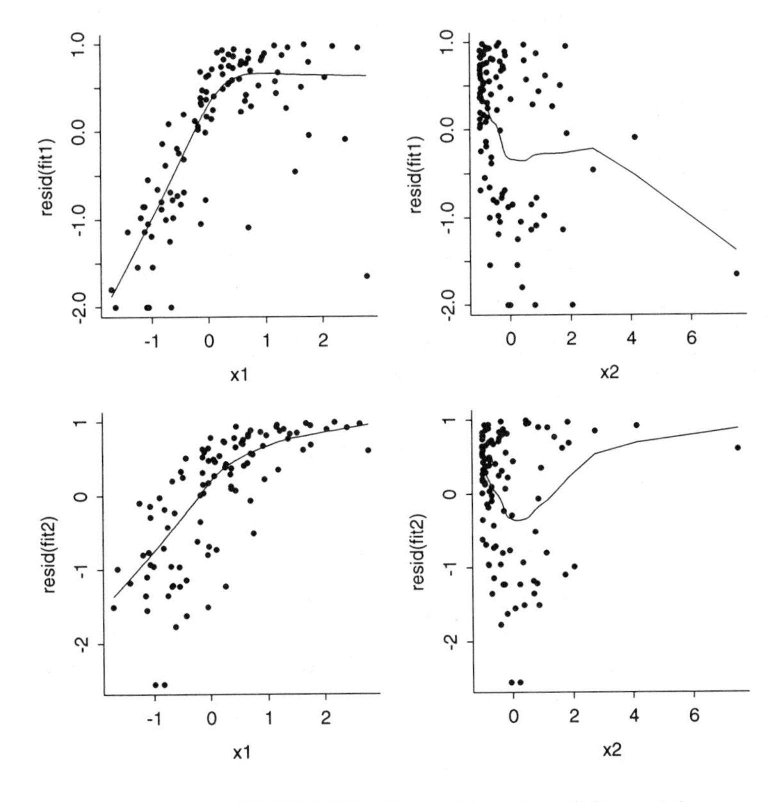

FIGURE 5.7: *"Survival" version of Figure 5.6*

5.2 Correlated predictors

The simple method based on null model residuals works well when the data are uncorrelated, but may fail when correlations are present. The same failure occurs for ordinary scatterplots in uncensored data: if $y = 2x_1 + 0x_2$ and $\text{cor}(x_1, x_2) = .9$, then a plot of y versus x_2 will show a spurious relationship.

We illustrate some of these points with a simple simulated data set. Let x_1 and x_3 be bivariate normal $N(0, 1)$ with correlation 0.8 and $x_2 = x_3^2 - 1$, with x_1 and x_2 being the "observed" covariates. Both have mean 0. Let

- $y_1 = 3x_1 - 2x_2 + \epsilon$, where $\epsilon \sim N(0, 1)$ is an iid additive error. This is a simple additive model, and the ideal scatterplot would show linear trends for both x_1 and x_2;
- $y_2 = 2 * f(x_1) + x_2$, where $f(x) = \log\{1 + \exp(2x)\}$, which mimics a threshold type of function often found in biomedical data.

Figure 5.6 shows the scatterplots of the raw data, along with the true functional forms and a `lowess` smooth. For y_1, the scatterplot shows nonlinearity for x_1, when the true relationship is linear, and for y_2 it shows a linear relationship to x_1 when the true relationship has a lower threshold! More complex artifacts are introduced into the plot of y_2 versus x_2.

Now, consider a survival version of the above. Fit a survival model to the same covariates but with y replaced by `time = rank(-y)`. We use $-y$ to invert the relationship, since in the Cox model a large value of $X\beta$ predicts a *shorter* survival. Using the ranks is a simple way to guarantee a positive time value, which is required by many programs. (Since the Cox model depends only on the order of the death times, ranking does not introduce any distortions in the fit.) The censoring time was set as a random uniform between 50 and 100 so that approximately 25% of the subjects are censored.

```
> fit0 <- coxph(Surv(time1, status1) ~ x1)
> plot(x1, resid(fit0))
> lines(lowess(x1, resid(fit0)))
```

The results are shown in Figure 5.7. The correspondence with the ordinary scatterplot is remarkable.

5.2.1 Linear models methods

The problem of correlated data and their effect on ordinary scatterplots has been investigated by multiple authors. Several suggestions for correction of the figure in the linear models case have been made, including adjusted variable plots [108, 28], partial residual plots [48], adjusted partial residuals [98], constructed variable plots [34] and others. Some of these have been applied to the Cox model, with varying amounts of success.

One common idea that does not work is to select a single variable of interest, age say, and plot the residuals of a model with all but age versus age itself. Figure 5.8 shows the result of the residuals from a Cox model of `time1` fit to `x2`, plotted against `x1`. It has not improved upon the simple functional form plot to assess the effect of `x1` (Figure 5.6), and in fact seems to have introduced additional visual artifacts.

Adjusted variable plot

In linear regression, the adjusted variable plot uses the pairs $(y_{(k)}, x_{(k)})$ as plotting points, where $y_{(k)}$ is the residual from a regression of y on all of the x variables *except* the kth, and $x_{(k)}$ is the residual of a regression of the kth predictor x_k on the others. Thus both x and y are adjusted for the other predictors. If the model is linear in all predictors, then the adjusted variable plot will also be linear. Adjusted variable plots for x_1 in the constructed data set are shown in Figure 5.9. As predicted, the model that is linear is well recovered. The correct functional form for the non-linear model, however, is not made apparent.

This basic flaw of adjusted variable plots — that they can only validate that a linear term *is* correct — is a major deficit. More problematic is that extending the method to survival models is not as straightforward as one might hope. Figure 5.10 shows the result of the obvious (but incorrect) construction of an adjusted variable plot for survival form of the test data:

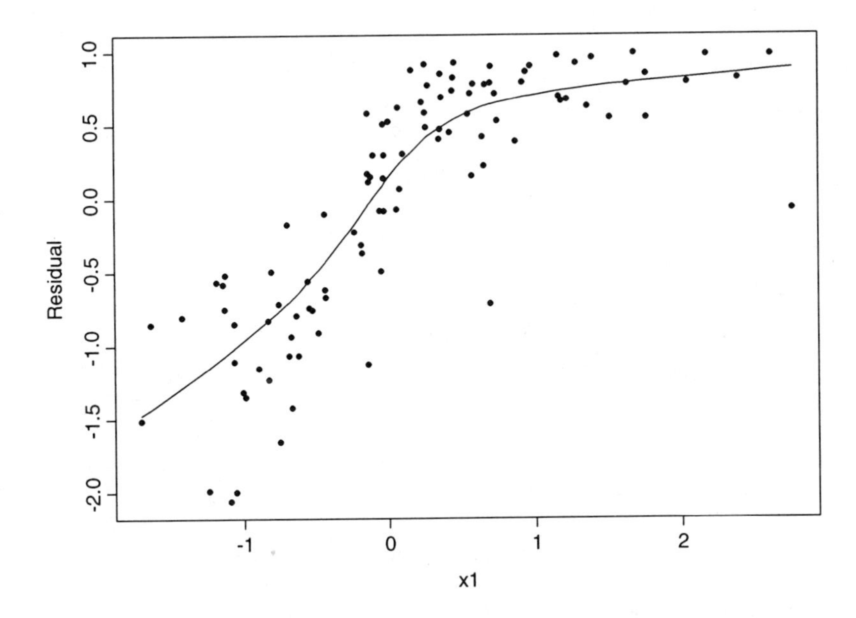

FIGURE 5.8: *Plot of x_1 versus the residuals from a fit of x_2*

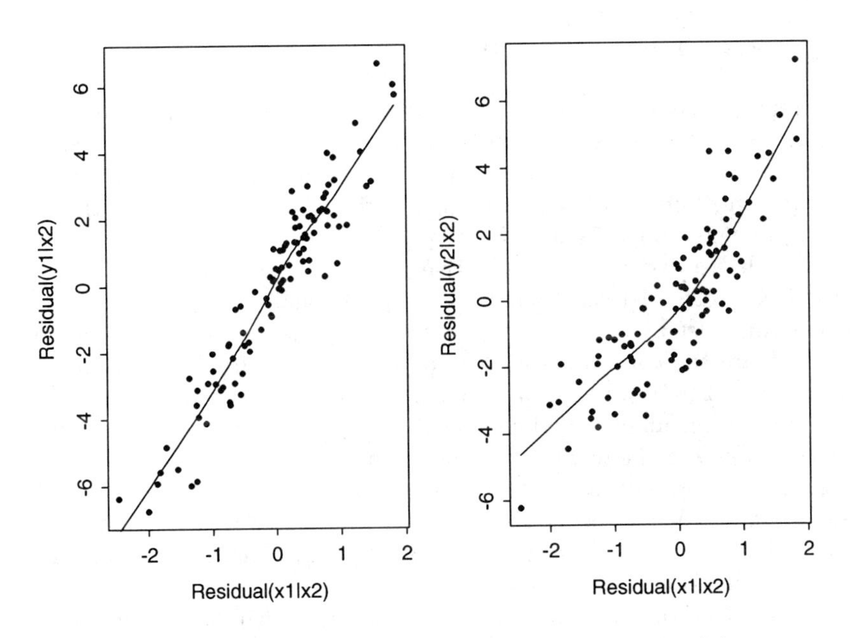

FIGURE 5.9: *Adjusted variable plots for the constructed data*

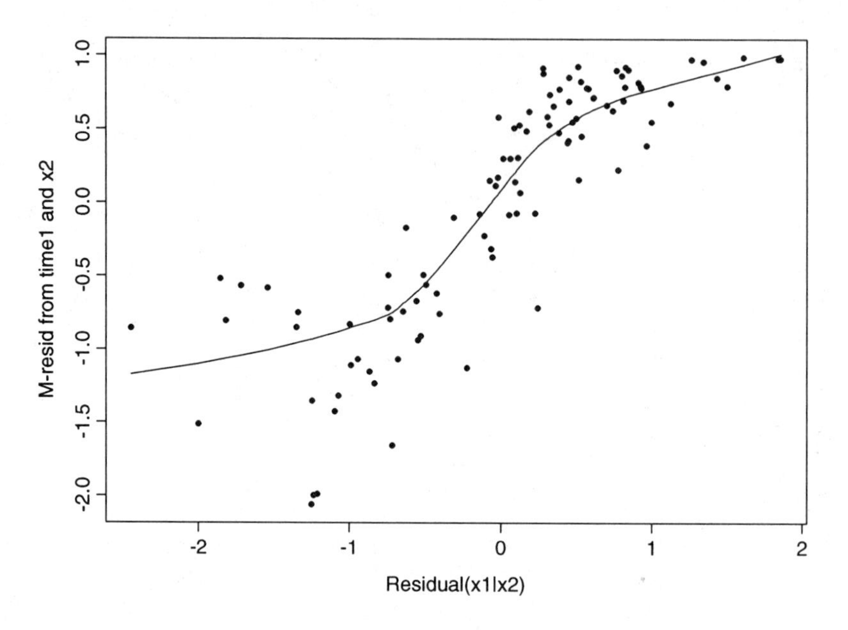

FIGURE 5.10: *Naive adjusted variable plot for the Cox model*

```
> cfit <- coxph(Surv(time1, status1) ~ x2)
> lfit <- lm(x1 ~ x2)
> plot(resid(lfit), resid(cfit))
```

A proper extension of the adjusted variable plot to the Cox model case requires that relative informativeness, as well as correlation of the predictors, be taken into account. For instance, a censored subject with very short followup contributes far less information to the fit than a subject with extensive time on study. Chen and Wang [32] use an analogy to a weighted linear model to derive a more effective result that accounts for differential followup. The derived formula is computationally complex, however. In particular, let Q be the $n \times n$ matrix such that $X'QX = \mathcal{I}$, where X and $\mathcal{I}$ are the covariate and information matrices from a Cox model without x_k. There is an explicit formulation for Q, but it requires approximately the same amount and complexity of computation as $\mathcal{I}$ itself; that is, it would need to be done in the underlying computer code of the `coxph` or `phreg` program. Given Q, the ordinate for the plot is a "standardized residual" $Q^{-1/2}M$, M being the vector of martingale residuals, and the abscissa is $x_{(k)} = (I - Q^{1/2}X(X'X)^{-1}Q^{1/2})Q^{1/2}x_k$. Further development of these methods is given in Hall et al. [60].

Since the focus of this monograph is on methods that can be employed using available statistical packages, however, the linear models approaches are not pursued further.

5.3 Poisson approach

As stated above, improving on the the simple residual plot requires that two issues be addressed: potential correlation between the predictors, and appropriate weighting of the observations to account for differential follow-up time. The second facet may often be more important than the first. A third issue, closely related to the weighting, is the proper handling of a subject who has been artificially broken into multiple observations in order to deal with a time-dependent covariate.

Grambsch et al. [55] extended the basic martingale method to address both linear and nonlinear relationships using a Poisson regression approach. Let $f(x)$ denote the p-vector whose jth component is $f_j(x_j)$, the "true" functional form for the covariate. Then we can compactly write the multivariate model with time-fixed covariates as

$$\lambda_i(t) = \exp(f(x)\beta)\lambda_0(t).$$

Recall

$$\mathcal{E}(N_i|x) = \exp(f(x)\beta) \int_0 Y_i(s)\lambda_0(s)ds. \tag{5.1}$$

Note that if we knew $\lambda_0(s)$, this is just a Poisson regression model with $\int_0 Y_i(s)\lambda_0(s)ds$ standing in the stead of the familiar "observation time." We do not know $\lambda_0(s)ds$, but we can get a reasonable estimate by fitting a Cox model using plausible transformations for the f_js, and in fact a simple model based on the untransformed data will usually suffice. We can then take advantage of any sophisticated modeling tools available in Poisson regression programs to help tease out the appropriate functional form. In S-Plus for instance this might involve the `gam` function, which implements the generalized additive models of Hastie and Tibshirani [63]. In SAS, Poisson regression/residuals based on the `genmod` procedure can be combined with known methods for Poisson residuals. We illustrate with the PBC data.

```
> pbcfit2 <- coxph(Surv(futime, status==2) ~ age + edema + bili +
                   protime  + albumin, data=pbc)
> print(pbcfit2)

           coef exp(coef) se(coef)     z       p
    age  0.0383      1.04  0.00806  4.75 2.0e-06
  edema  0.9351      2.55  0.28186  3.32 9.1e-04
   bili  0.1158      1.12  0.01302  8.90 0.0e+00
protime  0.2006      1.22  0.05661  3.54 3.9e-04
albumin -0.9682      0.38  0.20533 -4.72 2.4e-06

Likelihood ratio test=182  on 5 df, p=0  n=416
(2 observations deleted due to missing)
```

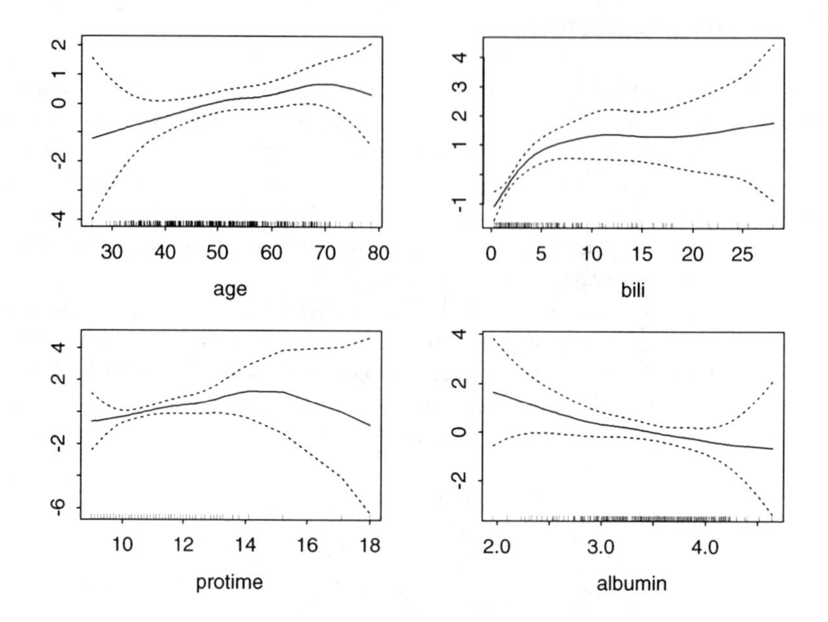

FIGURE 5.11: *PBC Data, functional form using Poisson approach*

```
> exp.fit <- predict(pbcfit2, type="expected")
> xbeta   <- predict(pbcfit2, type="lp")
> newtime <- exp(-xbeta) * exp.fit
> count   <- 1*(pbc$status==2)
> gfit <- gam(count ~ s(age) + edema + s(bili) + s(protime) +
                   s(albumin) + offset(log(newtime)),
               data=pbc, family=poisson)
> anova(gfit)

DF for Terms and Chi-squares for Nonparametric Effects

            Df Npar Df Npar Chisq    P(Chi)
(Intercept)  1
     s(age)  1     2.8    5.56682 0.1175459
      edema  1
    s(bili)  1     2.8   49.13039 0.0000000
 s(protime)  1     2.8    8.27830 0.0352276
 s(albumin)  1     2.8    1.68804 0.5959896

> plot(gfit, se=T, rug=T)
```

The `predict` function has options to return both the overall expected number of events E_i and the linear predictor for each subject $X_i\hat{\beta}$. The result of the `predict` function for `type='expected'` is the E_i part of the martingale residual, $\exp(X_i\hat{\beta})\hat{\Lambda}_0(T_i)$ for the ith individual, where (recall) T_i is the followup time. As a result, `newtime` is $\hat{\Lambda}_0(T_i)$, the estimate of $\int_0 Y_i(s)\lambda_0(s)$, used as an offset in Poisson regression. In the `gam` function, `s(age)` indicates that a nonlinear fit to the age coefficient is desired, using a default four degrees of freedom. The anova function prints out per term tests for nonlinearity; only bilirubin and prothrombin time show a significant curvature. The plots are shown in Figure 5.11 (a linear plot for edema is also produced by the plot command, but is omitted here). We can see the logarithmic form clearly for bilirubin. The rug option to the plot command produces the set of tick marks along the bottom of the plot, one at the location of each of the x-values for the data. One can see that the apparent downturn at the right extreme of the protime plot is based on only two data points. Extended illustration of GAM models or the genmod function is beyond the scope of this book, see Hastie and Tibshirani [63] for further exposition.

The SAS example below obtains the baseline hazard estimate by using the fact that $E_i = N_i - M_i$, and that N_i in this data set is equal to the count variable. As with S-Plus, newtime is $\hat{\Lambda}_0(T_i)$. It uses proc genmod to do Poisson regression.

```
proc phreg data=pbc noprint;
    model futime * status(0 1) = age edema bili protime albumin
                                            /ties=efron;
    output out=temp1 xbeta=xbeta resmart=mresid /order=data;

data temp2; merge pbc temp1;
    count = 1*(status=2);
    expect= count - mresid;
    newtime = expect * exp(-1*xbeta);
    ltime  = log(newtime);

proc genmod data=temp2;
    model count = bili / offset=ltime dist=poisson;
    ...
```

An interesting example in this vein is the application of tree-based models, as described in Breiman et al. [20], to survival data.(These are also known as classification and regression trees or CART based on the book title, recursive partitioning, automatic interaction detection (AID) models, and by several other labels.) Therneau et al. [143] suggest in passing that the null martingale residuals could be used as input to a tree model that expected a single continuous response variable. LeBlanc and Crowley [82] developed a direct incorporation of survival data into tree-based programs, with splits based on a local likelihood. Their method is equivalent to using a tree-based method for Poisson data, with splits based on the Poisson deviance statistic (available for instance in the rpart software for tree models; see the Statlib library), with time replaced by E_i from a null Cox model. The method shows improved performance over the Therneau et al. suggestion. Using E_i from a linear Cox model fit might be expected to do even better.

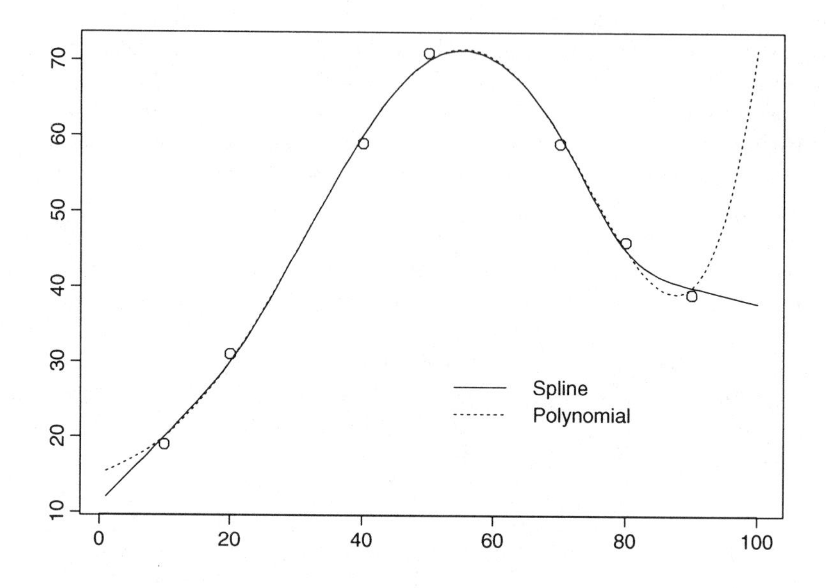

FIGURE 5.12: *Spline and polynomial fits to a set of control points*

5.4 Regression splines

An alternative to more complex residual manipulations is to model the functional form directly in the `coxph` or `phreg` functions themselves by using special variables such as indicator functions or polynomials. A particularly useful class of functions for this purpose is regression splines. The use of both regression and smoothing splines as a flexible fitting function, and their advantages over other methods such as polynomials, binning, and running averages is discussed in Chapter 2 of Hastie and Tibshirani [63].

Polynomials are of course one of the easiest smooth functions to fit: just add x, x^2, $x^3, \ldots$ as variables to the right-hand side of the model equation. Polynomials have major flaws, however. First, the data fits are not *local.* Picture a scatterplot of data with a high-order polynomial fit superimposed on the graph. Now imagine that you are allowed to select one of the data points in the right-hand portion of the plot, and move it up or down. One would like the fitted function to move up or down in the area of the disturbed point, and the fit on the left-hand portion of the graph to change very slightly if at all. This is not true of polynomials, and it makes them unstable as a general smoother. Second, although considerably less worrisome with modern computing packages, is that the fitting process for polynomials can be numerically ill-conditioned.

A better tool for exploring nonlinear relationships is splines. Spline curves fit by the computer have a natural approximate analogue: imagine one were to outline a shape by placing a small number of nails onto a wooden board, and then interpolating them with a thin flexible metal strip or *spline.*

Figure 5.12 shows a set of interpolation points and the resultant curve. Spline curves have several important properties. The first is locality of influence. Looking at the figure, imagine slowly moving the leftmost control point (or nail) upwards. This will affect the curve locally, from $x = 0$ to 40, but have almost no effect on the fit later in the curve. This is a desirable property of a smoother, and one not shared with polynomials. The second useful property is that the curve can be constrained to be linear beyond the last control point. Compare the spline and polynomial fits in Figure 5.12 for instance. Last, the spline can be fit using existing programs simply by creating an appropriate set of dummy variables, based on the prespecified horizontal locations of the control points (the nails). These *cubic splines* are a close approximation to the physical spline. The control points are called knots and the dummy variables are basis functions. One can then regress the data on the dummy variables. (Linear splines are a set of connected line segments, a continuous function with discontinuous first derivative at the knots. Quadratic splines have a continuous first derivative, cubic splines continuous first and second derivatives, and so on. Linear splines are obviously too rough an approximation to a physical spline, a cubic spline is adequate, quartic and higher order splines are possible but require more computation.)

In Figure 5.12, there is a knot at each data point; for larger data sets, there are typically far fewer knots than data points. This form of spline fit is often called "regression splines" or, if the computer version also obeys the constraint of linearity beyond the range of the control points, "natural splines" or "restricted cubic splines." The degrees of freedom for the fit is given by the number of basis functions, equal to the number of fitted regression coefficients. For regression splines, the degrees of freedom equals the number of knots plus 1; for natural splines, it is one fewer than the number of knots. One degree of freedom corresponds to a straight line. Increasing the degrees of freedom corresponds to more complicated curves. The natural spline curve in Figure 5.12 has seven knots and six degrees of freedom; fitting the curve required six predictor variables plus an intercept term. In Cox regression, of course, the intercept is subsumed in the underlying hazard function and no explicit intercept term is needed. The basis functions needed can be created using the `ns` function in S-Plus or the supplied `%daspline` macro in SAS.

We illustrate fitting natural splines in both predictors to the simulated survival data introduced in Section 5.2.

```
> fit1 <- coxph(Surv(time2, status2) ~ ns(x1, df=4) +ns(x2, df=4))
> print(fit1)
                    coef exp(coef) se(coef)      z       p
ns(x1, df = 4)1  -6.460  1.57e-03    7.888 -0.819 0.41000
ns(x1, df = 4)2  -0.808  4.46e-01    4.929 -0.164 0.87000
ns(x1, df = 4)3  -4.159  1.56e-02   16.029 -0.259 0.80000
ns(x1, df = 4)4  11.195  7.28e+04    3.409  3.284 0.00100
ns(x2, df = 4)1  -1.326  2.66e-01    0.502 -2.642 0.00820
ns(x2, df = 4)2  -5.965  2.57e-03    2.733 -2.183 0.02900
```

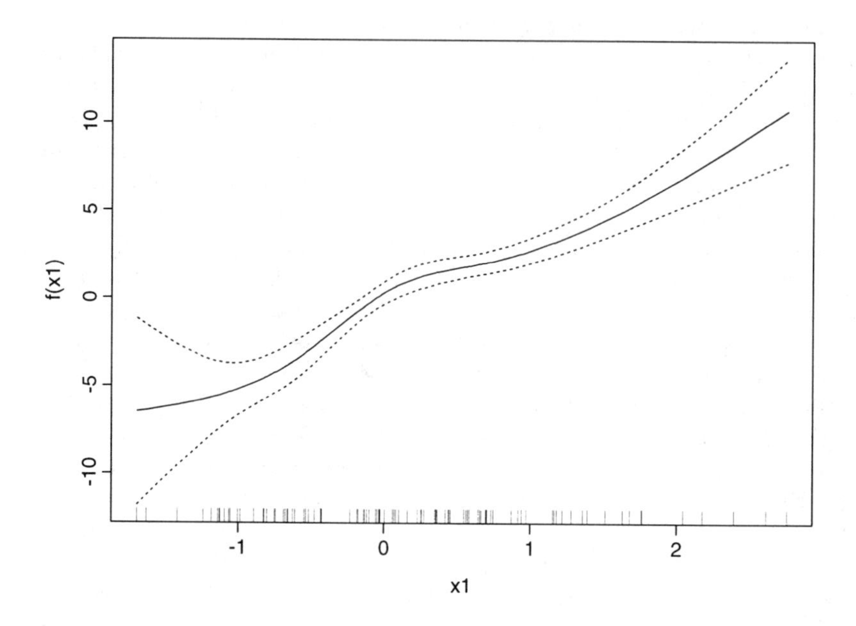

FIGURE 5.13: *Functional form for x_1, using natural splines*

```
ns(x2, df = 4)3 -22.675  1.42e-10    6.453 -3.514 0.00044
ns(x2, df = 4)4 -37.291  6.38e-17   14.577 -2.558 0.01100

Likelihood ratio test=97  on 8 df, p=0  n= 100

> temp <- predict(fit, type='terms')
> plotterm(fit1, 1)
```

The `ns` function automatically generates the necessary dummy regressor variables to accomplish a fit using natural splines. To achieve four degrees of freedom, knots are placed at the 25th, 50th, and 75th percentiles of x_1, along with two knots at the extremes of the data. The fitted coefficients are not particularly useful (they do not correspond to the y-coordinates of the control points), but two other functions make it easy to visualize the spline fits. The `predict` function, when asked for `type='terms'`, produces a matrix with one column for each term in the original model. In this case the matrix will have two columns. The first is `-6.46*ns1 -0.808*ns2 -4.159*ns3 +11.195*ns4 +c1`, where `ns1`–`ns4` are the four dummy variables for the natural spline fit of `x1`, that is, the fitted predictor for x_1, and `c1` is a constant that centers the plot at 0. Similarly, the second column is `-1.636*ns1 -5.965*ns2 -22.675*ns3 -37.291*ns4 + c2`. The `plotterm` function is listed in the Appendix. It is mostly bookkeeping, needed to produce the graph efficiently when x has many duplicate points.

As shown in Figure 5.13, the spline fit has been successful in recovering the true linear form of the relationship between x_1 and survival. Because the spline fit is just Cox regression on constructed regressors, pointwise confidence intervals are immediate. On the horizontal axis is a "rug," a tick mark at each location of an x_1 datapoint. The sparseness of datapoints at the edges of the plot, revealed by the rug fibers, accounts for the wider confidence intervals there.

We now examine some spline fits with the PBC data. In SAS we first use the `daspline` macro to create a pair of macro variables; these variables are then used within a data statement to create the set of dummy variables for the fit.

```
%daspline(bili  age, nk=5, data=save.pbc);
data temp; set save.pbc;
    &_bili;
    &_age;

proc phreg data=temp covout outest=fit;
    model futime* fustat(0) =age age1 age2 age3 bili bili1 bili2
                                    bili3;

-----------

                Analysis of Maximum Likelihood Estimates

                Parameter   Standard      Wald        Pr >         Risk
Variable DF      Estimate      Error  Chi-Square  Chi-Square      Ratio

AGE       1       0.08900     0.0613      2.1056      0.1468      1.093
AGE1      1      -0.10030     0.2675      0.1405      0.7078      0.905
AGE2      1       0.30553     1.0969      0.0775      0.7806      1.357
AGE3      1      -0.45119     1.6474      0.0750      0.7842      0.637
BILI      1       1.17847     1.3502      0.7617      0.3828      3.249
BILI1     1     106.35573   388.8674      0.0748      0.7845  1.548E46
BILI2     1    -218.62873   602.1344      0.1318      0.7165      0.000
BILI3     1     131.41991   220.2676      0.3559      0.5507  1.188E57

----
data plot1; set temp;
   s_bili = 1.178*bili + 106.356*bili1 -218.629*bili2 +
                                          131.420*bili3;
proc plot;
   plot s_bili * bili;
```

```
> fit1 <- coxph(Surv(futime, status ==2) ~ ns(bili,4) + ns(age,4),
                                 data=pbc)
```

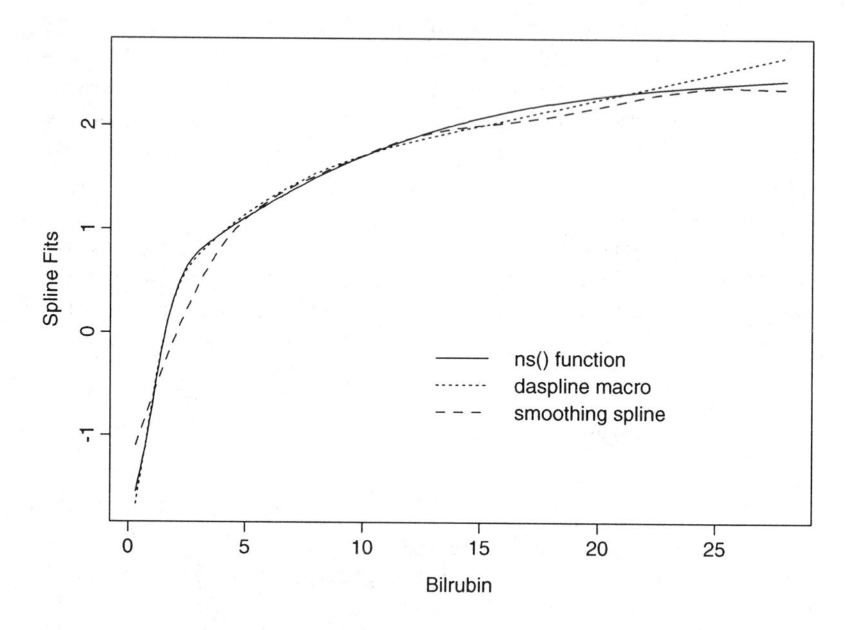

FIGURE 5.14: *Spline fits for bilirubin*

```
> print(fit1$coef)
 ns(bili, 4)1 ns(bili, 4)2 ns(bili, 4)3 ns(bili, 4)4 ns(age, 4)1
     2.234721     3.719024     4.344353      3.69994    1.917283
 ns(age, 4)2 ns(age, 4)3 ns(age, 4)4
    2.041127    3.793016    1.800988
> plotterm(fit, 2)
```

The coefficients of the models fit in S-Plus and SAS appear to be very different, but the fits are in actuality nearly identical. The difference is in the choice of basis functions for the splines, for which there are an infinite number of mathematically equivalent sets. The `ns` function uses B-splines, which are known to have excellent numerical (computational) properties; the `daspline` macro uses a truncated power basis, which is easier to create and manipulate. This latter leads to dummy variables that are highly collinear, hence the large coefficients of mixed sign in the above fit. However, the amount of collinearity is not normally severe enough to cause numerical difficulties in the fit.

The two fits above were chosen to have the same number of terms; `nk = 5` gives 5 knots, equal to four degrees of freedom. When plotted, the fits are almost identical, differing only slightly due to the choice in knot placement. The `ns` function chooses interior knots at the three quartiles; the `daspline` macro uses a more sophisticated rule based on simulation results [139]. Figure 5.14 shows the two fitted functions for the PBC bilirubin variable.

5.5 Smoothing splines

One issue with regression splines is the arbitrary choice of control point (knot) locations. Are the default quantiles good values, would the curve change significantly if other knot locations were selected, or can knot position be optimized? For a data set that contains a sudden feature, such as a changepoint, the choice of particular knot locations may either enhance or mask the feature.

An alternative to the regression spline is a *smoothing* spline. Let $f(x, \beta)$ be a spline based on a large number of knots, and choose the coefficients β for the basis functions to minimize the combined criterion

$$\theta \sum_{i=1}^{n} [y_i - f(x_i, \beta)]^2 + (1 - \theta) \int [f''(x, \beta)]^2 dx,$$

where the first term is the usual residual sum of squares and the second term is the integral of the squared second derivative of the function wrt x. The second term will be minimal for a straight line ($f''(x) = 0$) and will be large for a function with large curvature. θ is a tuning parameter for the problem: as $\theta \to 0$ minimizing the curvature dominates and the optimal solution will converge to the least squares line (two degrees of freedom, including the intercept); as $\theta \to 1$ the solution will converge to an interpolating curve that passes through every point (n degrees of freedom).

For small degrees of freedom (3–6), Hastie and Tibshirani [63][Section 2.8] show that a smoothing spline has better properties than a regression spline with respect to locality of influence [63]. For automatic selection of the amount of smoothing it has the additional advantage that the df parameter is continuous, making the problem more "friendly" to computer maximization functions.

Smoothing splines are simpler than regression splines from the user's point of view; for the latter both the knot positions and the number of knots (df) must be specified, but only the degrees of freedom for a smoothing spline. Computationally, smoothing splines are more difficult than regession splines and require special software routines. They are supported in S-Plus as a special case of penalized proportional hazards models, but not (at the time of this writing) in SAS.

Figure 5.14 shows a 4 df smoothing spline fit to the bilirubin covariate in the PBC data, along with the natural splines. It has "spent" slightly more of its degrees of freedom on the right-hand portion of the graph, and has a less sharp curvature on the leftmost quarter than did the natural spline fit. This is not surprising: the three interior knots for the natural spline are at 0.8, 1.4, and 3.4 (the three quartiles of the bilirubin distribution), leading to the sharp bend at a bilirubin value of 3.4. Below is the code and output for the fit; both the linear and the nonlinear components of the fit are highly significant.

```
> coxph(Surv(futime, status==2) ~ age + pspline(bili, df=4),
                data=pbc)

                          coef se(coef)      se2 Chisq   DF       p
                    age 0.0432 0.00748  0.00746  33.5 1.00 7.3e-09
pspline(bili), linear 0.1492 0.01446  0.01435 106.4 1.00 0.0e+00
pspline(bili), nonlin                            57.4 3.07 2.4e-12

Iterations: 4 outer, 11 Newton-Raphson
     Theta= 0.776
Degrees of freedom for terms= 1.0 4.1
Likelihood ratio test=185  on 5.06 df, p=0  n= 418
```

A more detailed discussion of the mathematical and computational basis for penalized Cox models is found in Section 5.8, including their connection to smoothing splines. The first component of the printout is a Wald test for significance of the smoothing spline term, split into linear and nonlinear portions. Four iterations were required to set the smoothing parameter: the program works internally on the θ scale rather than degrees of freedom, and although the relationship between them is monotone there is not an exact formula: the line for iteration count shows that four guesses at θ were required to achieve the specified degrees of freedom for the spline term, with about three Newton–Raphson iterations to complete the computation for each guess. The likelihood ratio test compares the unpenalized loglikelihood values at the initial and final parameter values.

Let us look at a slightly more complex example. The Multicenter Post-Infarction Project [107, 106] collected baseline and followup data on 866 patients, gathered after hospital admission for a myocardial infarction. A goal of the study was to ascertain which factors, if any, were predictive of the future clinical course of the patients. Four variables from the study are used below.

- VED, ventricular ectopic polarizations per hour, obtained from analysis of a 24-hour Holter monitor. A large number of these irregular heartbeats is indicative of high risk for fatal arrhythmia.
- New York Heart Association class, a measure of the amount of activity that a subject is able to undertake without angina, ranging from 1 to 4.
- Presence of pulmonary rales on initial examination.
- Ejection fraction, the proportion of blood cleared from the heart on each contraction.

VED is very skewed; it has a mean value of 19.1, a median of .45, a maximum value of 733, and 14% of the subjects have a value of 0. The minimum

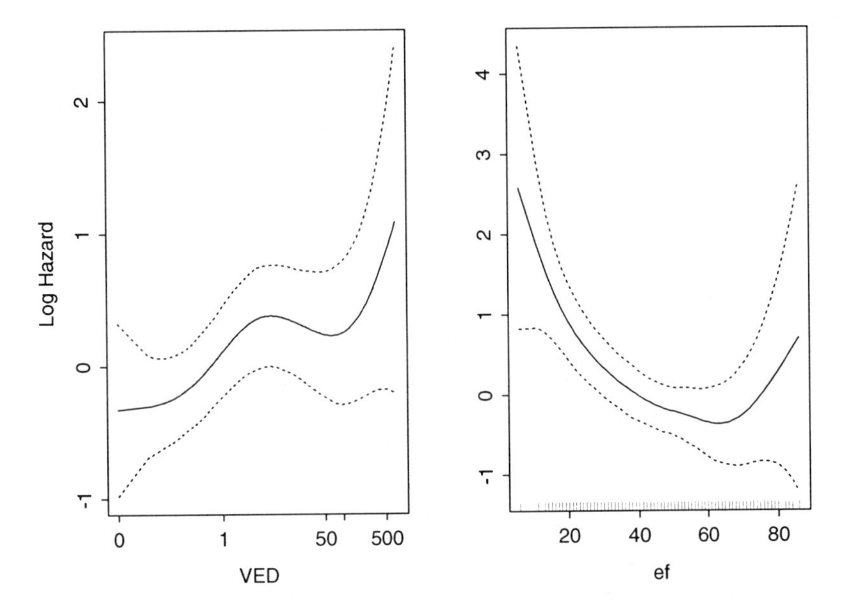

FIGURE 5.15: *Smoothing spline fits for log(ved) and ejection fraction, MPIP data*

nonzero value is 0.042, so we use `lved = log(ved+.02)` as a derived covariate. It is still a skewed variable, but is not unmanageably so.

A simple linear fit of the four variables shows them all to be highly significant.

```
> fit1 <- coxph(Surv(futime, status) ~ lved + nyha + rales +ef,
                     data=mpip)
> print(fit1)
          coef exp(coef) se(coef)     z       p
 lved   0.1007     1.106  0.04266  2.36 1.8e-02
 nyha   0.3707     1.449  0.09379  3.95 7.7e-05
rales   0.4535     1.574  0.10528  4.31 1.7e-05
   ef  -0.0265     0.974  0.00833 -3.18 1.5e-03

Likelihood ratio test=79.4  on 4 df, p=2.22e-16  n=764
  (102 observations deleted due to missing)
```

Next, let us explore more complicated forms for the effect of the covariates. Rales is a binary covariate, so no transformation is necessary; `nyha`, with four levels, is entered as a factor variable; and `lved` and `ef` are modeled as smoothing splines with the default (four) degrees of freedom.

```
> fit2 <- coxph(Surv(futime, status) ~ pspline(lved) +factor(nyha)
                     + rales + pspline(ef), data=mpip)
```

```
>print(fit2)
                              coef se(coef)     se2 Chisq   DF       p
pspline(lved), linear   0.0982 0.04384 0.04359  5.02 1.00 0.02500
pspline(lved), nonlin                           2.59 3.06 0.47000
       factor(nyha)2 -0.0615 0.31835 0.31780  0.04 1.00 0.85000
       factor(nyha)3  0.6971 0.31853 0.31729  4.79 1.00 0.02900
       factor(nyha)4  1.0151 0.29218 0.29113 12.07 1.00 0.00051
               rales  0.4204 0.10816 0.10761 15.11 1.00 0.00010
  pspline(ef), linear -0.0256 0.00738 0.00737 12.03 1.00 0.00052
  pspline(ef), nonlin                           8.06 3.01 0.04500

Iterations: 4 outer, 11 Newton-Raphson
 Penalized terms:
        Theta= 0.767
        Theta= 0.658
Degrees of freedom for terms= 4.1 3.0 1.0 4.0
Likelihood ratio test=92.5  on 12.04 df, p=1.69e-14  n=764
   (102 observations deleted due to missing)

> plotterm(fit2, 1, xaxt='n')                # leave off x axis
> xx <- c(0, 1, 50, 100, 500)                # x labels to be added
> axis(1, log(xx+.02), as.character(xx)) # add the axis

> plotterm(fit2, 4)  #plot of the ef term
```

A plot of the fitted spline functions is shown in Figure 5.15. The printed output showed no significant nonlinear effect for `lved`, and in the plot a straight line fit would lie within the confidence bands. (Since `lved` is not precisely a log scale, an extra `axis` command is needed to create a properly labeled x-axis.) Risk falls with increasing ejection fraction, up to a value of approximately 65 to 70%. The apparent rise after 70% is not significant based on the wide confidence intervals and this agrees with the conventional wisdom of the physicians that the instrumentation was not able to reliably distinguish values above this level. The function is quite smooth, and although it is certainly not linear (1 df), four degrees of freedom seems to be more than is necessary and the overfit may be contributing to the right-hand side's upturn. The `pspline` function will use Akaike's information criteria, AIC = LR test $-2*$df, to select a "best" degrees of freedom for the term if `df=0` is specified.

```
> fit3 <- coxph(Surv(futime, status) ~ lved + factor(nyha) +
                rales + pspline(ef, df=0), mpip)
> fit3
                               coef se(coef)    se2 Chisq   DF       p
                     lved  0.0991 0.0429  0.0429  5.33 1.00 2.1e-02
            factor(nyha)2 -0.0375 0.3169  0.3168  0.01 1.00 9.1e-01
            factor(nyha)3  0.6475 0.3159  0.3157  4.20 1.00 4.0e-02
            factor(nyha)4  1.0360 0.2870  0.2857 13.03 1.00 3.1e-04
                    rales  0.4304 0.1066  0.1063 16.29 1.00 5.4e-05
pspline(ef, df=0), line -0.0263 0.0077  0.0077 11.63 1.00 6.5e-04
pspline(ef, df=0), nonl                         3.82 1.05 5.4e-02
```

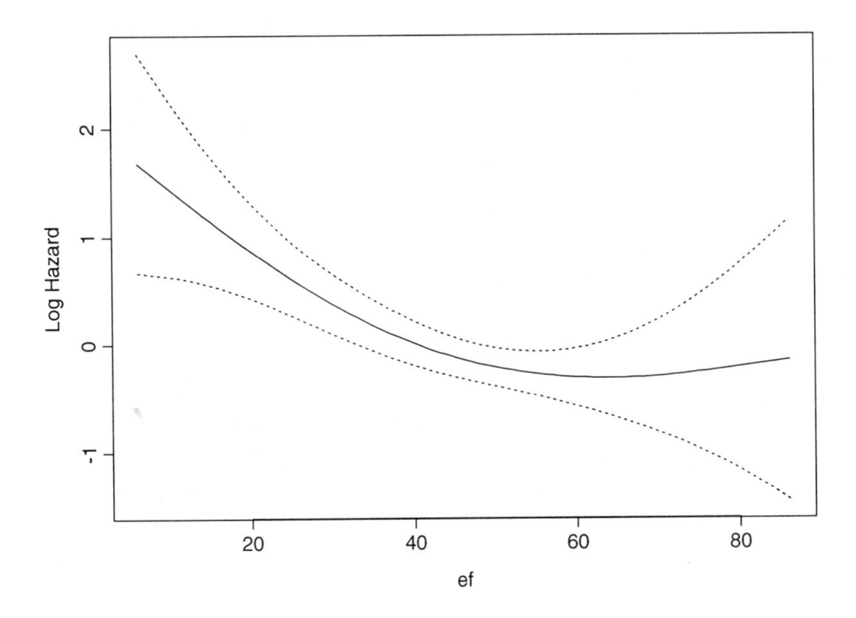

FIGURE 5.16: *Smoothing spline fit to EF, with degrees of freedom chosen by AIC*

```
Iterations: 10 outer, 30 Newton-Raphson
     Theta= 0.991
Degrees of freedom for terms= 1 3 1 2
Likelihood ratio test=86.1  on 7.03 df, p=7.77e-16
  n=764 (102 observations deleted due to missing)

> plotterm(fit3, term=4, ylab='Log Hazard')
```

The AIC criterion has chosen two degrees of freedom for the spline term. The corresponding plot is shown in Figure 5.16; the upward turn in the right-hand tail has disappeared.

5.6 Time-dependent covariates

If a subject with one or more time-dependent covariates is represented using the counting process style, the martingale residual is still easily computed. The patient will be represented as one or more observations, each consisting of a time interval, the status, and *fixed* covariate values over that interval. Assume that there are n subjects and $m > n$ observations in the data set; the programs will return the m per-observation martingale residuals. The per-subject residual for a given subject i is then the sum of residuals for his or her observations. When a time-dependent covariate is computed via programming statements, as is possible with SAS, the martingale resdiual is still well defined, but the computation of an overall residual requires considerably more internal bookkeeping by the fitting routine.

As an example we use a follow-up data set to the original PBC study. The data set `pbcseq` contains sequential laboratory measurements on the 312 protocol patients of the study. Patients were scheduled to return at 6 months, 12 months, and yearly thereafter; most patients have these visits, and many also have one or two "extra" (in connection with a Mayo Clinic appointment for another indication, for instance). Selected variables for a particular subject are shown below.

```
id  start  stop  event  drug ascites  edema  bili  albumin  ...
4      0    188    0      1     0      0.5    1.8   2.54
4    188    372    0      1     0      0.5    1.6   2.88
4    372    729    0      1     0      0.5    1.7   2.80
4    729   1254    0      1     0      1.0    3.2   2.92
4   1254   1462    0      1     0      1.0    3.7   2.59
4   1462   1824    0      1     0      1.0    4.0   2.59
4   1824   1925    2      1     0      1.0    5.3   1.83
```

In years, the visit times are 0, .5, 1, 2, 3.4, 4, and 5, so other than a delayed visit in year 3 this patient was compliant with the protocol. The subject died after 5.3 years on study (event is 0:alive, 1:transplant, 2:death) preceded by a steady worsening in bilirubin levels.

There is a total of 1,945 visits for the 312 patients in the trial. For these data, the age at randomization is a time-fixed covariate. Figure 5.17 compares the plot of the martingale residuals from the null model against age on a per-observation basis (left panel) versus on a per-subject basis (right panel). The latter is clearly preferable: breaking a subject into many intervals has generated multiple observations with a small E_i for the interval, leading to a bolus of 0 or near 0 points clogging the center of the plot. The events, being associated with a small interval at the end of followup, also have a small E_i and thus a martingale residual near 1. The code below generated the plots. Remember that the `pbc` data set contains the baseline data values on the 312 protocol patients followed by the 106 eligible but not enrolled nonprotocol patients.

```
> fit0 <- coxph(Surv(start, stop, event==2) ~ 1, data=pbcseq)
> rseq <- resid(fit0)                         # per observation
> rid  <- resid(fit0, collapse=pbcseq$id)     # per subject

> par(mfrow=c(1,2))
> plot(pbcseq$age, rseq, ylim=c(-1,1), pch='.',
        xlab="Age", ylab="Residual, per Observation")
> lines(lowess(pbcseq$age, rseq, iter=0))

> plot(pbc$age[1:312], rid, ylim=c(-1,1),
        xlab="Age", ylab="Residual, per Subject")
> lines(lowess(pbc$age[1:312], rid,iter=0))
```

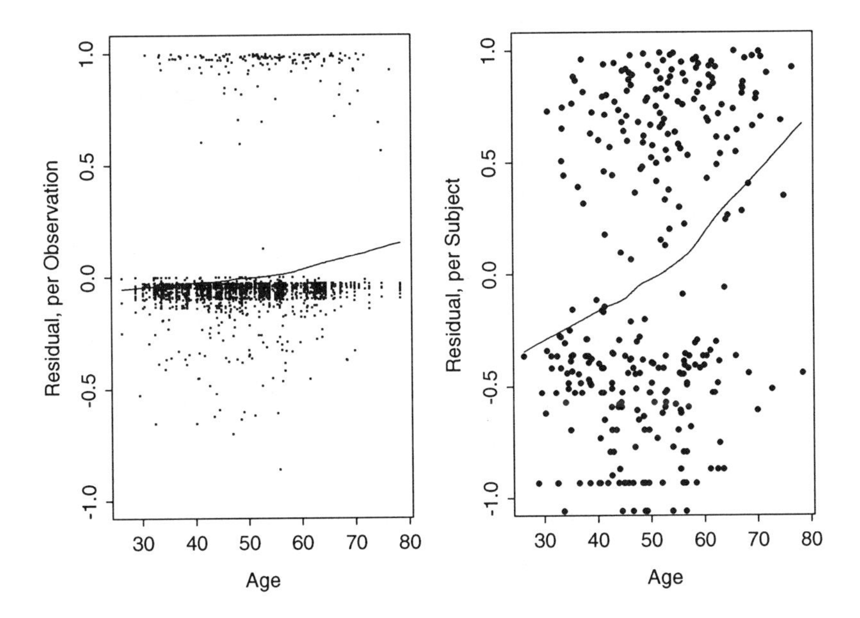

FIGURE 5.17: *Sequential PBC data, null model martingale residuals*

For time-dependent covariates such as bilirubin, one could in theory explore functional form by the usual null martingale residual plot, as was done above for age. There is a problem, however. If the martingale residuals are collapsed to one per subject, against which of the multiple bilirubin values for the subject should it be plotted? Using one residual per observation, the plot is subject to the distortions of the left panel in Figure 5.17 and rarely works well in practice.

Also, the conditions leading to bias in the martingale residual plots discussed in Section 5.7 are much more likely to be met in situations with time-dependent covariates. For example, consider a study of a progressive disease where the time-dependent covariates are blood chemistry values that increase as the disease progresses. Small values of x would tend to occur in the earlier observations for each individual and thus be related to censored observations, whereas larger x values would be associated with the later measurements and thus more likely to go with failures. We would expect that the per-observation $\mathcal{E}(N|x)$ would be heavily dependent on x, Plots of null model martingale residuals basically show a noisy version of $f(x)\mathcal{E}(N|x)$ (cf. equation (5.9)) and since $\mathcal{E}(N|x)$ is not constant in this situation, the plots do not show $\approx f(x)c$ (with c the proportion uncensored), which is often the case with time-fixed covariates.

The Poisson and spline-based methods, however, control for this by incorporating both the covariates and the estimated baseline hazard and can be used without modification in such a data set. The right panel in Figure (5.18) shows the smoothing spline fit for bilirubin, in a model controlling for age. A plot based on a Poisson/GAM approach is nearly identical, but

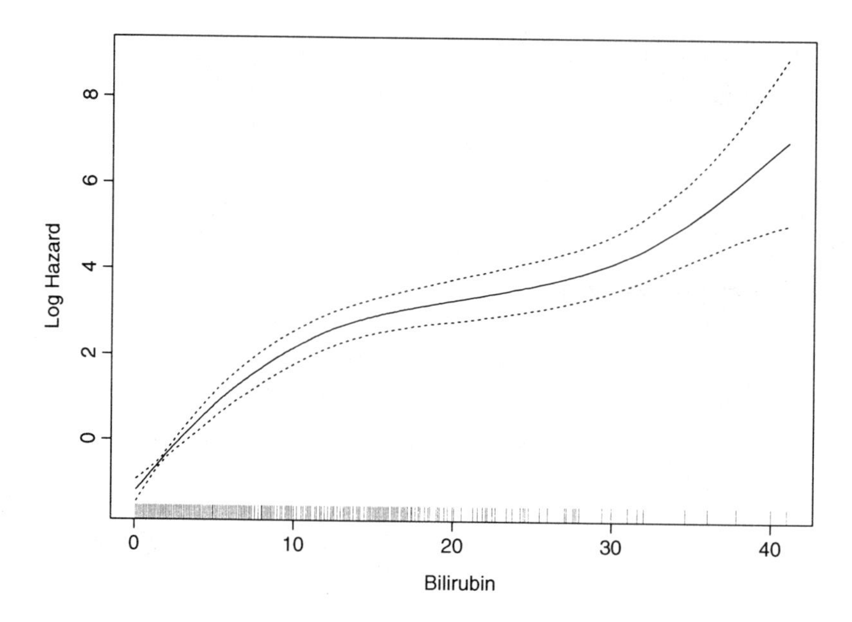

FIGURE 5.18: *Sequential PBC data, smoothing spline fit*

one using the natural splines misses the upturn at the right because there are no knots there.

Unlike the earlier plots based on the bilirubin value at study entry, this plot does not suggest the log transformation as the best transformation of bilirubin, at least for bilirubin values above 25 where the smooth turns up. There were very few such large values in the baseline data set; it is possible that there is a different risk with very high bilirubin values. A more intriguing possibility is associated with the fact that a small minority of the visits do not appear to be protocol visits; the table below shows the distribution of the number of missing covariates for each observation. All of those with >4 missing covariates are the last for a subject, and most are not spaced at the expected interval.

Number of Missing Values						
0	1	2	3	4	5	6
1113	761	11	3	0	1	56

(The cost of laboratory tests was covered by the study, but for protocol visits only. On a nonprotocol visit only selected tests were obtained.) If the 57 visits missing more than four measurements are removed from the database, the upturn virtually disappears (see Figure 5.19), as well as the two largest bilirubin values. It is likely that many of these visits were prompted by crises or sudden worsening in the patient condition.

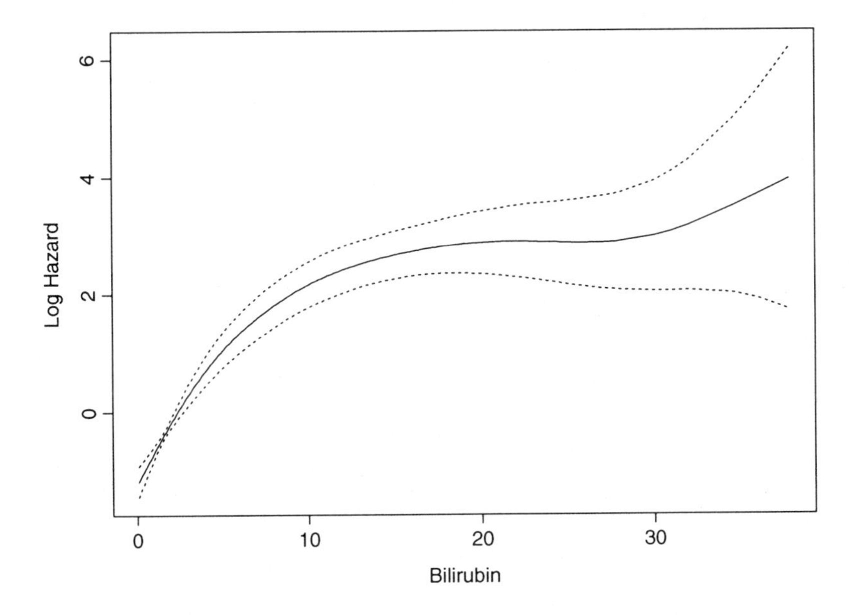

FIGURE 5.19: *Sequential PBC data, protocol visits only*

5.7 Martingale residuals under misspecified models

5.7.1 *Theoretical considerations*

Definition of problem

To develop the properties of martingale residuals under misspecified models, we expand equation (4.4).

$$\begin{aligned} \widehat{M}_i(t) &= N_i(t) - E_i(t) + E_i(t) - \widehat{E}_i(t) \\ &= M_i(t) + [E_i(t) - \widehat{E}_i(t)]. \end{aligned} \quad (5.2)$$

If the model is correct, then $E_i(t) - \widehat{E}_i(t)$ is asymptotically negligible and for most practical purposes, the $\widehat{M}_i(t)$ processes behave like the counting process martingales they are estimating. However, if the model is incorrect, the processes $E_i(t) - \widehat{E}_i(t)$ contain useful information. We consider a simple but illustrative case, a model based on a single time-fixed covariate. The same ideas are applicable for a multivariate model, but the notation and details are considerably more complex. We sketch them in briefly at the end. After we show the properties of $\widehat{M}_i(t)$s and $E_i(t) - \widehat{E}_i(t)$s, we discuss various useful diagnostic plots.

Theory for a single covariate

Suppose the true model is $\lambda_i(t) = \lambda_0(t)e^{f(X_i)}$ but we fit the model $\lambda_i(t) = \lambda_0(t)e^{X_i\beta}$. This includes the null model, $\beta = 0$. Under regularity conditions, there is a finite β^* such that $\hat\beta$ converges to β^* in probability. Define

$$\overline{rr}(t) = \frac{E(Y(t)e^{f(x)})}{E(Y(t)e^{x\beta^*})} = \frac{E(e^{f(x)}|Y(t)=1)}{E(e^{x\beta^*}|Y(t)=1)}$$

to be the ratio of the average risk scores at time t, for the true and misspecifed models. Then,

$$\begin{aligned}\widehat{E}_i(t) &= \int_0^t Y_i(s)e^{X_i\hat\beta}d\hat\Lambda_0(s) &(5.3)\\ &= \int_0^t Y_i(s)e^{X_i\beta^*}\overline{rr}(s)\lambda_0(s)ds + o_p(1), &(5.4)\end{aligned}$$

under regularity conditions. To justify (but not prove) this asymptotic approximation, note that

$$\begin{aligned}d\hat\Lambda_0(s) &= \frac{\sum_j dN_j(s)}{\sum_j Y_j(s)e^{x_j\hat\beta}}\\ &= \frac{\sum_j dM_j(s) + dE_j(s)}{\sum_j Y_j(s)e^{x_j\hat\beta}}.\end{aligned}$$

Divide numerator and denominator by n and take the limit as $n \to \infty$. Since $\sum_j dM_j(s)/n \to 0$, we get

$$d\hat\Lambda_0(s) \approx \frac{\sum_j Y_j(s)e^{f(X_j)}\lambda_0(s)ds}{\sum_j Y_j(s)e^{X_j\beta^*}} \approx \overline{rr}(s)\lambda_0(s)ds.$$

Applying equation (5.2),

$$\begin{aligned}\widehat{M}_i(t) \approx M_i(t) &+ e^{f(X_i)}\int_0^t Y_i(t)\lambda_0(s)ds\\ &- e^{X_i\beta^*}\int_0^t Y_i(t)\overline{rr}(s)\lambda_0(s)ds. \qquad (5.5)\end{aligned}$$

Using these properties, we show that the shape of $f(x)$ can often be found by plotting estimates of the mean martingale residuals $\mathcal{E}(\widehat{M}_i|X_i = x)$ scaled by estimates of $\mathcal{E}(\widehat{E}_i|X_i = x)$ or variants against x and discuss situations leading to distortions in these plots. Suppose the experiment occupies the time period $(0, \tau]$, so that $N_i = N_i(\tau)$, $\widehat{M}_i = \widehat{M}_i(\tau)$, and $\widehat{E}_i = \widehat{E}_i(\tau)$. Let $\mathcal{E}(N|x)$ denote $\mathcal{E}(N_i|X_i = x)$ and $\mathcal{E}(\widehat{M}|x)$ denote $\mathcal{E}(\widehat{M}_i|X_i = x)$ with similar notation for $\mathcal{E}(\widehat{E}|x)$. Then,

$$\mathcal{E}(\widehat{M}|x) \approx e^{f(x)}\int_0^\tau \pi(x,s)\lambda_0(s)ds - e^{x\beta^*}\int_0^\tau \pi(x,s)\overline{rr}(s)\lambda_0(s)ds,$$

where $\pi(x,s) = \mathcal{E}(Y_i(s)|X_i = x)$, the probability of being at risk at time s for covariate value x. In addition, from (5.4),

$$\mathcal{E}(\widehat{E}|x) \approx e^{x\beta^*} \int_0^\tau \pi(x,s)\overline{rr}(s)\lambda_0(s)ds.$$

Given estimates of $\mathcal{E}(\widehat{M}|x)$ and $\mathcal{E}(\widehat{E}|x)$ (discussed below), we can estimate the ratio of means, as suggested by Grambsch et al. [55]:

$$\frac{\mathcal{E}(\widehat{M}|x)}{\mathcal{E}(\widehat{E}|x)} \approx \frac{e^{f(x)}}{e^{x\beta^*}} \frac{1}{\overline{\overline{rr}}(x)} - 1, \tag{5.6}$$

where

$$\overline{\overline{rr}}(x) = \frac{\int_0^\tau \overline{rr}(s)\pi(x,s)\lambda_0(s)ds}{\int_0^\tau \pi(x,s)\lambda_0(s)ds}.$$

If $\overline{\overline{rr}}(x)$ depends only weakly, if at all, on x, so that we can treat it as a constant c, then equation (5.6) becomes

$$\log\left[\frac{\mathcal{E}(\widehat{M}|x)}{\mathcal{E}(\widehat{E}|x)} + 1\right] \approx f(x) - \beta^* x + \log(c) \tag{5.7}$$

and a plot of $\log[\mathcal{E}(\widehat{M}|x)/\mathcal{E}(\widehat{E}|x)+1] + \hat\beta x$ *versus* x would show $f(x)$ up to an additive constant. A simpler, but similar plot has $\mathcal{E}(\widehat{M}|x)/\mathcal{E}(\widehat{E}|x) + \hat\beta x$ as ordinate; a one-term Taylor expansion of $\log[\mathcal{E}(\widehat{M}|x)/\mathcal{E}(\widehat{E}|x) + 1]$ gives $\mathcal{E}(\widehat{M}|x)/\mathcal{E}(\widehat{E}|x)$. Note that

$$\frac{\mathcal{E}(\widehat{M}|x)}{\mathcal{E}(\widehat{E}|x)} = \frac{\mathcal{E}(N(\tau)|x)}{\mathcal{E}(\widehat{E}|x)} - 1.$$

Therefore, explicit computation of the average martingale residual or of any martingale residuals is not necessary to explore the issue of functional form. A variant standardization was suggested by Therneau et al. which is particularly useful for residuals from null models:

$$\frac{\mathcal{E}(\widehat{M}|x)}{\mathcal{E}(N|x)} \approx 1 - \frac{e^{x\beta^*}}{e^{f(x)}}\overline{\overline{rr}}(x) \tag{5.8}$$

When is $\overline{\overline{rr}}(x)$ approximately constant? Certain conditions are obvious from the definition.

1. $\pi(x,s)$ is independent of x. This would hold precisely in a study of multiple nonfatal events where the observation time did not vary with x and approximately in a survival study where the censoring time was independent of x and the hazard was only weakly dependent on x.

2. $\overline{r}(t)$ does not vary with t. If $f(x)$ is approximately linear or, in the case of fitting a null model, $f(x)$ does not vary much with x, then $\overline{rr}(t) \approx 1$.

Although equation (5.6) suggests that $\overline{\overline{rr}}(x)$ can introduce distortions into diagnostic plots, we have found both in practice and in simulation studies [55] that, except in extreme situations, these distortions are rather minor. Typically, $\overline{\overline{rr}}(x) \approx 1$.

Multiple covariates

The situation is a bit less favorable with multiple covariates. To keep notation simple, we only consider two; extensions to more than two are straightforward. Suppose the true model is $\lambda_i(t) = e^{f(X_i)+g(Z_i)}\lambda_0(t)$ and we fit a loglinear model $\lambda_i(t) = e^{X_i\beta+Z_i\gamma}\lambda_0(t)$. Under regularity conditions, there are finite values β^* and γ^* such that $\hat{\beta}$ converges to β^* and $\hat{\gamma}$ converges to γ^* in probability. Define

$$\overline{rr}(t) = \frac{E(Y(t)e^{f(x)+g(z)})}{E(Y(t)e^{x\beta^*+z\gamma^*})}.$$

Then, by the same reasoning as above, we can show:

$$\widehat{E}_i(t) = \int_0^t Y_i(s)e^{X_i\beta^*+z\gamma^*}\overline{rr}(s)\lambda_0(s)ds + o_p(1).$$

Suppose we are interested in determining the correct functional form for the x variable. As above, we examine the ratio of conditional means and following the same steps obtain

$$\frac{\mathcal{E}(\widehat{M}|x)}{\mathcal{E}(\widehat{E}|x)} \approx \frac{e^{f(x)}}{e^{x\beta^*}} \frac{\int_0^T \mathcal{E}(Y(s)e^{g(z)}|x)\lambda_0(s)ds}{\int_0^T \mathcal{E}(Y(s)e^{z\gamma^*}|x)\overline{rr}(s)\lambda_0(s)ds} - 1.$$

If x and z are uncorrelated, not only at $t = 0$, but also throughout the entire experiment, then the above equation reduces to equation (5.6). Otherwise, the presence of other covariates can introduce distortions into diagnostic plots for x. We have not found these to be particularly serious unless the correlations are at least moderately high and the model fit assumes functional forms for the other covariates that are clearly in error. Of course, this problem is not unique to Cox regression; it is apparent even in multiple linear normal theory regression.

5.7.2 Relation to functional form

What should one plot to reveal functional form for covariate x? If the data set has a large number of individuals all with the same value of x for many possible x_is in the range of x, the answer is clear. Let $\widehat{M}_{ij}$ denote the martingale residual for the jth individual whose x covariate has value x_i, $j = 1, \ldots, n_i$, with a similar notation for $\widehat{E}_{ij}$. One would plot either $\log(\sum_j \widehat{M}_{ij}/\sum_j \widehat{E}_{ij} + 1) + \hat{\beta}x_i$ or $\sum_j \widehat{M}_{ij}/\sum_j \widehat{E}_{ij} + \hat{\beta}x_i$ against x_i. This situation is unusual, although it does occur. An example is in staging of a disease or grading of a tumor, where the stage or grade will take one of a small number of integer values. It is typically thought that higher stages or grades are associated with worse prognoses, but the precise relationship is unknown and may be worth investigating.

More frequently with quantitative variates, one has at most a few instances of replicate values, typically due to rounding. It is tempting to consider a plot of $\widehat{M}_i/\widehat{E}_i$ against x_i, but that is not a good idea in general. First, we have the principle that the mean of a ratio is not the same as the ratio of the means. In particular, $\mathcal{E}(\widehat{M}_i/\widehat{E}_i)$ need not be approximately 0 when the model fit is correct. Second, the quantities $\widehat{M}_i/\widehat{E}_i$ are very poorly behaved. Since $\widehat{E}_i$ is the "estimated expected number of events," it is natural to think of it as behaving as a fitted value from a model, with a variance $O(1/n)$, much smaller than the variance of $\widehat{M}_i$. However, that is not the case; the numerator and denominator have comparable variability. As a result, the mean may not even be defined or the variance finite. What to plot? A simple approach is to consider a weighted smooth of the plot of $\widehat{M}_i/\widehat{E}_i + \hat{\beta}x_i$ against x_i with weights $\widehat{E}_i$. Note that in the case of replicate covariate values discussed above, this becomes $\sum_j \widehat{M}_{ij}/\sum_j \widehat{E}_{ij} + \hat{\beta}x_i$, the appropriate ordinate. Of course, the individual plotting points $\widehat{M}_i/\widehat{E}_i$ are poorly behaved and one may wish to replace the $\widehat{M}_i$s by the corresponding deviance residuals for a more visually appealing plot. A somewhat more complicated approach is based on the relationship

$$f(x_j) \approx \log\left\{\frac{\text{smooth}(N)}{\text{smooth}(\widehat{E})}\right\} + \hat{\beta}_j x_j$$

which follows from equation (5.7) and the fact that

$$\frac{\mathcal{E}(\widehat{M}|x)}{\mathcal{E}(\widehat{E}|x)} + 1 = \frac{\mathcal{E}(N(\tau)|x)}{\mathcal{E}(\widehat{E}|x)}.$$

Simulations presented in [55] suggested that this approach performs somewhat better, at the expense of having to fit two smooths and the potential for numerical difficulties if the event rate is small since smooth($\widehat{E}$) may not always be nonnegative. Finally, one may take advantage of the Poisson connection. In the case of two covariates, one has

$$\mathcal{E}(N_i|x,z) = \exp(f(x)\beta + g(z)\gamma)\mathcal{E}(\int_0^\tau Y_i(s)\lambda_0(s)ds|x,z).$$

If $\lambda_0(s)$ were known, one could treat this as a Poisson regression model with $\log(\int_0^\tau Y_i(s)\lambda_0(s))ds$ as the known observation time, to be fit via an offset term. One can often get a reasonable estimate of λ_0 by fitting a Cox model using a priori plausible transformations of the covariates. One can use any of the tools available for Poisson regression to suggest the functional form for the covariates.

At the other extreme, the simplest possible approach is a plot of the martingale residuals from a null model against x with a scatterplot smooth superimposed. If there is only one covariate at issue then equation (5.8) becomes

$$\begin{aligned} \frac{\mathcal{E}(\widehat{M}|x)}{\mathcal{E}(N|x)} &\approx 1 - \frac{\overline{\overline{r}}(x)}{e^{f(x)}} \\ &\approx [f(x) - \log(\overline{\overline{r}}(x))] \end{aligned} \tag{5.9}$$

by a one-term Taylor expansion. The conditions under which $\overline{\overline{r}}(x)$ is approximately constant and the Taylor expansion valid are those under which $\mathcal{E}(N|x)$ does not vary much with x. In particular, we need the censoring and event rate only weakly dependent on x. So, with $\mathcal{E}(N|x) \approx \mathcal{E}(N)$, we get

$$\mathcal{E}(\widehat{M}|x) \approx f(x)\mathcal{E}(N) + c. \tag{5.10}$$

This suggests plotting the martingale residuals against x and smoothing the plot to reveal $f(x)$. If there are several covariates, but not highly correlated, the same approach will work.

5.8 Penalized models

This section defines the relationship between penalized Cox models and smoothing splines, as implemented in the S-Plus `coxph` and `pspline` functions. It is not essential reading for use of the functions. More detail about the penalized code can be found in the online complements.

5.8.1 Definition and notation

Consider a Cox model with both constrained and unconstrained effects

$$\lambda_i(t) = \lambda_0(t)e^{X_i\beta + Z_i\omega}, \tag{5.11}$$

where X and Z are covariate matrices of dimension $n \times p$ and $n \times q$, and β and ω are the unconstrained and constrained coefficients, respectively. Estimation is done by maximizing a penalized partial loglikelihood

$$PPL = \ell(\beta, \omega) - g(\omega; \theta) \tag{5.12}$$

over both β and ω. Here $\ell(\beta, \omega$ is the log of the usual Cox partial likelihood of equation (3.3), and g is some constraint function that assigns penalties to "less desirable" values of ω. For the moment assume that θ, a vector of tuning parameters, is known and constant.

Consider testing the set of hypotheses $z = C(\beta', \omega')' = 0$, where $(\beta', \omega')'$ is the combined vector of $p+q$ parameters, and C is a $k \times (p+q)$ matrix of full row rank k, $k \le p+q$. Following Gray [56], let $\mathcal{I}$ be the usual Cox model information matrix, and

$$H = \mathcal{I} - \begin{pmatrix} 0 & 0 \\ 0 & -g'' \end{pmatrix} \equiv \mathcal{I} + G \tag{5.13}$$

be the second derivative matrix for the penalized loglikelihood PPL. (G is a positive definite matrix.) Gray suggests that

$$V = H^{-1}\mathcal{I}H^{-1} \tag{5.14}$$

be used as the covariance estimate of the parameter estimates. He recommends a Wald-type test statistic, $z'(CH^{-1}C')^{-1}z$, with generalized degrees of freedom

$$\text{df} = \text{trace}[(CH^{-1}C')^{-1}(CVC')]. \tag{5.15}$$

The total degrees of freedom for the model (i.e., when $C = I$), simplifies to

$$\begin{aligned} \text{df} &= \text{trace}[HV] \\ &= \text{trace}[H(H^{-1}(H-G)H^{-1})] \\ &= (p+q) - \text{trace}[GH^{-1}]. \end{aligned} \tag{5.16}$$

Under H_0, the distribution of the test statistic is asymptotically the same as $\sum e_i X_i^2$, where the e_i are the k eigenvalues of the matrix

$$(CH^{-1}C')^{-1}(CVC')$$

and the X_i are iid standard Gaussian random variables. In nonpenalized models, the e_i are all either 0 or 1, and the test statistic has an asymptotic chi-square distribution on $\sum e_i$ degrees of freedom. In penalized models, the test statistic has mean $\sum e_i$ and variance $2\sum e_i^2 < 2\sum e_i$. Because $0 \le e_i \le 1$, using a reference chi-square distribution with df $= \sum e_i$ will tend to be conservative.

Verweij and Van Houwlingen [153] discuss penalized Cox models in the context of restricting the parameter estimates. They use H^{-1} as a "pseudo standard error," and an "effective degrees of freedom" identical to (5.16) above. With this variance matrix, the test statistic $z'(CH^{-1}C')^{-1}z$ is a usual Wald test. To choose an optimal model they recommend either the Akaike information criterion (AIC), which uses the degrees of freedom described above, or the cross-validated (partial) loglikelihood (CVL), which uses a degrees of freedom estimate based on a robust variance estimator.

The variance estimate H^{-1} also has an interpretation as a posterior variance in a Bayes setting. It tends to be larger than V and thus more conservative. Wahba [154] showed it had good frequentist coverage properties for pointwise intervals for the smoothing spline curve fit to noisy data. In the context of smoothing, Hastie and Tibshirani [63, p. 60] compare confidence intervals based on the analogue of V with those based on the analogue of H and show that H has a component of bias built into it. They further suggest that with small degrees of freedom for the smoother, the two are likely to be very similar but differ more as there are more degrees of freedom.

The S-Plus function returns both `var`$=H^{-1}$ and `var2`$=H^{-1}\mathcal{I}H^{-1}$. Significance tests are based on `var` as the more conservative choice. A very limited amount of experience suggests to the authors that H^{-1} is the more reliable choice for tests, but we do not claim definitive advice.

5.8.2 S-Plus functions

Penalized likelihoods for the Cox model have been implemented in S-Plus in a very general way. The iteration depends on two functions, a control function `cfun` and a penalty function `pfun`, both of which can be user-defined. If there are multiple penalized terms (e.g., smoothing splines on two distinct variables), then each term has its own pair of functions, but for the moment assume only a single penalized term. The algorithm is as follows.

1. On the initial call (with `iteration=0`) the control function `cfun` returns an initial value for θ.

2. The penalized likelihood is solved, for fixed θ, using Newton–Raphson iteration. Repeated calls to the penalty function `pfun` are used to obtain necessary values of g and its first and second derivatives.

3. The control function `cfun` is called to obtain both the next value for θ and a flag indicating whether iteration is complete. If iteration is not complete, return to step 2.

The algorithm thus consists of an outer and an inner loop, and the returned value of `iter` is a vector of length 2 giving the number of outer and inner iterations, respectively. There are at least three distinct types of outer loop: θ fixed, in which the control function does nothing (e.g., the user has directly specified θ); calibration problems, where the parameter is fixed by the user but is on a different scale from the internal θ; and iterative maximization, such as the use of generalized cross-validation (GCV) to choose an optimal θ. The variance formula used by the routine assumes a fixed value of θ, and so is not correct for the third case. Nevertheless, it seems to be fairly accurate in several instances. For many of the problems considered here, the program is fast enough that more reliable variance estimates could be obtained via resampling techniques such as the bootstrap.

Let $g(\omega, \theta) = (\theta/2)\sum \omega_j^2$, a penalty function that will tend to shrink coefficients towards zero. The same penalty in a linear model yields the well-known ridge regression estimate. The online complements use this as an example to show how users can add their own penalty functions to the S-Plus code, and create a penalty function `ridge`. Below is a simple example using a data set from Edmonson et al. [44], on the survival time of 26 women with advanced ovarian carcinoma, randomized to two treatments. Important covariates are the patient's age and performance score. The latter is a measure of physical debilitation with $0 =$ normal and $4 =$ bedridden. The value of $\theta = 1$ used for the shrinkage parameter was chosen arbitrarily.

```
> fit0 <- coxph(Surv(futime, fustat) ~ rx + age + ecog.ps,
                   data=ovarian)
> fit1 <- coxph(Surv(futime, fustat) ~ rx +
                   ridge(age, ecog.ps, theta=1), data=ovarian)

> print(fit0)
               coef exp(coef) se(coef)     z      p
          rx -0.815     0.443   0.6342 -1.28 0.2000
         age  0.147     1.158   0.0463  3.17 0.0015
     ecog.ps  0.103     1.109   0.6064  0.17 0.8600

> print(fit1)

                  coef  se(coef)    se2  Chisq DF      p
          rx -0.8124  0.6333   0.6327   1.65  1  0.2000
  ridge(age)  0.1468  0.0461   0.0461  10.11  1  0.0015
ridge(ecog.ps)  0.0756  0.5177   0.4429   0.02  1  0.8800

Iterations: 1 outer, 4 Newton-Raphson
Degrees of freedom for terms= 1.0 1.7
Likelihood ratio test=15.9  on 2.73 df, p=0.000875  n= 26
```

The printed likelihood ratio test is twice the difference in the Cox partial loglikelihood between the null model $\beta = \omega = 0$ and the final fitted model $\beta = -0.8124$, $\omega = (0.1468, 0.0756)$. The p-value is based on comparing this to a chi-square distribution with 2.73 degrees of freedom. As mentioned earlier, this comparison is somewhat conservative (p too large). The eigenvalues for the problem, `eigen(solve(fit1$var, fit1$var2))`, are 1, 0.9156, and 0.8486. The respective quantiles of this weighted sum of squared normals (the proper reference distribution) and the chi-square distribution `qchisq(q, 2.73)` used in the program printout are

	80%	90%	95%	99%
Actual sum	4.183	5.580	7.027	10.248
$\chi^2_{2.73}$	4.264	5.818	7.337	10.789

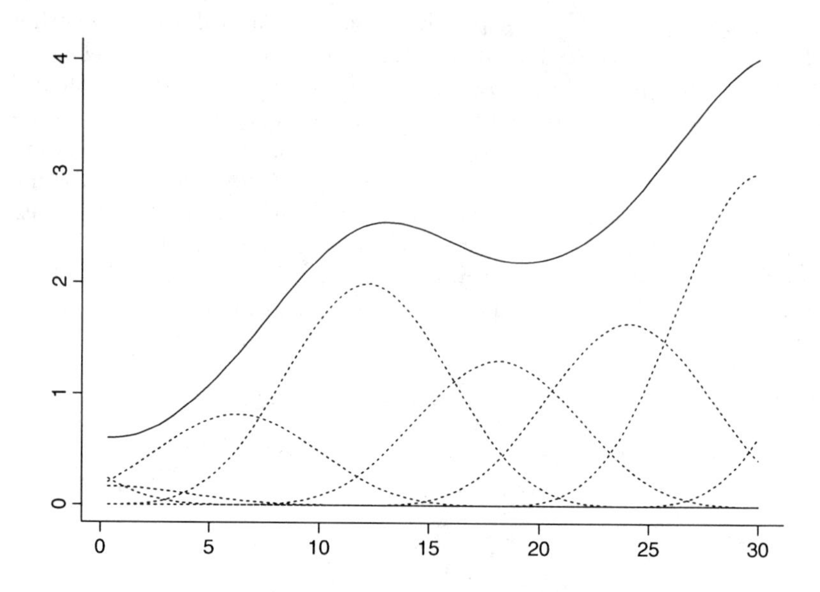

FIGURE 5.20: *A representative set of weighted P-splines, with their sum*

from which we see that the actual distribution is somewhat more compact than the chi-square.

A comparison of `fit0` and `fit1` shows that the coefficient for the ECOG score is noticeably smaller in the penalized fit, but the age coefficient is virtually unchanged. This difference is readily explained. Although the unpenalized coefficients for the two covariates are of about the same magnitude, the standard error for the age coefficient is much smaller than for the ECOG score coefficient. In maximizing the penalized partial loglikelihood, equation (5.12), shrinking the age coefficient reduces the loglikelihood portion $\ell(\beta, \omega)$ more than shrinking the ECOG coefficient, while having an equivalent impact on the penalty term. The age coefficient is "harder to change."

5.8.3 *Spline fits*

We now explore a more complicated example, which is to fit a smoothing spline term. The method we use is P-splines [47]. Start by spanning the range of x with a B-spline basis, such that the basis functions are evenly spaced and identical in shape. This differs from the traditional B-spline basis for smoothing splines, which has an asymmetric basis function (knot) for each data point. An example using eight basis functions is shown in Figure 5.20; the heights of the basis functions are the coefficients, and the sum of the basis functions (solid line) is the fit.

Several authors have noted that for moderate degrees of freedom, a smaller number of basis functions give a fit that is nearly identical to the standard smoothing spline. Gray [56] suggests that there is little advantage to using more than 10 to 20 knots and uses 10 knots for his three degree of freedom simulations and examples. Hastie [62] uses a more sophisticated eigenvector approach to find a nearly optimal approximating set of basis functions, adding more terms in an adaptive way. For several examples with four to five degrees of freedom his basis set has seven to eight terms. The functions below use `round(2.5*df)` terms by default, but the user can adjust this parameter.

P-splines have several attractive properties, one of which was the key reason for their use in adding smoothing spline capabilities to `coxph`. Because of the symmetry of the basis functions, the usual spline penalty $\theta \int [f''(x)]^2 dx$ is very close to the sum of second differences of the coefficients, and this last is very easy to program. Let T be the matrix of second differences; for example, for six coefficients T is

$$\begin{pmatrix} 1 & -2 & 1 & 0 & 0 & 0 \\ 0 & 1 & -2 & 1 & 0 & 0 \\ 0 & 0 & 1 & -2 & 1 & 0 \\ 0 & 0 & 0 & 1 & -2 & 1 \end{pmatrix}.$$

Then with $P \equiv T'T$ the P-spline penalty is $g(\omega, \theta) = \theta\omega' P\omega$. The first derivative of the penalty is $2\theta P\omega$ and the second derivative is $2\theta P$. Other properties of note are as follows.

- The penalty does not depend on the values of the data x, other than for establishing the range of the spline basis.
- If the coefficients are a linear series, then the fitted function is a line. Thus a linear trend test on the coefficients is a test for the significance of a linear model. This makes it relatively easy to test for the significance of nonlinearity.
- Since there are a small number of terms, ordinary methods of estimation can be used; that is, the program can compute and return the variance matrix of $\hat{\beta}$. Contrast this to the classical smoothing spline basis, which has a term (knot) for each unique x value. For a large sample, storage of the $n \times n$ matrix H becomes infeasible.

A P-spline fit to the ovarian data gives the following.

```
> coxph(Surv(futime, fustat) ~ rx + pspline(age, df=4),
                 data=ovarian)
                              coef se(coef)    se2 Chisq   DF      p
                          rx -0.373 0.761    0.749 0.24  1.00 0.6200
pspline(age, df=4), linear  0.139 0.044    0.044 9.98  1.00 0.0016
pspline(age, df=4), nonlin                         2.59  2.93 0.4500

Iterations: 3 outer, 13 Newton-Raphson
         Theta= 0.26
Degrees of freedom for terms= 1.0 3.9
Likelihood ratio test=19.4  on 4.9 df, p=0.00149  n= 26
```

There are actually 13 coefficients associated with the four degree of freedom spline for age. These have been summarized in the printout as a linear and nonlinear effect. Because of the symmetry of the P-spline basis functions, the chi-square test for linearity is a test for zero slope in a regression of the spline coefficients on the centers of the basis functions, using `var` as the known variance matrix of the coefficients. The linear coefficient that is printed is the slope of this regression. This computation is equivalent to an approximate "backwards stepwise" elimination of the nonlinear terms for age. (By fitting a nonspline model $\sim$ `rx + age` we find that the true linear coefficient is .147 and the chi-square statistic for nonlinearity is 3.5.; the approximation is reasonably good.)

The degrees of freedom for the terms are the trace of the appropriate matrix (equation (5.15)), computed for both the penalized and the unpenalized terms. This gives a value of 0.9 df for the `rx` term, when we know that the "true" df for this term is 1 since it is unpenalized. However, the treatment and age covariates in the data set are not perfectly uncorrelated, which allows these general fits to "borrow" degrees of freedom from one term to another.

5.9 Summary

The simple method based on null model residuals is the most useful technique for exploring functional form, at least in the early stages of an analysis. All of the usual tools in the package's arsenal for ordinary plotting: smoothers, 3-D methods such as rotation, projection pursuit, and the like can be brought to bear, *without special programming.* Shortcomings of the ordinary scatterplot are inherited as well, in particular the plots for correlated data will be distorted. Differences in the followup for each observation also affect the reliability (variance) of each point, and this is not adjusted for in the plot. Computationally, only one fit to the data is required, with the resultant martingale residual used for all the plots. Because no predictors are used in the Cox model fit, missing values in one predictor do not affect the plot for another.

Linear model analogues for extending the simple method, such as adjusted variable plots, do not work all that well. The Poisson method is reasonably accurate, and may be attractive if good tools exist for analyzing Poisson data. However, the direct use of either natural splines or smoothing splines is perhaps the most reasonable next step after the simple null residual plots. The splines are easy to fit, and because they are computed within the Cox model standard tests of hypothesis can be used to test for "significant" nonlinearity. Confidence intervals are easily added as well.

6

Testing Proportional Hazards

6.1 Plotting methods

A key assumption of the Cox model is proportional hazards. That is, with time-fixed covariates, the relative hazard for any two subjects i and j obeys the relationship

$$\frac{\lambda_0(t)e^{X_i\beta}}{\lambda_0(t)e^{X_j\beta}} = \frac{e^{X_i\beta}}{e^{X_j\beta}}$$

which is independent of time. Furthermore, the relationship holds individually for each variable in the model, as can be seen by choosing hypothetical subjects such that X_i and X_j differ in a single variable. With time-varying covariates, the relative hazard for two given subjects

$$\frac{e^{X_i(t)\beta}}{e^{X_j(t)\beta}}$$

is not independent of time, but the relative impact of any two given *values* of a covariate, a cholesterol value of 200 versus 250, for example, is still summarized by a single coefficient β.

For time-fixed variables that have a small number of levels, a simple graphical test of the assumption can be made by looking at the survival curves. If proportional hazards hold, then the log survival curves should steadily drift apart. Since the survival function under the model satisfies $S_i(t) = \exp(-\Lambda_0(t)\beta X_i)$, $\log[-\log(S_i(t))] = \log[\Lambda_0(t)] - X_i\beta$, then if the Cox model is correct the Kaplan–Meier curves for the levels should be

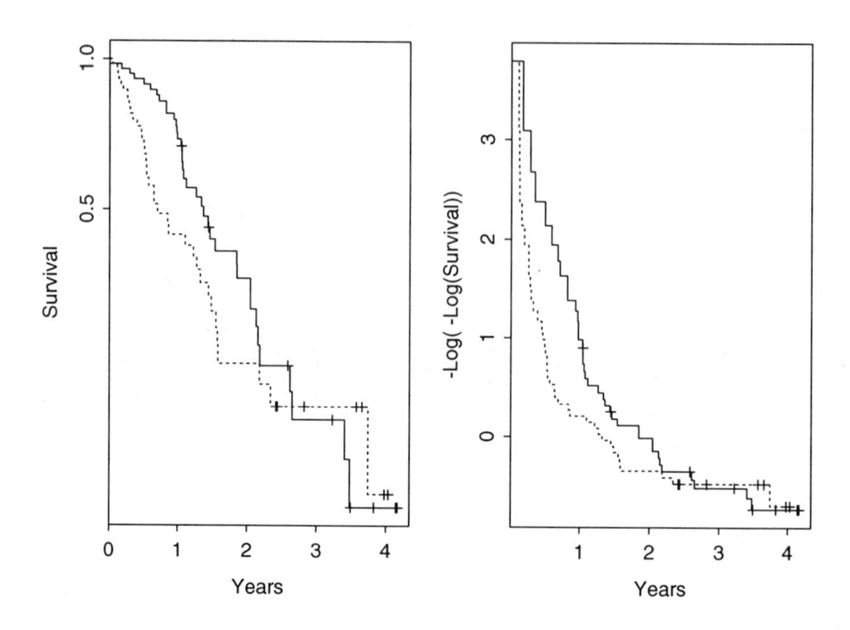

FIGURE 6.1: *Survival curves for the gastric cancer data*

approximately parallel if plotted on log–log scale. Figure 6.1 shows the standard Kaplan–Meier and log–log plots for the gastric cancer data set used in Stablein et al. [138]. These were data from a clinical trial of survival in patients with locally advanced nonresectable gastric carcinoma, comparing chemotherapy plus radiation to chemotherapy alone. It is clear that the impact of treatment on hazard is nonproportional, even without using the log–log scale.

When the covariate has many levels or is continuous, however, the Kaplan–Meier plot is not useful for discerning either the fact or the pattern of non-proportional hazards. Figure 6.2 shows the survival curves by Karnofsky status for the well-known Veteran's lung cancer trial. A common test of proportional hazards, corresponding to the *Z:ph* test printed by the SAS `phglm` procedure (since retired) shows that proportional hazards is badly violated, but how? Kaplan–Meier plots, whether transformed or not, have additional shortcomings. The curves become sparse at longer time points, there is not a good estimate of how close to parallel is "close enough," and there is not a clear relationship between the plots and standard tests of proportional hazards.

Another graphical approach is the use of cumulative sums of Schoenfeld residuals. An example is shown in Figure 6.3 for both the gastric and Veteran data sets. Under proportional hazards each curve should be a Brownian bridge (a random walk starting and ending at 0). Both of the curves appear to be predominantly on one side of the horizontal, too much so for a random walk. Wei et al. [88] have shown how to create confidence bands for the plots, which allow an accurate test of significance. Nevertheless, it is difficult to visualize the actual pattern and consequences of the

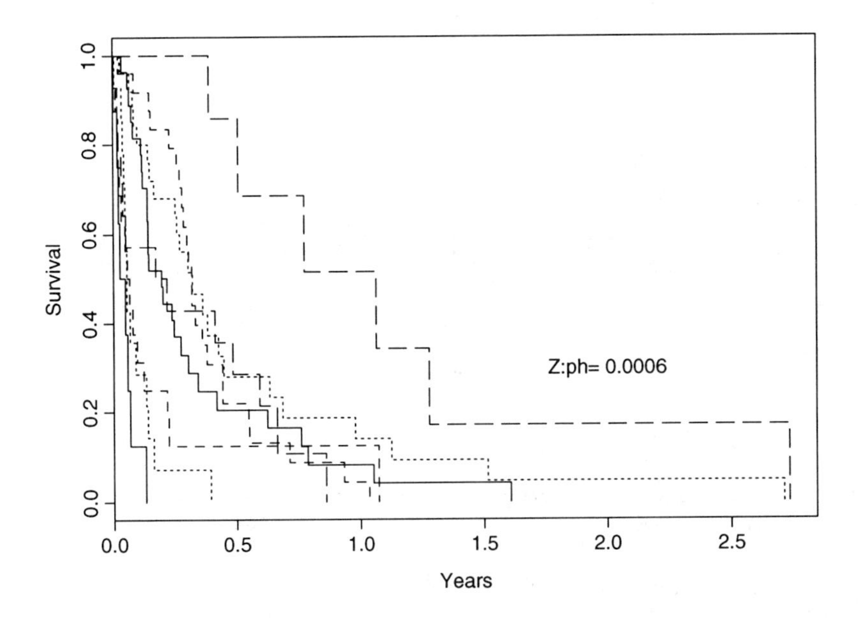

FIGURE 6.2: *Survival curves for the Veteran's cancer trial, by Karnofsky score*

Karnofsky Score	20	30	40	50	60	70	80	90+
Count	8	14	16	14	27	25	25	8

TABLE 6.1: *Group counts for the Karnofsky plot*

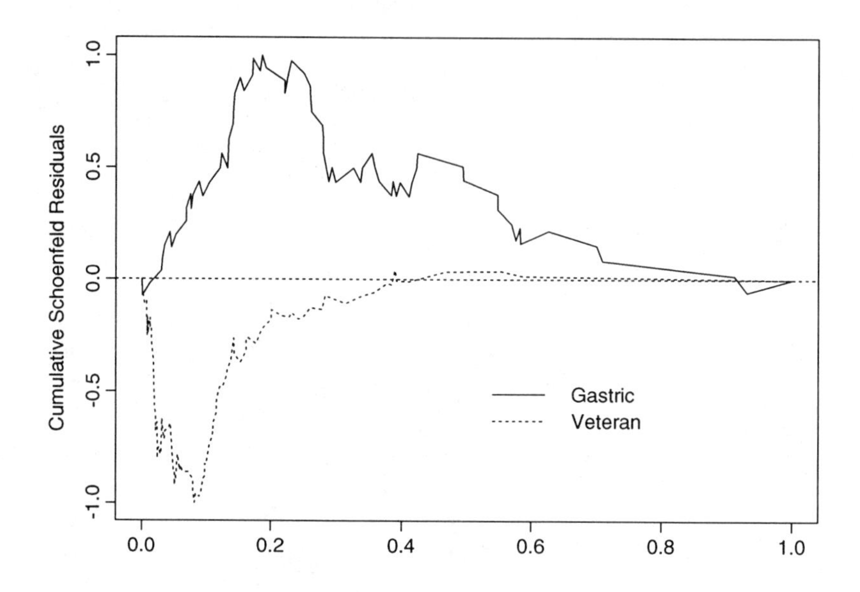

FIGURE 6.3: *Cumulative Schoenfeld residuals for two studies, with the total study time scaled to (0,1)*

underlying violation of proportional hazards. The plot is very difficult for most people to read.

6.2 Time-dependent coefficients

One easily expressed alternative to proportional hazards is provided by models with a *time-dependent coefficient*

$$\lambda(t) = \lambda_0(t)\exp\{X\beta(t)\}\,.$$

When $\beta(t)$ is not constant, the impact of one or more covariates on the hazard may vary over time. For example, a treatment may gradually lose effectiveness, leading to $\beta(t)$ for treatment decreasing with t. Or a treatment may have a latent period of minimal effectiveness before the required cumulative dose is attained. The restriction $\beta(t) = \beta$ implies proportional hazards; if proportional hazards holds then a plot of $\beta_j(t)$ versus time will be a horizontal line.

Let $0 < t_1 < \cdots < t_k < \cdots t_d$ denote the $d = \overline{N}(\infty)$ event times in the study; s_k be the $p \times 1$ Schoenfeld residual for the kth event as defined in equation (4.9), and $V(\beta, t)$ the variance matrix of X at time t as defined in equation (3.7). Grambsch and Therneau [54] show that if $\hat\beta$ is the coefficient from an ordinary fit of the Cox model, then

$$E(s^*_{kj}) + \hat\beta_j \approx \beta_j(t_k)\,,$$

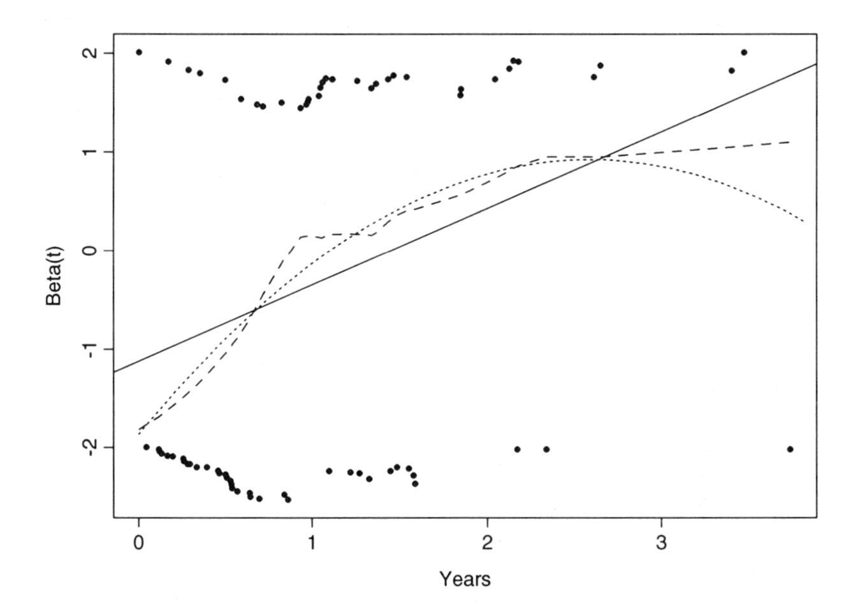

FIGURE 6.4: *Time-dependent coefficient plot for the gastric data*

where s^*_k is the *scaled Schoenfeld residual* $V^{-1}(\hat\beta, t_k)s_k$. This suggests plotting $s^*_{kj} + \hat\beta_j$ versus time, or some function of time $g(t)$, as a method for visualizing the nature and extent of nonproportional hazards. A line can be fit to the plot followed by a test for zero slope; a nonzero slope is evidence against proportional hazards.

Figure 6.4 shows the plot of the scaled Schoenfeld residuals versus time for the gastric cancer data whose Kaplan–Meier plot was shown in Figure 6.1. The plot is augmented with three lines: the linear regression of the s^*_ks on t_k, the quadratic hazard function computed by Stablein et al. [138] using specialized software, and a simple `lowess` scatterplot smooth to the data-points. We see that the scatterplot smooth has nearly reconstructed the parametric functional estimate. The fit suggests that the treatment coefficient is negative for the first 9 to 12 months of treatment, which corresponds to a lower death rate for treatment and an increasing separation of the survival curves in Figure 6.1, a roughly 0 coefficient for the next few months (parallel curves), followed by a positive treatment coefficient or increased death rate. The test for zero slope gives a p-value = .005.

Different choices of the time-scale g lead to somewhat different least-squares lines and thus to different tests. For example, replotting the gastric data on a log(time) scale gives a less extreme linear slope with a p-value of .05; Based on the quadratic shape of the smoothed curve, replotting on sqrt(time) would be expected to yeild a stronger association, and indeed has a p-value of .005.

The test statistic can be motivated heuristically by an analogy to generalized least squares. Write $\beta(t)$ as a regression on $g(t)$.

$$\beta_j(t) = \beta_j + \theta_j(g_j(t) - \bar g_j),\ j = 1, \ldots, p, \tag{6.1}$$

where $\bar{g}_j$ is the mean of the $g_j(t_k)$s. The null hypothesis of proportional hazards corresponds to $\theta_j \equiv 0$, $j = 1, \ldots, p$. Let G_k be a $p \times p$ diagonal matrix whose (j,j) element is $g_j(t_k) - \bar{g}_j$, let

$$Q = \sum G_k \widehat{V}_k G_k - (\sum G_k \widehat{V}_k)(\sum \widehat{V}_k)^{-1}(\sum G_k \widehat{V}_k)', \tag{6.2}$$

where $\widehat{V}_k = V(\hat{\beta}, t_k)$, and estimate θ by

$$\tilde{\theta} = Q^{-1} \sum G_k s_k.$$

To justify this estimator, note that $\hat{\beta}_j$ is a good approximate estimator of β_j and so $E(s_k^*) \approx G_k \theta$. Grambsch and Therneau [54] have shown that $\mathrm{Var}(s_k^*) \approx V^{-1}(\beta, t_k)$. If the s_k^*s were independent, multivariate generalized least squares would estimate θ by

$$\hat{\theta} = (\sum G_k \widehat{V}_k G_k')^{-1} \sum G_k \widehat{V}_k s_k^* = (\sum G_k \widehat{V}_k G_k')^{-1} \sum G_k s_k.$$

Equation (6.2) adds a correction term to $\sum G_k \widehat{V}_k G_k'$, which takes into account the covariance among the s_k^*s resulting from the fact that $\sum s_k = 0$. The matrix Q^{-1} gives a consistent estimator of the variance of $\tilde{\theta}$ under H_0 and a standard test of the null hypothesis is

$$\begin{aligned} T(G) &= \tilde{\theta}' Q \tilde{\theta} \\ &= \left(\sum G_k s_k\right)' Q^{-1} \left(\sum G_k s_k\right). \end{aligned} \tag{6.3}$$

It has an asymptotic χ_p^2 distribution when the proportional hazards assumption holds.

The estimator and test statistic can also be derived from standard partial likelihood arguments: $\tilde{\theta}$ is a one-step Newton–Raphson algorithm update starting from $(\beta, \theta) = (\hat{\beta}, 0)$ and $T(G)$ is the Rao efficient score test of $H_0 : \theta = 0$. The asymptotic distribution of $T(G)$ under H_0 follows from the properties of score processes of partial likelihoods using martingale asymptotics.

Interestingly, nearly all of the tests for proportional hazards that have been proposed in the literature are $T(G)$ tests and differ only in their choice of the time transform $g(t)$.

1. If $g(t)$ is a specified function of time, then T is a score test for the addition of the time-dependent variable $g(t) * X$ to the model, a test initially suggested by Cox [35]. That is, the test of proportional hazards obtained by the addition of $\log(t) * X$ to the Cox model is equivalent to a plot of the scaled Schoenfeld residuals against log(time). Chappell [31] describes the relationship between this test and the test of Gill and Schumacher [53].

2. If g is piecewise constant on nonoverlapping time intervals with the intervals and constants chosen in advance, T is the score test proposed by O'Quigley and Pessione [116], which generalizes and extends goodness-of-fit tests proposed by Schoenfeld [128] and Moreau et al. [105]. This test has the disadvantage that the investigator must choose a partition of the time axis, but they suggest guidelines for doing so.

3. If $g(t) = \overline{N}(t-)$ then T is based on a plot of the residuals versus the rank of the event times. This is equivalent to the test of Breslow et al. [24] which uses rank scores as a time-dependent variate in the Cox model, and is similar to one proposed by Harrell [61], who uses the correlation between the unscaled residuals and rank of the event times. This latter test is familiar to users of the (now discontinued) SAS `phglm` procedure.

4. Lin [85] suggests comparing $\hat\beta$ to the solution $\hat\beta_g$ of a weighted Cox estimating equation

$$\sum_i \int g(t)\,[X_i(t) - \bar{x}(t)] dN_i(t) = 0$$

with $g(t)$ one of the scalar weight functions commonly chosen for weighted log rank tests. Lin shows that $\hat\beta - \hat\beta_g$ is asymptotically multivariate normal with mean ~ 0 and a variance matrix derived from martingale counting process theory. If the estimator $\hat\beta_g$ were based on a one-step Newton–Raphson algorithm starting from $\hat\beta$, his test would be identical to T. Lin suggested a monotone weight function such as $\widehat{F}(t)$, the left-continuous version of the Kaplan–Meier estimator for the survivor function of the entire data set, to detect monotone departures from proportionality and a quadratic function such as $\widehat{F}(t)\{1 - \widehat{F}(t)\}$ for nonmonotone trends.

5. Nagelkerke et al. [110] suggest using the serial correlation of the Schoenfeld residuals for a univariate predictor or for multivariate covariates, the serial correlation of a weighted sum. They suggest $\hat\beta$ as a natural choice for the weights, followed by examination of individual covariates if the test is significant. This is equivalent to using the lagged residuals as $g(t)$.

The key point is that each of the above tests can be directly visualized as a simple trend test applied to the plot of the scaled residuals versus $g(t)$. The ability to "see" the test is a powerful tool, particularly to ensure that a small subset of points has no undue influence on the result.

In reality, the $\hat{V}_k$s may be unstable, particularly near the end of follow-up when the number of subjects in the risk set is not much larger than the number of rows of $\widehat{V}_k$. For most data sets, $V(\hat{\beta}, t)$ changes slowly, and is quite stable until the last few death times. Combining this observation with the fact that

$$\sum_k \widehat{V}_k = \mathcal{I}(\hat{\beta})$$

suggests the use of the average value $\overline{V} = \mathcal{I}/d$. With this substitution,

$$Q = d^{-1} \sum G_k \mathcal{I} G_k$$

and test statistics simplify. Let S be the $d \times p$ matrix of unscaled Schoenfeld residuals and $S^* = dS\mathcal{I}^{-1}$, the matrix of scaled Schoenfeld residuals under the simplifying assumption of constant variance. Assume further that $g_j(t) \equiv g(t)$, that is, the same test is being used for all covariates in a given model. Then the global test of proportional hazards over all p covariates is

$$T = \frac{(g-\bar{g})' S \mathcal{I}^{-1} S' (g-\bar{g})}{\sum (g_k - \bar{g})^2 / d} = \frac{(g-\bar{g})' S^* \mathcal{I} S^{*'} (g-\bar{g})}{d \sum (g_k - \bar{g})^2}. \tag{6.4}$$

Let $\mathcal{I}^{jk} = \mathcal{I}^{-1}_{jk}$, the (j,k) element of $\mathcal{I}^{-1}$. Then the univariate test for non-proportionality for the jth covariate is based on

$$\tilde{\theta}_j = \frac{\sum_k (g_k - \bar{g}) s^*_{kj}}{\sum_k (g_k - \bar{g})^2} = \frac{\sum_k (g_k - \bar{g})(s^*_{kj} - \bar{s}^*_j)}{\sum_k (g_k - \bar{g})^2}, \tag{6.5}$$

the least squares slope for regressing the s^*_{kj}s on the g_ks, and the test statistic is

$$T_j = \frac{d \{\sum_k (g_k - \bar{g}) s^*_{kj}\}^2}{\mathcal{I}^{jj} \sum_k (g_k - \bar{g})^2}. \tag{6.6}$$

Note that this test is almost identical to the standard test for assessing the correlation of a scatterplot of s^*_{kj} on g_k, $k = 1, \ldots, d$, but has $\mathcal{I}^{jj}/d$ instead of the regression mean square error.

To aid in detecting the possible form of departure from proportional hazards, a smooth curve with confidence bands is added to the plot of the scaled Schoenfeld residuals versus $g(t)$. For both the S-Plus and SAS functions this has been done using a spline fit. Let X be the matrix of basis vectors for the spline fit of the scaled residuals on the $g(t_k)$s and B the matrix for the same spline functions, but evaluated at the plotting points. (B will usually be based on 30 to 40 points evenly spread over the range of $g(t)$.) Suppose there are q plotting points. The plotted values of the spline curve for the jth covariate will be

$$\hat{y} = 1\hat{\beta}_j + B(X'X)^{-1} X' S^*_j \equiv 1\hat{\beta}_j + H S^*_j,$$

where 1 is a q-vector of ones and S^*_j is the jth column of S^*. Under our simplifying assumption of constant variance over time and controlling for the fact that the Schoenfeld residuals sum to 0, the variance matrix of S_j^* is consistently estimated under proportional hazards by

$$\mathcal{I}^{jj}[dI_d - J_d],$$

where I_d is the $d \times d$ identity matrix and J_d is the $d \times d$ matrix of ones. The Schoenfeld residuals and therefore the scaled Schoenfeld residuals are asymptotically uncorrelated with $\hat{\beta}$. So

$$\text{Var}(\hat{y}) = \mathcal{I}^{jj} J_q + \mathcal{I}^{jj} dHH' - \mathcal{I}^{jj} HJ_d H'.$$

For the spline, as for most smoothers, smooth(constant) = constant so that $HJ = J$ and the first and third terms cancel.

$$\text{Var}(\hat{y}) = d\mathcal{I}^{jj} HH'. \tag{6.7}$$

Formula (6.7) is equivalent to the standard linear model formula for the variance of predicted values except that dI^{jj} replaces the usual estimator of σ^2. Confidence intervals can be formed by standard linear model calculations, for example, Scheffé intervals using the rank of $\text{Var}(\hat{y})$ for simultaneous confidence bands or simple z-intervals for pointwise estimates.

6.3 Veterans Administration data

As an example consider the Veterans Administration lung cancer data as found in Kalbfleisch and Prentice [73, pp. 223–224] from a clinical trial of 137 male patients with advanced inoperable lung cancer. The endpoint was time to death and there were six covariates measured at randomization: cell type (squamous cell, large cell, small cell, and adenocarcinoma), Karnofsky performance status, time in months from diagnosis to the start of therapy, age in years, prior therapy (yes/no), and treatment (test chemotherapy versus standard).

```
> fit.vet <- coxph(Surv(futime, status) ~ trt + celltype + karno+
                     months + age + prior.rx, data=veteran)
> print(fit.vet)
                        coef exp(coef) se(coef)       z       p
             trt  0.319242     1.376  0.20949  1.5239    .13
    celltypelarge -0.799691     0.449  0.30305 -2.6388    .008
celltypesmallcel -0.328601     0.720  0.27632 -1.1892    .23
celltypesquamous -1.236709     0.290  0.30491 -4.0560    .0005
           karno -0.032886     0.968  0.00553 -5.9471  <.0001
          months -0.000269     1.000  0.00914 -0.0295    .98
             age -0.009646     0.990  0.00932 -1.0346    .30
        prior.rx  0.084866     1.089  0.23312  0.3640    .72
```

```
Likelihood ratio test=62.7  on 8 df, p=1.39e-10  n= 136

> zph.vet <- cox.zph(fit.vet, transform='log')
                      rho   chisq        p
              trt -0.01561  0.0400 0.841485
    celltypelarge  0.00942  0.0121 0.912556
celltypesmallcel -0.11908  2.2200 0.136235
celltypesquamous -0.16278  3.8950 0.048430
            karno  0.29329 11.8848 0.000566
           months  0.11317  1.6952 0.192913
              age  0.20984  6.5918 0.010245
         prior.rx -0.16683  3.9874 0.045842
           GLOBAL       NA 27.5320 0.000572

> plot(zph.vet[5])  # plot the effect of Karnofsky score
```

For these data, we have chosen $g(t) = \log(t)$ by using the option `transform = 'log'`. Other common possibilities are `transform = 'identity'` for $g(t) = t$, and `transform = 'rank'` for the rank of the event times. The default choice of the function is `tranform = 'km'`, which uses the left-continuous version of the Kaplan–Meier survival curve (without covariates) to scale the horizontal axis. (Consider a plot of t versus $(1 - KM(t-))$, and replace each time point by its vertical position on the plot.) There is usually very little difference between the '`km`' and '`rank`' transformations, but the former is less sensitive to censoring patterns. The reason for choosing the K–M transform as the default is that it tends to spread the residuals s_k^* fairly evenly across the plot from left to right, avoiding potential problems with outliers. The other scales are easier for an audience to interpret, however. For long-tailed survival distributions, such as in this data set, $\log(t_k)$ is often a good choice.

The three columns of the `cox.zph` output are fairly self-explanatory. The column `rho` is the Pearson product-moment correlation between the scaled Schoenfeld residuals and $g(t_k)$ for each covariate; the column `chisq` gives the test statistics, equation(6.6); and the last row `GLOBAL` gives the global test, equation (6.4). The column `p` gives the p-values. There is strong evidence for nonproportionality as shown by the large global test statistic.

The Karnovsky score has the largest test statistic for nonproportionality and is also the most significant predictor in the model. Figure 6.5 shows the scaled Schoenfeld residuals for the Karnofsky score, along with the fitted least squares line. The slope is $\tilde{\theta}_j$, equation (6.5), and the test statistic tests whether $\theta_j = 0$. Also shown is a spline smooth with 90% confidence intervals. The impact of the Karnofsky score clearly changes with time. Early, a low score is protective. However, the effect diminishes over time and is effectively zero by 100 days. Another way of interpreting this would be that a three-to-four month-old Karnofsky score is no longer medically

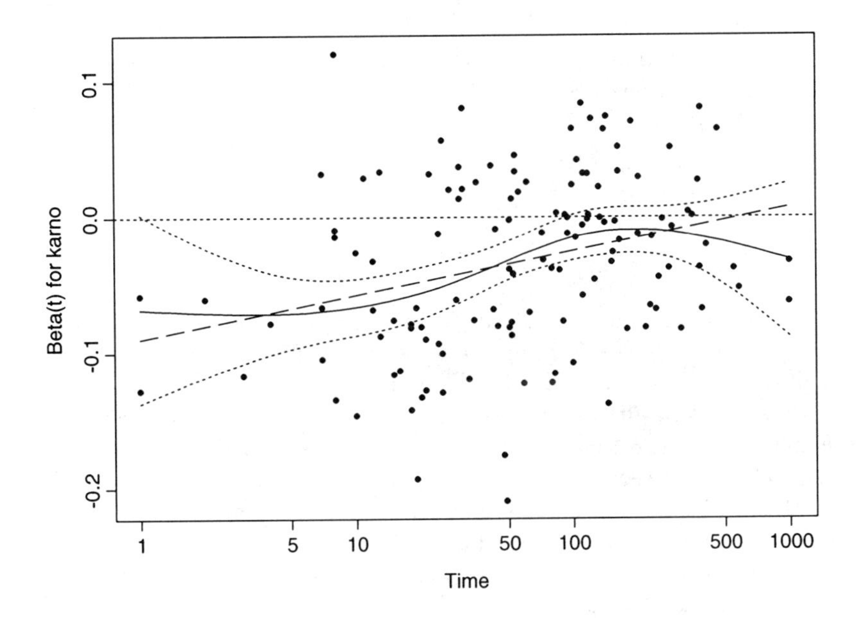

FIGURE 6.5: *Veteran data, test of PH for Karnofsky score*

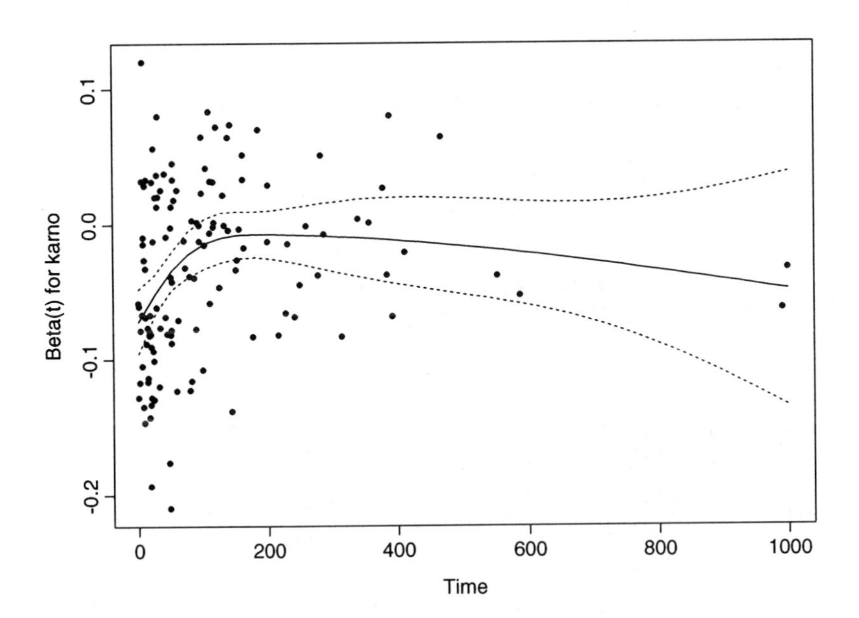

FIGURE 6.6: *Veteran data, test of PH for Karnofsy score using* $g(t) = t$

useful. The downturn at the right end of the plot is likely an artifact of small numbers and disappears if the last four points are excluded.

The effect of the time transformation function $g(t)$ can be substantial. The code below produces Figure 6.6, a plot on the identiy scale. different scales using SAS.

```
> zph.vet2 <- cox.zph(fit.vet, transform='identity')
> plot(zph.vet2[5])
> print(zph.vet2[5])
          rho chisq      p
karno 0.149  3.08 0.0793
```

When drawn on the identity scale the test for nonproportionality is not significant; with a p-value of .07. The two isolated datapoints at the very right of the plot have a tremendous influence on the least-squares line. The SAS code below shows results for all three of the identity (`futime`), rank(`rtime`), and Kaplan–Meier (`probevt`) scales. The macro uses `proc corr` to compute the correlations between the x and y points of the plot and their significance. The correlation is correct, but the resultant p-value is somewhat conservative; it corresponds to equation (6.6) but with the regression mean square error substituted for $\mathcal{I}^{jj}$. The amount of conservatism introduced by the approximation is normally small.

```
data temp; set veteran;
    cell1 = (celltype='large');
    cell2 = (celltype='smallcel');
    cell3 = (celltype='squamous');

%schoen(data=temp, time=futime, event=status,
        xvars= rx cell1 cell2 cell3 karno months age prior_rx,
        plot=n);
```

	FUTIME	RTIME	PROBEVT
RX	-0.03755	-0.02416	-0.02682
	0.6739	0.7866	0.7638
CELL1	0.04398	0.01084	0.01369
	0.6220	0.9033	0.8781
CELL2	-0.08760	-0.13838	-0.13872
	0.3255	0.1193	0.1184
CELL3	-0.06096	-0.14758	-0.14470
	0.4943	0.0964	0.1032
KARNO	0.14846	0.31089	0.30753
	0.0944	0.0004	0.0004
...			

Cell type was the other significant predictor in the Cox model and there is some evidence for nonproportionality, particularly in the squamous versus

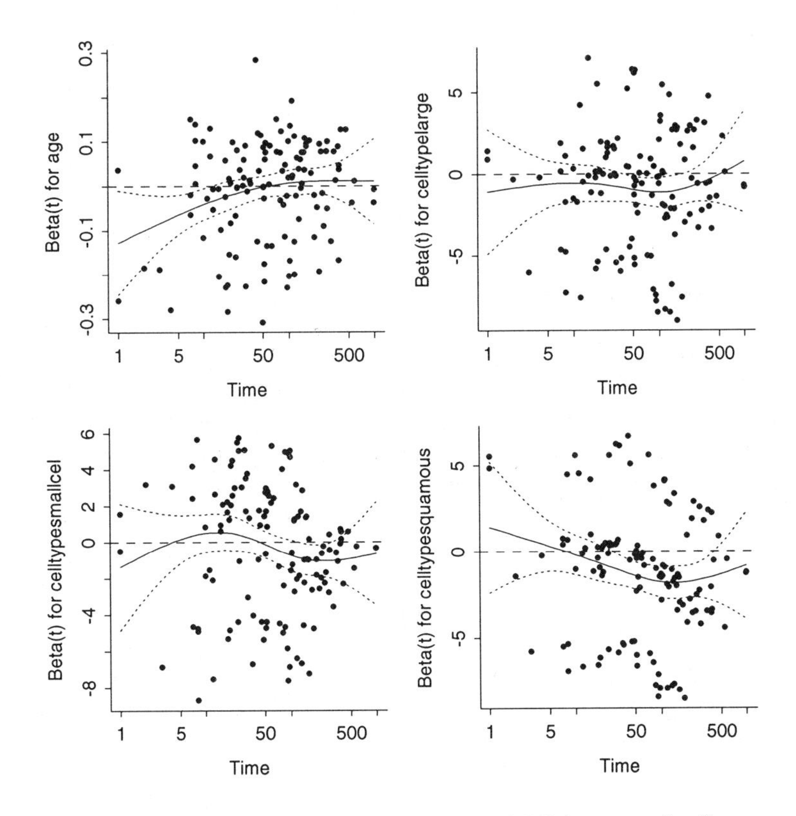

FIGURE 6.7: *Veteran data, test of PH for age and cell type*

adenomatous (reference type) contrast. The standard output lists only the single tests for each of the three dummy variables in the fit. The returned object **zph.vet** also contains the x and y coordinates to be used in the plot; the latter is a 128×8 matrix with one column for each covariate. To test the overall effect of **celltype** on proportionality, a three degree of freedom test for all three coefficients can be constructed as shown below. There is also a suggestion of nonproportionality for age.

```
> xx <- zph.vet$x - mean(zph.vet$x)     # g - mean(g)
> temp1 <- xx %*% zph.vet$y[,2:4]       # times scaled Schoen
> temp2 <- solve(fit.vet$var[2:4,2:4]) # matrix inverse
> test <- temp1 %*% temp2 %*% t(temp1) /
             (sum(veteran$status) * sum(xx^2))
> round(c(test=test, p=1-pchisq(test,3)), 2)
 test    p
 7.42 0.06
```

Smoothed scaled Schoenfeld residual plots for these predictors are shown in Figure 6.7 and provide an interpretation of the nonproportionality. There is little pattern in the large or small cell plots. The protective effect of squamous cell type as compared to the adenomatous seems to develop slowly and is not fully effective until long-term survivors (beyond 50 days).

The beneficial effect of older age wears off quickly. For those who have survived at least 50 days, age has little predictive value.

6.4 Limitations

6.4.1 *Failure to detect non-proportionality*

The plots and tests based on time-dependent coefficients are a powerful tool for testing and understanding proportional hazards. There are other forms of nonproportionality, however, and the tests and plots discussed above may fail to detect them.

A simple example is a quadratic shape for $\beta(t)$. It might be apparent on the plot, but be undetected by the test for linear slope. More general tests of this nature can be proposed, for example, fitting a quadratic function to the plot followed by a two degree of freedom test. The choice of how many degrees of freedom to use along with the flexibility in time scale provided by $g(t)$ leads to a wide array of possible tests.

In the case where there is a single, time-fixed binary covariate, such as the treatment arm in a clinical trial, the time-varying coefficient model includes all possible instances of nonproportionality, and one could in principle test for, or at least visualize, all reasonable alternatives. But in all other situations, it encompasses only a subset of the possible nonproportionality. For a more general case, one could have

$$\lambda_i(t) = \lambda_0(t)e^{X_i\beta(X_i,t)},$$

where there is an interaction between the time-varying covariate effects and the value of the covariates. In theory, every value of every covariate (except the reference value) could have its own time-varying relative risk function — rising with time for patientss who weigh 153 pounds, decreasing for weight 156, sinusoidal for those over 200. It would be quite possible for the tests and plots proposed here to have little, if any power, to detect nonproportionality of this sort, depending on the precise nature of the interaction. Of course, with a large enough data set, one could always do separate Schoenfeld plots and tests for subsets of the covariates (e.g., low, medium, and high values) to detect interaction of this sort.

6.4.2 *Sample size*

The nonproportionality for the Karnofsky score in the Veterans data set was clear and interpretable. This will not always be the case. Many clinical trials, for instance, are conducted with just enough sample size for 90 or even 80% power to detect the treatment effect. That is, the studies are barely able to detect that the fit of the best horizontal line to one of the

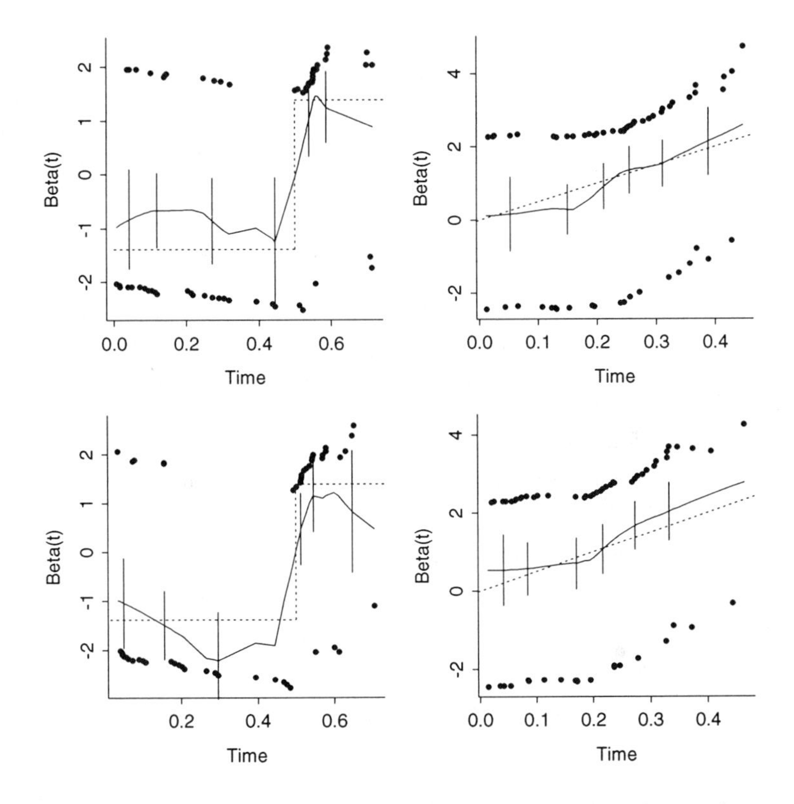

FIGURE 6.8: *Four simulations of a non-proportional model. The true form is shown as a dotted line.*

figures (6.7 for instance) is significantly better than a line at $\beta = 0$. In this context, it is unrealistic to expect that the PH plot for the treatment coefficient will show fine detail about the actual functional form. Figure 6.8 shows the result of four simulations. Each is based on a single binary covariate, with 50% censoring and n chosen so as to have 80% power to detect a 50% decrease in death rate, for a two-sided test with $\alpha = .05$. In the left two panels, the true $\beta(t)$ is a step function at $t = 0.5$; for the right two panels $\beta(t)$ is linear. Although the proposed test for proportional hazards can detect "not horizontal" in both instances, it is not possible to distinguish between a linear and a discrete increase.

6.4.3 Stratified models

Both S-Plus and SAS currently return the scaled Schoenfeld residuals based on an overall estimate of variance $V(t) \approx \mathcal{I}/d$. This average over the risk sets is appropriate if the variance matrix is fairly constant over those risk sets. If two strata differ substantially in their overall covariate pattern (e.g., two institutions with quite different patient populations) then this average might not be justified. Another case is if there are strata by covariate interactions, for which the averaging is almost certainly unwise. Consider the following example: assume that trt1 is defined as follows.

$$\text{trt1} = \begin{cases} \text{treatment arm} & \text{if center} = 1 \\ 0 & \text{otherwise.} \end{cases}$$

Assume trt2, trt3, and trt4 are defined similarly and that center has values 1, 2, 3, and 4 for four participating centers in the study. The model could be

```
coxph(Surv(time, status) ~ age + gender + trt1 + trt2 + trt3 +
                              trt4 + strata(center))
```

Clearly, the variable trt1 is identically zero in stratum 2 and so has variance 0 within that stratum. The information matrix $\mathcal{I}$ for stratum 1 will be identically 0 for variables trt2, trt3, and trt4, and should not be averaged with that for other strata.

An option to do within-stratum variance computation important but as yet missing feature in both the cox.zph function and the %schoen macro. A "by hand" work around is

1. fit the overall model to the data;
2. refit each stratum separately, using the iter=0 and initial options to force the same $\hat{\beta}$ as the overall fit. Extract and save the scaled Schoenfeld residuals;
3. combine the saved residuals into a single matrix, and proceed with the usual tests and plots.

6.5 Strategies for nonproportional data

Suppose the Schoenfeld residual plot or other diagnostic technique gives strong evidence of nonproportionality for one or more covariates. What should one do? The first two questions to ask are "does it matter" and "is it real;" it will often turn out that nothing is required.

A "significant" nonproportionality may make no difference to the interpretation of a data set, particularly for large sample sizes. Figure 6.9 shows a plot of $\hat{\beta}(t)$ from a study of the occurrence of deep vein thrombosis (DVT) or pulmonary embolism following a stroke. DVT is the formation of a blood clot, typically in the large vessels of the lower extremities. It can be a significant medical problem in conditions that result in long periods of immobility, such as traumatic spinal cord injury or stroke. If the thrombus detaches before being detected and treated, it may travel to the lungs and cause a pulmonary embolism (PE), an event with significant associated mortality. During the course of the study there were 771 DVT/PE events observed in 1,649 patients; followup time averaged about 9 years with a maximum of 27 years. Patient age at the time of stroke is an important predictor of DVT risk; age ranged from under 1 to 97 years with median age of 61.

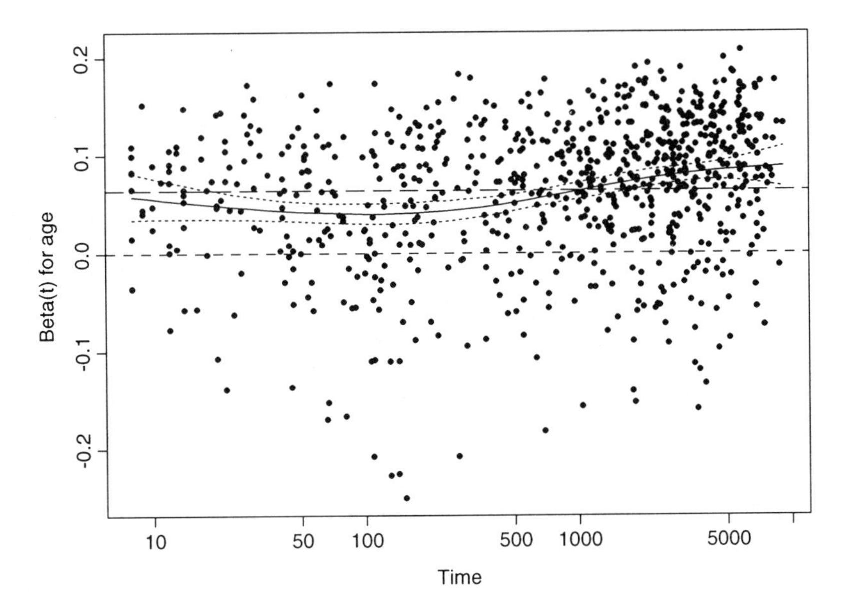

FIGURE 6.9: *DVT/PE data, test of PH for age*

```
> fit <- coxph(Surv(time, event) ~ age + male + var.vein, stroke)
> print(fit)
            coef exp(coef) se(coef)      z       p
     age  0.0662     1.068  0.00271 24.377 0.0e+00
    male  0.3962     1.486  0.07356  5.386 7.2e-08
var.vein -0.0446     0.956  0.08082 -0.552 5.8e-01

> zfit <- cox.zph(fit, transform='log')
> print(zfit)
            rho chisq        p
     age 0.1884  28.5 9.58e-08
    male 0.0456   1.6 2.05e-01
var.vein 0.1327  13.6 2.31e-04
  GLOBAL     NA  43.5 1.95e-09

> plot(zfit[1], xlab="Days post stroke")
> abline(h=0, lty=3)
> abline(h=coef(fit)[1])
```

There is a profound effect of age on the risk of DVT/PE, and the test shows the effect to be significantly nonproportional. However, the smoothed residual plot shows that the variation in $\hat{\beta}(t)$ is small relative to $\hat{\beta}$. The plot includes horizontal reference lines at 0 and at $\hat{\beta}$, the Cox model's estimate of a best "overall" age effect. The impact of age is fairly constant for the

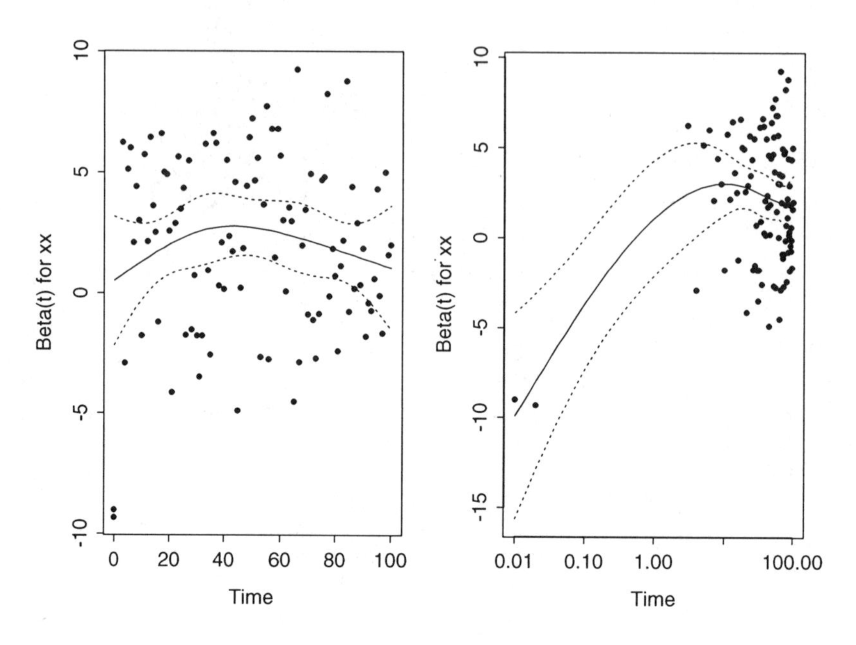

FIGURE 6.10: *Outliers and test for PH*

first year or two following the stroke and then increases slightly. However, the change is small and makes little difference to the conclusion.

It is also possible to have a "significant" test for nonproportionality that is unreliable upon further examination. The next example shows the impact of a few outlying points and reinforces the importance of examining plots, rather than just relying on test statistics. One of the authors received the following query: "Why does your procedure accept PH, but if I put an `x * log(time)` term into SAS `phreg` it rejects PH?" Upon request, the data creating the problem were also sent, a modification of which (for confidentiality reasons) is shown below and in Figure 6.10.

```
> fit <- coxph(Surv(time, status) ~ xx)
> cox.zph(fit, transform = 'identity')
                         rho chisq    p
                  xx 0.0384 0.159 0.69

>cox.zph(fit, transform='log')
                       rho chisq       p
                 xx 0.26  7.29 0.00694

>plot(cox.zph(fit, transform='identity'))
>plot(cox.zph(fit, transform='log'))
```

The SAS test based on adding `x * log(time)` as a time-dependent covariate is essentially identical to the `zph` test and plot based on a log transformation. The plots show that the significant test for nonproportionality is due entirely to the two very early event times that show up as outliers in the log scale. On the identity or Kaplan–Meier scale, both of which space the points much more evenly from left to right, the test is (appropriately) not significant.

But if the nonproportionality is large and real, what then? Numerous approaches are possible. Several are particularly simple and can be done in the context of the Cox model itself, using available software.

1. Stratify. The covariates with nonproportional effects may be incorporated into the model as stratification factors rather than regressors. This approach is completely effective in removing the problem of nonproportionality and is simple to do, but has some drawbacks.

    (a) Because stratum effects are modeled nonparametrically, there are no immediate tests of the null hypothesis of no association between a stratification factor and survival.

    (b) Stratification works naturally for categorical variables. Quantitative variables can always be discretized, but it is not always obvious how to do so. A too coarse categorization leaves residual bias in the beta coefficients for the regressors and a too fine division loses efficiency.

    (c) As we have discussed in Section 3.6.1, stratified analyses are less efficient.

2. Partition the time axis. The proportional hazards assumption may hold at least approximately over short time periods, although not over the entire study. For example, we can consider the Veterans data over the first 60 days, a time point suggested by the residual plots and by the fact that the median of the event times is 61 days. This is accomplished by censoring everyone still at risk at 60 days.

```
data temp; set save.veteran;
    if (futime > 60) then do;
        futime = 60;
        status =0;
        end;

    cell1 = (celltype='large');
    cell2 = (celltype='smallcel');
    cell3 = (celltype='squamous');

%schoen(data=temp, time=futime, event=status,
                   xvars=karno age cell1 cell2 cell3, plot=n);
 ...
                Analysis of Maximum Likelihood Estimates
```

```
                   Parameter  Standard      Wald         Pr >        Risk
Variable DF        Estimate     Error   Chi-Square Chi-Square   Ratio

KARNO      1   -0.049487   0.00704     49.39906       0.0001   0.952
AGE        1   -0.025719   0.01211      4.51128       0.0337   0.975
CELL1      1   -0.894996   0.47940      3.48530       0.0619   0.409
CELL2      1   -0.017949   0.31998      0.00315       0.9553   0.982
CELL3      1   -0.635774   0.40047      2.52038       0.1124   0.530

 ...
                     FUTIME                 RTIME                PROBEVT

 KARNO              0.10623               0.12891                0.13134
                     0.4073                0.3140                 0.3049
 ...
```

In this analysis, the evidence for nonproportionality is much weaker; none of the `zph` test statistics are significant at the conventional .05 level, although the power is less because of fewer event times. Many, but not all, of the covariate effects are stronger than in the original analysis of the entire time period. Note particularly the coefficient for age which was negligible in the original analysis but in this truncated data set suggests a decided beneficial effect. Similarly the Karnovsky score impact has increased. Both changes are in accord with our expectations from the original plots.

One can also consider the later data, for those still at risk after 60 days.

```
> fit2 <- coxph(Surv(futime, status) ~ karno + age + celltype,
                data= veteran, subset=(futime > 60))
> print(fit2)
                       coef exp(coef) se(coef)      z       p
           karno -0.00931     0.991  0.00989 -0.941 0.35000
             age  0.01568     1.016  0.01477  1.062 0.29000
    celltypelarge -1.26747     0.282  0.40419 -3.136 0.00170
celltypesmallcel -1.01245     0.363  0.47927 -2.112 0.03500
celltypesquamous -1.80772     0.164  0.43348 -4.170 0.00003

> cox.zph(fit2)
                     rho  chisq     p
           karno  0.0344 0.0988 0.753
             age -0.0212 0.0361 0.849
    celltypelarge  0.0890 0.4970 0.481
celltypesmallcel -0.0795 0.5953 0.440
celltypesquamous -0.0583 0.2385 0.625
          GLOBAL      NA 4.7331 0.449
```

In the later part of the experiment there is also little evidence for nonproportionality. The effect of the Karnovsky score has virtually disappeared. On the other hand, the protective effect of the nonadenomatous cell types is noticeably greater than in the first period, particularly for large and squamous.

3. Model nonproportionality by time-dependent covariates. To model a time-varying effect, one can always create a time-dependent covariate $X^*(t)$ so that

$$\beta(t)X = \beta X^*(t).$$

   $X^*(t)$ could be based on theoretical considerations or could be a function inspired by the smoothed residual plot. In fact, the smooth itself could serve as $X^*(t)$.

   The functions $X_i^*(t)$ would usually vary continuously in time, which presents a computational challenge, as continuous functions do not lend themselves to the (start,stop] representation so useful in other contexts. This is one area where the computed time-dependent covariates of SAS `phreg` are useful. For instance

```
proc phreg data=veteran;
   model futime * status(0) = age + tage + karno /ties=efron;
   tage = futime*age;
```

   will fit a model where the age coefficient is a linear function $\beta(t) = a + bt$. For more general effects the `%daspline` macro can be used to create a set of basis functions in the `futime` variable. A decaying effect of the regressor of the form $\beta(t) = \beta\exp(-\rho t)$ has sometimes been suggested, but cannot be fit by the SAS formulation unless ρ is prespecified.

   However, using data-based functions as time-varying covariates is subject to caveats. The inferential statistics from `phreg` are valid only under the assumption that the model was specified independently of the data values actually realized; using functions inspired by the appearance of residual plots may nearly guarantee "significant" p-values and narrow confidence intervals. Using the smooth itself suffers from the additional technical difficulty of nonpredictability; the value of the smooth at any point in time is a function of residuals from the future relative to that point.

4. Use a different model. An accelerated failure time or additive hazards model might be more appropriate for the data.

6.6 Causes of nonproportionality

There are several possible model failures that may appear as time-varying coefficients but would be dealt with more fruitfully by another approach. These include the omission of an important covariate, incorrect functional form for a covariate, and the use of proportional hazards when a different survival model is appropriate.

There are many other possible models for survival data. Two that are often worth investigating are accelerated failure time (AFT) and additive models. In the standard (time-fixed) accelerated failure time model, the covariates (time-fixed) act by expanding or contracting time by a factor $e^{X\beta}$. This creates a linear model for the log of the failure time:

$$\log T = \mu_0 - X\beta + \varepsilon,$$

where μ_0 is the mean log time for $X = 0$ and ε is a mean zero random variable whose distribution does not depend on X. The cumulative hazard function is

$$\Lambda_i(t) = \Lambda_0(te^{X_i\beta}). \tag{6.8}$$

AFT models are common in industrial applications, and multiplicative time scales often make sense. As a trivial example, assume that a photocopier has a hazard function that is actually a function of the total number of copies made, but that the data on their failures were recorded in calendar time. Covariates that were related to the number of copies per day might be very successful in an ACF model. If the underlying hazard function had a particular form, say a sharp upturn after 20,000 cycles, a proportional hazards model would not fit as well. A similar argument can be made for biological data related to cumulative toxicity or other damage.

Both SAS and S-Plus can fit a range of parametric AFT models, that is, with ε from a gamma, Gaussian, extreme value, or a small set of other specified distributions. AFT models based on a nonparametric error term, such as proposed in Wei et al. [156], have appeal but are not yet a part of the standard release.

The linear regression model for hazard is

$$\lambda_i(t) = \lambda_0(t) + \beta X_i. \tag{6.9}$$

Aalen [2, 3] suggested a time-dependent coefficient form using $\beta(t)$ along with a computationally practical estimator of the cumulative coefficient $\int \beta(t)$ and its variance. The model is often attractive in epidemiologic applications, where λ_0 is taken to be the baseline mortality of the population and β measures excess risk for the patients under study. For instance, in a study of diabetic patients the proportional hazards model might not be appropriate if the measured covariates predict severity of disease and its downstream mortality/morbidity, but have no impact on independent causes of death such as malignancy: one does not want to multiply *all* components of λ_0 by the disease severity.

The two models may not be as different from the time-varying coefficient model as their formulae suggest, however. A Taylor expansion argument due to Pettitt and Bin Daud [119] can be used to show that when the coefficient effects are not too big, either of them may be approximated by a time-varying coefficient Cox model. For the accelerated failure time model, let

$$f(x) = e^x \lambda_0(e^x).$$

Then, we can rewrite the hazard as

$$\lambda(t) = t^{-1} f(\log t + X\beta). \tag{6.10}$$

A one-term Taylor expansion of $\log f(\log t + X\beta)$, fixing $\log t$, about the point $X\beta = 0$, yields

$$\log f(\log t + X\beta) \approx \log f(\log t) + X\beta g(t),$$

where $g(t) = f'(\log t)/f(\log t)$. Substituting into (6.10) gives

$$\lambda(t) = t^{-1} f(\log t) \exp\{X\beta g(t)\}. \tag{6.11}$$

This has precisely the form of a time-varying coefficient Cox model where there is a common time modulation for all covariates, given by g. This is the structure that the global test in `cox.zph` is designed to detect. For the Aalen model, we can write

$$\begin{aligned} \lambda(t) &= \lambda_0(t)[1 + \beta(t)X/\lambda_0(t)] \\ &\approx \lambda_0(t)e^{\beta(t)X/\lambda_0(t)}. \end{aligned}$$

This is again a time-varying coefficient Cox model. Thus the tests and plots for nonproportionality can also be taken as indicating that one of these models may hold.

The appearance of nonproportionality may indicate a misspecified model in other ways; that is, the data may follow a proportional hazards model with hazard

$$\lambda = \lambda_0 \exp(\omega_1 Z_1 + \omega_2 Z_2 + \ldots + \omega_p Z_p)$$

but the investigator fits

$$\lambda = \lambda_0 \exp(\beta_1 X_1 + \beta_2 X_2 + \ldots + \beta_q X_q)$$

in which some key covariates have been omitted, given the wrong functional form(e.g., $X = \log(Z)$ is used where Z is correct), or measured with error. Diagnostics applied to the residuals from the incorrect model, such as smoothed Schoenfeld residual plots, will suggest the presence of nonproportionality. We have already discussed diagnostics for the functional form for covariates; a finding of lack of proportionality should lead one to check functional form diagnostics.

The case of omitted covariates has been well studied [135, 136, 141, 87], particularly for a two-arm treatment comparison. We show the problems it can cause in another context later (multiple event models), so it is useful to give some detail here in a simpler situation of a single event per subject. Suppose that the true model is:

$$\lambda(t) = \lambda_0(t) \exp(x_1\beta_1 + x_2\beta_2),$$

where x_1 is a 0–1 binary treatment indicator and x_2 is an important predictor. One might omit x_2 when modeling the data (a large simple trial is a case in point) and fit the model:

$$\lambda(t) = \lambda_0(t) \exp x_1\beta.$$

This misspecified model suffers from some drawbacks.

- When X_2 is omitted, proportional hazards does not hold.
- The partial likelihood estimate of β based on the misspecified model is biased as an estimate of β_1.

This bias exists even when X_2 is perfectly balanced between the two treatment groups at the start of the study. This fact sets Cox regression modeling of survival data apart from linear or logistic regression. With those methods, ignoring a perfectly balanced covariate (one that is statistically independent of treatment) does not lead to biased estimation. However, the Cox estimator is biased towards 0 when a perfectly balanced covariate is ignored.

When a covariate is ignored, the operative hazard is the average hazard of those at risk at each time point, a mixture of hazards. Let $\lambda(t|x_1)$ denote the marginal hazard for treatment group x_1, $x_1 = 0, 1$. One can show:

$$\lambda(t|x_1) = \lambda_0(t) \exp(\beta_1 x_1)\mathcal{E}(e^{\beta_2 x_2}|Y(t) = 1, X_1 = x_1). \tag{6.12}$$

Let $G(x_2)$ denote the distribution function of X_2 at study start and $C(t; x_2)$ denote the survival function for the censoring variable. C may even depend on x_2, but not on x_1 and is thus conditionally independent of failure given x_2. Then,

$$\mathcal{E}(e^{\beta_2 x_2}|Y(t) = 1, X_1 = x_1) = \frac{\int e^{\beta_2 x_2} \exp[\Lambda_0(t)e^{\beta_1 x_1 + \beta_2 x_2}]C(t; x_2)dG(x_2)}{\int \exp[\Lambda_0(t)e^{\beta_1 x_1 + \beta_2 x_2}]C(t; x_2)dG(x_2)}. \tag{6.13}$$

This same result for censoring independent of x_2 is in Appendix 3 of Lagakos and Schoenfeld [79] and there is a closely related development in

Omori and Johnson [115]. In terms of the time-varying coefficient model $\lambda_0(t)e^{x_1\beta(t)}$, we have

$$\begin{aligned} e^{\beta(t)} &= \frac{\lambda(t|x_1=1)}{\lambda(t|x_1=0)} \\ &= e^{\beta_1}\frac{\mathcal{E}(Y(t)e^{\beta_2 x_2}|X_1=1)}{\mathcal{E}(Y(t)e^{\beta_2 x_2}|X_1=0)}. \end{aligned} \tag{6.14}$$

The bias and nonproportionality in the estimation of β_1 result from the second factor in the equation, which is a ratio of expected values for the treatment group versus the control, for those still at risk. The treatment group means of $e^{\beta_2 x_2}$ are equal at $t = 0$ but move apart because there is differential survival for x_2 in the two treatment groups; the treatment that improves survival gives an edge to the poorer prognosis patients, those with an unfavorable x_2. The size of the bias and the extent of the nonproportionality increase with $|\beta_1|$, $|\beta_2|$ and the variability of x_2. The shape of $\beta(t)$ depends on the distribution of x_2, $\lambda_0(t)$, and on the censoring distribution if it varies with x_2.

The simplest case occurs when x_2 is binary and $C(t)$ is independent of x_2. Schumacher et al. [131] and Schoenfeld [130] considered this case. Suppose survival times are exponential with $\lambda_0(t) = \log(2)/3 = 0.231$, $\beta_1 = \log(2/3) = -0.405$, $\beta_2 = \log(4) = 1.386$, and the two levels of x_2 are equally represented in each treatment group at $t = 0$; the parameter values were used by Schoenfeld. Figure 6.11 shows a plot of the hazard ratio $e^{\beta(t)}$. The apparent effect of x_1 is decreasing (approaching 1) for the first 3.5 years, and then increases again. If one were unaware of the hidden covariate and had a four- or fewer-year study, it would be easy to misinterpret such a plot as suggesting that the treatment was becoming less effective over time.

In more complicated situations the plot of $\beta(t)$ versus t can take many shapes, depending on the distribution of the omitted covariates and on the dependence of censoring on the omitted covariates. It may even be multimodal. However, it has the following signature: $\beta(t)$ is dampened over time. It may change sign, but it is not enhanced; a bad treatment does not get worse nor a good one improve. However, this feature depends on using an additive model. If we allow the omitted covariate to interact with treatment, other behaviors are possible. Schumacher et al. give examples in which $\beta(t)$ increases from a positive value due to an omitted binary covariate in the model. In the most general case, unfortunately, there is no feature of the plots that will allow one to distinguish a time-varying coefficient from an omitted covariate.

If one erroneously interprets nonproportionality due to an omitted covariate as due to a time-varying effect of treatment, and then models the resulting $\beta(t)$, even modeling it correctly to match the true marginal hazard (6.14), one may gain virtually nothing in efficiency, at least as compared to the ideal of having the omitted covariate actually in the model. As Schoenfeld [130] pointed out, statistical tests such as the log–rank that ignore covariates other than treatment are less efficient than tests that use the covariates, often substantially less when the omitted covariates have greater

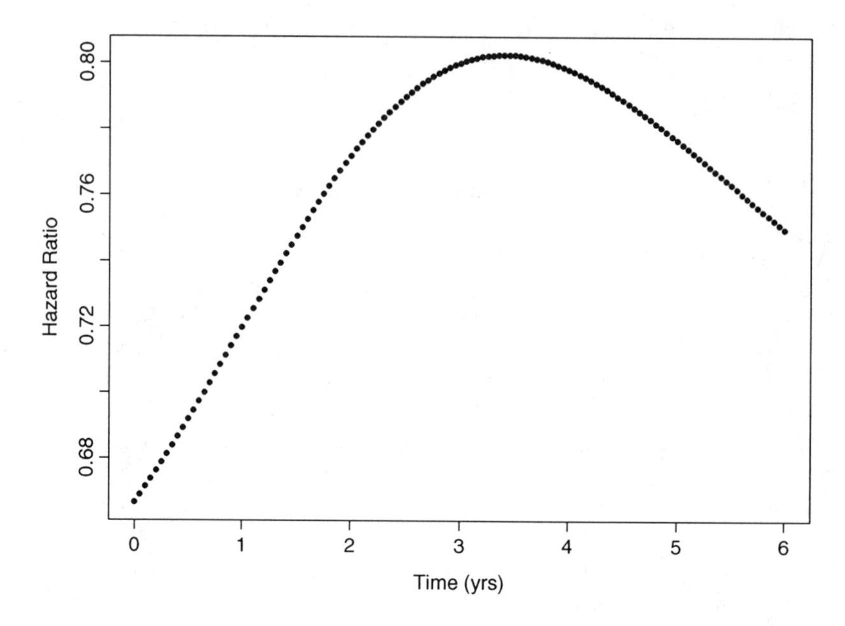

FIGURE 6.11: $e^{\beta(t)}$ *with binary covariate omitted from Cox model*

impact on hazard than the treatment (which is often the case). Schoenfeld considered the above parameters in a study with two years of accrual and two years of followup and showed that the log–rank test will have an efficiency of 61% compared to a test using the covariate. The optimally weighted log–rank test using $\beta(t)$ has an efficiency of only 63%.

7

Influence

7.1 Diagnostics

Our third important use for residuals is to assess *influence*, the impact of each point on the fit of a model. The most direct measure of influence is the jackknife value

$$J_i = \hat{\beta} - \hat{\beta}_{(i)} ,$$

where $\hat{\beta}_{(i)}$ is the result of a fit the includes all of the points except observation i. Because the jackknife involves a significant amount of computation, we would like to find an alternative approximate value that does not involve an iterative refitting of the model.

Figure 7.1 shows an ordinary least squares line fit to a scatterplot, with points a, b, and c labeled. Consider the influence of these points on the estimate of slope $\hat{\beta}$; they are 3.1, 0.2, and 0.4, respectively, on an overall slope estimate of -21.8. Points b and c have negligible effects on the slope of the fit, whereas a has a substantial one. In fact the actual influence of each point is proportional to $(x_i - \bar{x}) *$residual; a point must be both far from the mean x value and have a large residual to impart significant influence. For the Cox model then, we might expect that the influence would be related to the score residual

$$U_{ij} = \int [X_{ij}(t) - \bar{x}(\hat{\beta}, t)] \, d\widehat{M}_i(t) .$$

As we show below, this is correct.

The jackknife residual for a linear model can be computed in multiple ways, all giving the same result. In the Cox model, each of these computations leads to a slightly different residual.

One fairly simple way to proceed is to look directly at the Newton–Raphson iteration for the model. Experience has shown that the computa-

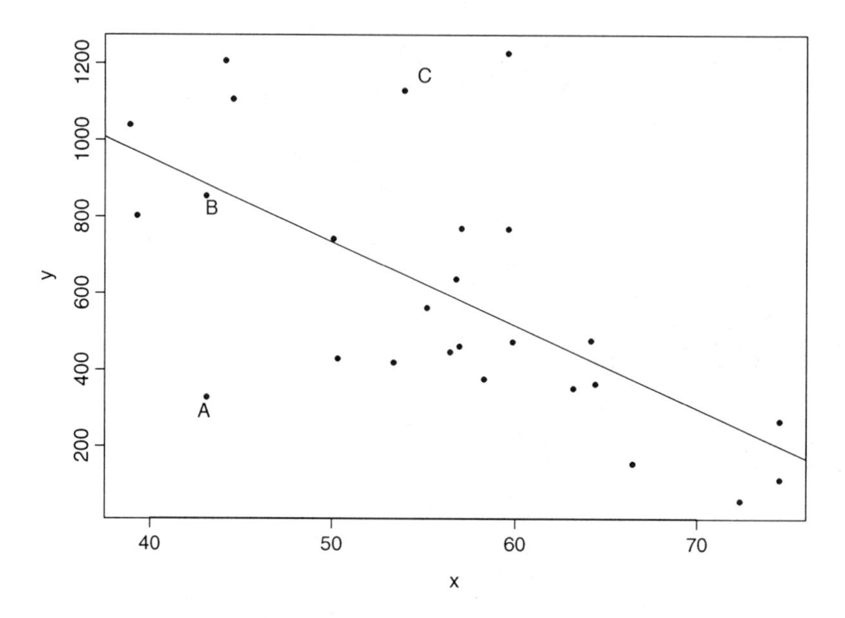

FIGURE 7.1: *Influence for a least squares plot*

tion converges very rapidly from a starting point of zero, usually in two to four iterations. Consider then the following iteratative scheme.

1. Iterate the model to convergence, using all of the data.

2. Delete observation i from the data set.

3. Perform one more NR iteration step.

We might expect the final answer from this procedure to be very close to $\hat\beta(i)$.

The Newton–Raphson procedure for a Cox model can be rewritten in the following way.

$$\begin{aligned}\Delta\beta &= 1'(U\mathcal{I}^{-1}) \\ &\equiv 1'D,\end{aligned}$$

where $\Delta\beta$ is the change in the estimated coefficient vector and U is the $n \times p$ matrix of score residuals. Thus the change in $\hat\beta$ at each iteration is the column sum of a matrix D, defined as the score residuals scaled by the variance of $\hat\beta$. (Note that in the earlier equation (3.8) U stood for the p element score vector obtained by summing over subjects, that is, the column sums of the $n \times p$ matrix form. We use the two forms interchangeably, as the proper choice is always clear from the context.)

At the conclusion of the iteration $\Delta\beta$ must be 0 by definition (otherwise the algorithm would continue to iterate). We now remove point i from the data set, and recalculate U while holding $\mathcal{I}$ fixed; this corresponds to the removal of row i from D. Step 3 of the above procedure would form the new column sum, which must, by construction, be equal to -1 times the row that has been removed. That is, $-D_i$, the ith row of D, is the approximate change in $\hat\beta$ if observation i is removed. The calculations necessary to form D are no different from those needed to perform the Cox model iteration itself. We call D the matrix of *dfbeta* residuals.

A more formal derivation that leads to the same residual is found in Cain and Lange [27]. They write down the Cox PL for a problem with case weights w_i as

$$l(\beta; w) = \sum_{i=1}^{n} \int_0^\infty \left[Y_i(t) w_i r_i(t) - \log\left(\sum_j Y_j(t) w_j r_j(t) \right) \right] dN_i(t).$$

One can then define the influence as

$$\text{influence}_i \equiv \left(\frac{\partial\hat\beta}{\partial U} \frac{\partial U}{\partial w_i} \right)_{w=1}$$

A straightforward application of the chain rule leads to $D = U\mathcal{I}^{-1}$. This is an example of Jaeckel's *infinitesimal jackknife* approach [71, 46]. A third approach based on functional derivatives is given by Reid and Crépeau [124]; it also leads to $D = U\mathcal{I}^{-1}$.

One possible failing of this approximation is that although it accounts for the change in U due to deleting an observation, it ignores the change in $\mathcal{I}$. Because a large outlier will normally increase the variance of $\hat\beta$, we might expect some underestimation in this approximation for the larger influence points. Figure 7.2 shows the results of the jackknife procedure (26 separate Cox model fits) and the dfbetas for the ovarian cancer data. As expected, the dfbetas underestimate the influence of the most influential points. Overall, however, they seem to do very well on this small data set. For larger data sets, where the influence of any single observation will be small, better performace would be anticipated.

Because of their adequate performance in actual data sets and their ease of computation, both SAS and S-Plus have implemented the dfbeta residuals. The example below computes and displays the dfbeta residuals for all variables in the PBC data set. The figures produced are similar to those in Fleming and Harrington [50], Figure 4.6.7, Section 4.6 but with the vertical axis reversed. (If the removal of an observation causes $\hat\beta$ to decrease, then the dfbeta residuals of SAS and S-Plus attribute a *positive* effect to the observation.)

```
attach(pbc[1:312,])     # use only the first 312 observations
par(mfrow=c(3,2))            # set the figures to 6 per page

fit <- coxph(Surv(futime, status==2) ~ age + edema + log(bili) +
                 log(albumin) + log(protime) )
rr <- resid(fit, type='dfbeta')
```

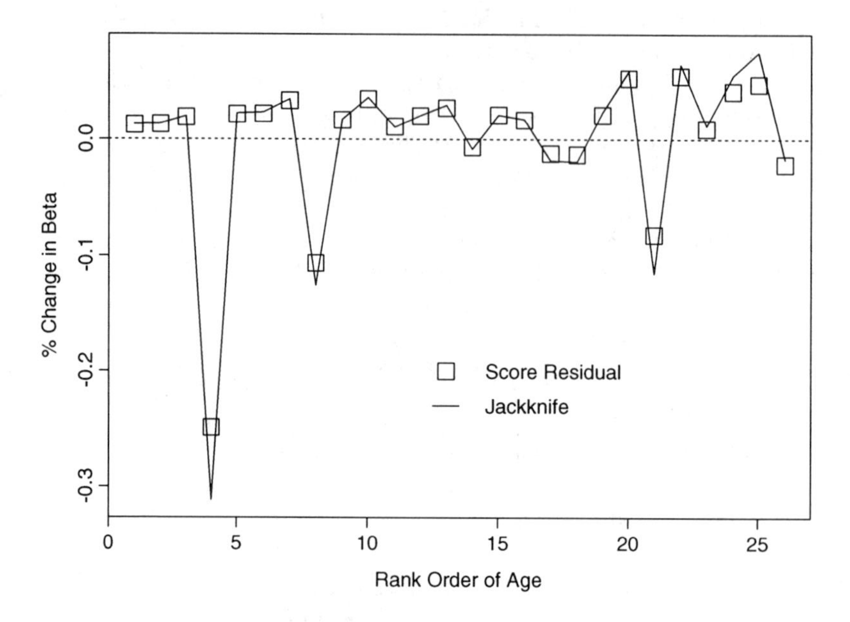

FIGURE 7.2: *Jackknife and dfbeta influences for the ovarian cancer data set*

```
plot(age, rr[,1], xlab='Age', ylab='Influence for Age')
plot(1:312, rr[,2], xlab='1 - 312', ylab='Influence for Edema')
plot(bili,  rr[,3], xlab='Bilirubin',
                  ylab='Influence for Bilirubin', log='x')
plot(albumin, rr[,4], xlab='Albumin',
                  ylab='Influence for Albumin', log='x')
plot(protime, rr[,5], xlab='Protime',
             ylab='Influence for Protime', log='x')
```

Points on four of the graphs in Figure 7.1 have been circled. These data had been checked and rechecked during the course of the analysis. Nevertheless, the study assistants were asked to take one more look at the four indicated values. The edema outlier corresponds to a patient with edema = 1 (the largest possible value), and moderately bad values for the other components of the risk score. Nevertheless, this patient survived longer than most of her cohort. The bilirubin value had a similar explanation.

Case 253 was discovered to have a true age of 54.4 years rather than 78.4 years, and case 107 to have `protime` of 10.7 rather than 17.1 seconds. In this case the influence residuals have pointed out problems in the data set.

The next example computes and plots dfbeta residuals using SAS, for the Stanford heart transplant data.

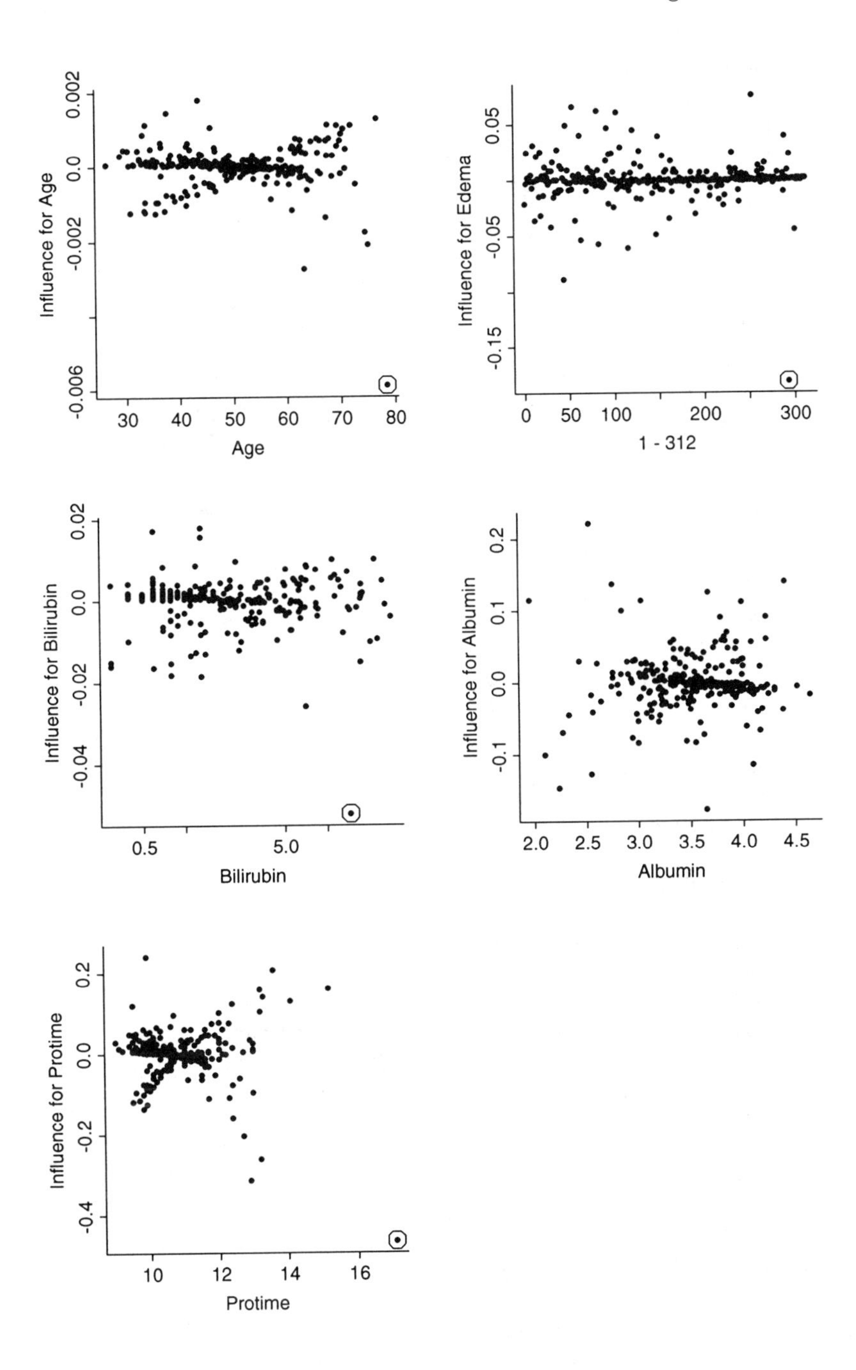

FIGURE 7.3: *Influences for the PBC data set*

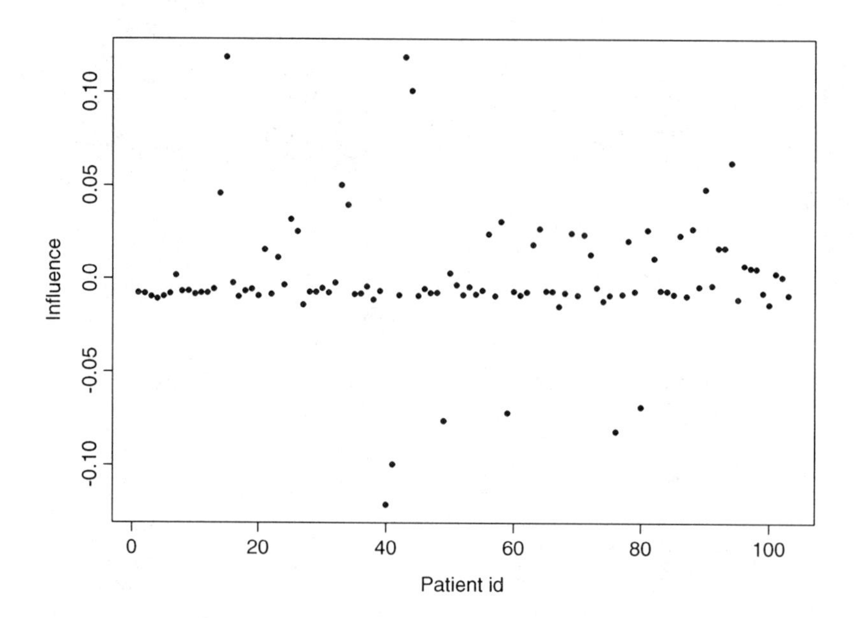

FIGURE 7.4: *Influence for the surgery variable*

```
proc phreg data=stanford;
    model (start, stop) * status(0) = age rx prior_sx /ties=efron;
    output out=temp1 dfbeta= age_inf rx_inf surg_inf;
    id id;

proc sort data=temp1; by id;

proc means noprint data=temp1;
    var age_inf rx_inf surg_inf;
    by id;
    output out=temp2 sum=age_inf rx_inf surg_inf;

data temp3; merge temp2 stanford;
    by id;
    if (first.id=1);
    dummy = _n_;          * Add a 1-n variable;

proc plot;
    plot age * age_inf;
    plot dummy * rx_inf;
    plot dummy * surg_inf;
```

In the `means` procedure, we sum up the influences for those subjects who have been represented by multiple observations. If this is not done, then the results will be *per-observation* influence rather than *per-subject* influence. The former are also useful, especially as a check for erroneous data; however we were interested in each subject's influence in this case. When we merge the residuals back into the original data set, in order to recover the `age` variable for plotting, it is necessary to ensure that the data set is not "reexpanded" from 103 subjects to 172 observations. This is done using the `first.id` conditional, which in effect pairs each residual with the age variable for the *first* of any multiple observations. (In this data set age is "age at entry" and does not vary among multiple observations for the same subject.)

Figure 7.4 shows the plot for the prior surgery variable. The estimate and standard error of the variable from the fitted model are -0.77 and 0.36, respectively. The influences are small, no more than about 1/3 of a standard error. Indeed, an alternative option is to request the `dfbetas` residuals, or "dfbeta scaled," which give the residuals with each column scaled by the standard error of the appropriate coefficient.

7.2 Variance

The jackknife can also be used to derive a robust estimate of variance for the Cox model. If J is the matrix of jackknife influence values (i.e., the ith row of J is $\hat\beta_{(i)} - \hat\beta$) then the jackknife estimate of variance can be written as the matrix product

$$V_J = \frac{n-1}{n}(J - \bar J)'(J - \bar J),$$

where $\bar J$ is the matrix of column means of J.

A natural approximation to this is $D'D$, the matrix product of the approximate jackknife variances (ignoring the $(n-1)/n$ term). Because the column sums of D are zero no recentering is necessary. In fact, the approximation $D'D$ may be preferable. Lipsitz et al. [93] examined the performance of three variance estimates in a logistic regression setting, using the six cities data. They used the jackknife, the approximate jackknife $D'D$ (which may be derived in the logistic regression setting by exactly the same Newton–Raphson argument as was used for the Cox model), and an improved approximation to the jackknife based on closer mimicry of the exact formula for a linear model. They found that for small n the jackknife variance significantly overestimated the variance, $D'D$ did quite well, and the "better" approximation also overestimated the variance (it is closer to the jackknife values), although not as severely as the true jackknife. For moderate n the jackknife did better but was still dominated by $D'D$.

Much of the problem could be traced to the most influential values. Since the variance estimate involves the squares of influence values, it appears that due to Jensen's inequality it is better to somewhat underestimate the larger influences!

The use of $D'D$ as an alternative variance for a Cox model is mentioned in the appendix of Reid and Crépeau [124], although it was not pursued further there. Writing $D'D = \mathcal{I}^{-1}(U'U)\mathcal{I}^{-1}$ we see that the variance can be viewed as a sandwich estimator ABA where A is the usual variance and B a correction term; sandwich estimates are familiar from robust variance estimation in parametric models and in generalized estimating equation (GEE) methods. Lin and Wei [87] derive a sandwich estimator appropriate to the Cox model. It turns out to be algebraically equivalent to $D'D$, although they do not make an explicit connection to the jackknife argument. Lin and Wei show that the estimate is consistent, and robust to several possible misspecifications in the Cox model including the lack of proportional hazards, incorrect functional form for the covariates, and omitted covariates.

For a linear regression Gaussian model, the infinitesimal jackknife approach leads to the estimate

$$D'D = (X'X)^{-1}X'RX(X'X)^{-1}$$

of White [157, 158], where R is a diagonal matrix containing the squared residuals. White recommends its use when the data are heteroscedastic. If one believed the data to be homoscedastic, then a natural step would be to replace R with $\hat{\sigma}^2 I$, the "average" squared residual times an identity matrix. The estimator then collapses down to the usual linear model variance estimate. We can rewrite $D'D$ in the sandwich form as well,

$$\hat{\sigma}^2(X'X)^{-1}\left[\hat{\sigma}^{-2}X'RX\hat{\sigma}^{-2}\right]\hat{\sigma}^2(X'X)^{-1},$$

a nonparametric variance estimator sandwiched between two copies of the inverse estimated information matrix $\hat{\sigma}^2(X'X)^{-1}$. The infinitesimal jackknife variance estimator and the famous sandwich estimator are usually one and the same.

In SAS the robust variance can be computed using the **phlev** macro, as found in Appendix B. This macro invokes **phreg**, obtains the dfbeta residuals, sums them within subject if necessary, computes the matrix product $D'D$, and then prints the results in a **phreg**-like format. The macro does not include a large number of the possible **phreg** options, but it can be easily modified. Below is an example using the Stanford heart transplant data (some columns are edited out of the SAS output to fit the page width).

```
%phlev(data=stanford, time=(start,stop), event=status,
       xvars=rx age, id=id, collapse=Y);
```

Variable	Parameter Estimate	SE	Robust SE	Chi-Square	DF	P
rx	-0.005499	0.31202	0.31292	0.000		0.9860
age	0.030736	0.01450	0.01516	4.110		0.0426
Wald				4.172	2	0.1242
robust score				5.591	2	0.0611

In S-Plus computation of the robust variance is even simpler. All that is necessary is to add the term "`+ cluster(id)`" to the model statement and all of the steps are carried out automatically by the `coxph` function.

```
> coxph(Surv(start, stop, status) ~ rx + age + cluster(id),
                    data=Stanford)

          coef exp(coef) se(coef) robust se        z     p
 rx -0.00418     0.996   0.3121    0.3142 -0.0133 0.990
age  0.03074     1.031   0.0145    0.0152  2.0249 0.043

Likelihood ratio test=5.17  on 2 df, p=0.0754  n= 172
```

In both packages, the printed tests are based on the robust variance estimate. For this data set, at least, the differences between the model-based and jackknife estimates of variance are slight.

The robust properties of the approximate jackknife estimate are not free, however. Below we present a simple simulation result. One thousand data sets were drawn from the simple model with two independent Gaussian (0,1) covariates, $\beta_1 = 0, \beta_2 = 0.5$, with exponential hazards. Each data set had 200 subjects and approximately 50% censoring; 90 to 100 events is a not an uncommon sample size in clinical data sets, and β_2 is chosen to give approximately 90% power. Figure 7.5 shows smoothed histograms for the ordinary Cox variance $\mathcal{I}^{-1}$ and for the sandwich estimate $D'D$. As we can see, the jackknife estimate, although unbiased, is much more variable. This is a common finding. It points to a disadvantage of the robust variance estimator and has implications for inference on the β coefficients. In small data sets, distortions caused by the occasional outlying robust variance estimator are problematic. Some authors have suggested that for small data sets, the gain in robustness for $D'D$ comes at too high a price. However, we still recommend examination of the sandwich estimate in cases where the Cox model assumptions are suspect.

7.3 Case weights

Both SAS and S-Plus allow for case weights in the Cox model fit. Two distinct uses for case weights (among many uses) need to be distinguished. The first is *frequency* weights; a weight of 3 means that 3 data points were actually observed, had the same values for all variables, and have been collapsed into a single observation to save space. The program should then treat an observation with a weight of k as if it had appeared k times in the input data set. The second is *sampling* weights. For instance, if 10% of the high-risk subjects for a condition were included in a study but only 1% of those with low or moderate risk, we would want to weight the observations inversely as the sampling fractions to reflect this design, giving case weights 10 times greater to the low/moderate-risk individuals than to the high-risk ones.

The SAS `phreg` procedure uses computations appropriate to frequency weights; this is emphasized by using a `freq` statement to specify the weights.

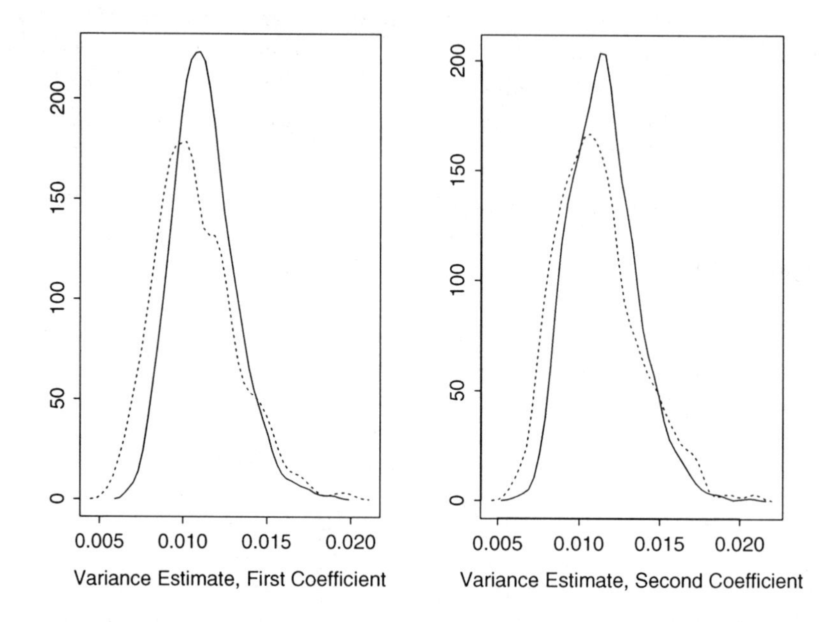

FIGURE 7.5: *Comparison of the variance estimators; solid line: model based, dashed line: sandwich estimate*

Weights are truncated to integer values before being applied, a necessity if one is to be precise in applying the various methods for handling tied event times. The S-Plus `coxph` function uses computations more appropriate to sampling weights. A single uncensored observation with a case weight of 2, for instance, would not cause the Efron computation for tied event times to be invoked. The weighted formulas for the score vector and information matrix are the obvious extensions of the unweighted formulae (3.4) and (3.6),

$$U'(\beta) = \sum_{i=1}^{n} w_i \int_0^\infty [X_i(s) - \bar{x}(\beta, s)]\, dN_i(s) \equiv \sum w_i U_i \qquad (7.1)$$

$$\mathcal{I}(\beta) = \sum_{i=1}^{n} w_i \int_0^\infty V(\beta, s) dN_i(s), \qquad (7.2)$$

with $w_i Y_i(t) r_i(t)$ replacing $Y_i(t) r_i(t)$ in the definitions of the weighted mean and variance $\bar{x}$ and V. For computation of $\hat{\beta}$ the actual magnitude of the weights is unimportant; for example, for the oversampling example given above using case weights of 1 and 10 or weights of .1 and 1 for the high and low/moderate-risk subjects, respectively, would yield precisely the same $\hat{\beta}$. The model-based variance estimate (7.2) is affected by the choice of weights, however. In particular, a uniform case weight of 3 for every subject in a data set will yield the same $\hat{\beta}$, but a variance matrix estimate that is 1/3 the prior value.

The appropriate dfbeta matrix is still $D = \mathcal{I}^{-1}U$. Binder [17] derives an appropriate variance estimate for the model with sampling weights as $\mathcal{I}^{-1}\tilde{U}'W\tilde{U}\mathcal{I}^{-1}$ where $\tilde{U}$ is the unweighted score residuals matrix; each row of the matrix is the U_i of equation (7.1). This reduces to $D'D$; thus a `cluster` term in the model is sufficient to produce an appropriate variance matrix for weighted Cox models in S-Plus.

As a contrived example, consider a subsampled version of the PBC data set. The new data set will contain 40/157 of the subjects with a bilirubin that is ≤ 1, the upper limit of normal. This mimics a protocol that enrolled all of the high-risk subjects but only a portion of the others. To make the example reproducible, we retained the 1st, 5th, 9th, /ldots , 157th subject in the data with normal bilirubin, and assigned a case weight to each of 157/40; all subjects with bilirubin > 1.0 were retained and given a case weight of 1.

```
> fit <- coxph(Surv(futime, status==2) ~ age + edema + log(bili) +
                  log(albumin) + log(protime)  + cluster(id),
                  data= wpbc, weights=casewt)
> summary(fit)
  n=300 (1 observations deleted due to missing)

                coef exp(coef) se(coef) robust se     z       p
          age  0.0373    1.0380  0.00775    0.0103  3.63 2.9e-04
        edema  0.8835    2.4193  0.26835    0.3172  2.79 5.4e-03
    log(bili)  0.9027    2.4663  0.08145    0.0955  9.45 0.0e+00
 log(albumin) -2.6841    0.0683  0.65804    0.6738 -3.98 6.8e-05
 log(protime)  2.8133   16.6641  0.78962    1.0937  2.57 1.0e-02

 Likelihood ratio test= 248  on 5 df,   p=0
 Wald test            = 189  on 5 df,   p=0
 Score (logrank) test = 325  on 5 df,   p=0,    Robust = 191  p=0

   (Note: the likelihood ratio and score tests assume independence
      of observations within a cluster, the Wald and robust score
      tests do not).
```

Note that the uncorrected standard errors are significantly deflated: since they are based on the sum of the weights they are essentially assuming a sample size of 418 rather than 300. The likelihood ratio and uncorrected score tests have the same bias. If we had used case weights of 1 for the low bilirubin and 40/157 for the high bilirubin subjects the coefficients would be unchanged, but the LR test would become an underestimate of the correct value.

Pugh et al. [123] show how to use derived sampling weights to deal more appropriately with missing covariate data than blind use of only the complete cases. *Complete case analysis*, that is, deletion of any observations with missing values for any of the covariates, is the common approach; it leads to reduced efficiency and frequently to biased inference. Pugh proposes a *propensity score* correction, which weights observations based on their likelihood of being incomplete. The underlying idea is to reweight cases from underrepresented groups. A hypothetical example helps illustrate the concept. Suppose there are two covariates, x_1, a clinic id for one of three clinical sites from which a patient was entered into a multicenter study, and x_2, a laboratory test result, missing on 20% of the subjects. Furthermore, suppose that the missingness depends on x_1: due to local practice patterns only 1/2 of the patients referred from clinic A have received the test, but it was ordered for all patients referred from B and C. If the choice of which patients received the test was random *within* clinic A, then a solution is a standard survey sampling approach. Site A patients have effectively been undersampled by a factor of 2 for any models that include x_2 because the analysis program will ignore all those with missing data, half of the site A group. Giving a case weight of 2 to those site A observations with an observed x_2 corrects for the undersampling.

In the more general case, let $y_i = 1$ if individual i has no missing covariates, and 0 otherwise. We can use logistic regression to estimate each subject's probability of complete data π_i or "propensity score," and use $1/\pi_i$ as a case weight in the Cox model. In the hypothetical case given above, this would exactly correct the problem if `clinic` were the only variable in the logistic regression model. A subject with complete data and a low propensity score is treated as the representative for a large cohort of similar subjects for whom data collection failed, and is thus given a correspondingly large weight.

The `lung` cancer data set contains the lung cancer subset of a prognostic variables study [95]. The study collected several simple measures of functional status for a cohort of advanced cancer patients, with the goal of testing their utility in prognosis and patient management. Values on the two dietary variables "weight loss in the last three months" and "calories eaten at regular meals" are missing for 25% of the 228 subjects in the study. Only 6 subjects are missing any one of the other important predictors: enrolling institution, age, sex, ECOG performance score (physician estimate), and Karnofsky status (physician and patient estimates). For simplicity below, a data set `lung2` has been created with these 6 removed. Institution codes greater than 25 are combined because of very small numbers.

```
> y     <- 1*(is.na(lung2$meal.cal) | is.na(lung2$wt.loss))
> inst2 <- pmin(lung2$inst, 25)
> lfit<- glm(y ~ time + status + age + sex + ph.karno +
                              pat.karno + ph.ecog + factor(inst2),
                 family=binomial, data=lung2)
> pscore <- 1- predict(lfit, type='response')
> hist(pscore, nclass=25, xlab='Propensity Score', ylab='Count')
```

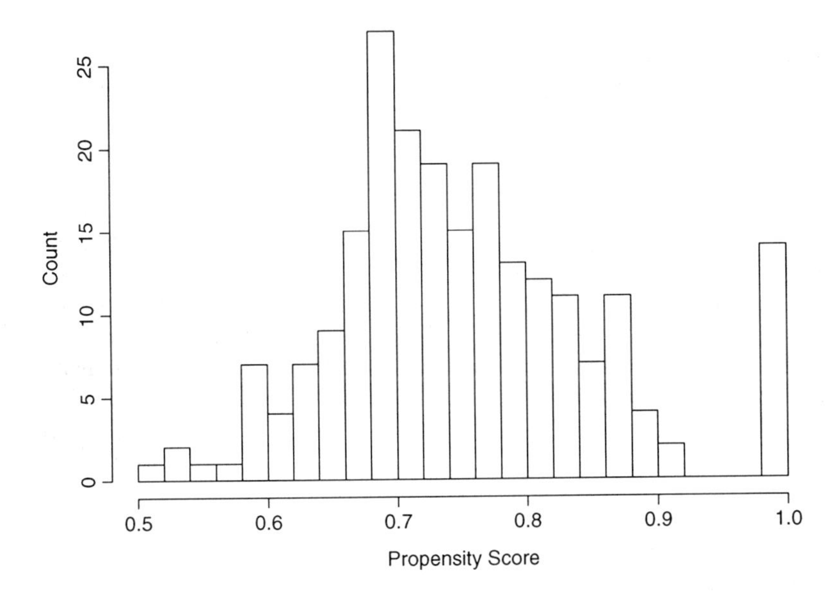

FIGURE 7.6: *Propensity score distribution for the lung cancer data*

We create the "observed missingness" variable and fit a logistic regression, then extract the predicted values. The histogram of the propensity scores is shown in Figure 7.6. Scores range from about 50 to 100%, the latter for one small institution with no missing values for the diet variables. The majority of the values are clustered between 65 and 85%; this is a modest range, and we would anticipate only a modest effect on the Cox model estimates.

```
> fit1 <- coxph(Surv(time, status) ~ sex + pat.karno +meal.cal +
                            wt.loss + strata(inst) + cluster(id),
                      data=lung2)
> print(fit1)
               coef exp(coef) se(coef) robust se      z       p
       sex -0.608183     0.544 0.229683  0.212978 -2.856 4.3e-03
 pat.karno -0.026979     0.973 0.008023  0.006830 -3.950 7.8e-05
  meal.cal -0.000217     1.000 0.000274  0.000263 -0.828 4.1e-01
   wt.loss -0.011118     0.989 0.008181  0.007725 -1.439 1.5e-01

 n=167 (55 observations deleted due to missing)

> fit2 <- coxph(Surv(time, status) ~ sex + pat.karno + meal.cal +
                            wt.loss + strata(inst) + cluster(id),
                    data=lung2, weights= 1/pscore)
> print(fit2)
```

```
                coef exp(coef) se(coef) robust se      z       p
       sex -0.624866     0.535 0.197595  0.210416 -2.970 3.0e-03
 pat.karno -0.026670     0.974 0.006878  0.006803 -3.920 8.8e-05
  meal.cal -0.000243     1.000 0.000239  0.000264 -0.922 3.6e-01
   wt.loss -0.011070     0.989 0.007125  0.007622 -1.452 1.5e-01
  n=167 (55 observations deleted due to missing)
```

Neither the estimates nor the appropriate robust standard errors have been much affected in this particular case. The standard errors from the weighted model given above are not technically correct, as they are based on the assumption of *known* case weights. To take account of the estimation of the propensity scores, Pugh [123] suggests the variance estimator $D'[I-T(T'T)^{-1}T']D$, where T is the matrix of dfbetas from the logistic regression model and D the dfbeta matrix from the weighted Cox model. This variance will be smaller than $D'D$ — Pugh et al.[123] point out that the estimation of the πs contains information from the incomplete cases which would otherwise be ignored. The S-Plus `glm` function does not directly return the dfbeta matrix, but a function to do so can be easily constructed using the code and suggestions in Chambers and Hastie [29, Section 6.3.4]. We also need a dfbeta matrix for `fit2` that has all 222 rows, with zeros for the 55 subjects not included in the fit, rather than one with 167 rows.

```
> dfbeta.glm <- function(model) {
        betas <- lm.influence(model)$coefficient
        betas - outer(rep(1, nrow(betas)), coef(model))
        }

> d1 <- resid(fit2, 'dfbeta', weighted=T)
> d1[is.na(d1)] <- 0    #will have all 0 rows for 55 subjects
> d2   <- dfbeta.glm(lfit)
> temp <- diag(222) - d2%*% solve(chol(t(d2) %*% d2), t(d2))
> newvar <-  t(d1) %*% temp %*% d1
> print(sqrt(rbind(diag(fit2$var), diag(newvar))))
        sex    pat.karno   meal.cal   wt.loss
[1,] 0.2104   0.006803   0.0002638  0.007622
[2,] 0.2086   0.006626   0.0002566  0.007538
```

The final lines compare the unadjusted standard errors of `fit2` to new values correcting for the uncertainty in the weights. The difference in this case is small. The adjustment produces smaller standard errors, as would be anticipated from the formula. Note that if the logistic regression is completely uninformative ($\hat{\pi}_i$ = constant), then the weighted model reduces to the unweighted fit, and the adjusted variance reduces to the ordinary sandwich estimate.

A cautionary note is in order: the propensity score method need not improve on complete case analysis and may do worse. The relative performance of the two approaches depends on the mechanism leading to the

Scenario	Complete Case $\hat{\beta}_1$	$\hat{\beta}_2$	Pugh $\hat{\beta}_1$	$\hat{\beta}_2$
1	0.97	1.02	0.79	0.92
2	0.75	0.80	0.97	1.02
3	0.76	1.15	0.79	1.19

TABLE 7.1: *Missing covariates*

missing data [123]. If the probability of a particular covariate datum being missing depends on the (possibly unobserved) value of the covariate, but not on other covariates or data, then the complete case approach is consistent, but the propensity score method need not be. On the other hand, if the probability of missingness depends on the values of completely observed variables, but not on the value of the missing covariate itself, then Pugh's method is consistent, but complete case analysis need not be so. If missingness depends on both of these factors, both methods may be inconsistent. We illustrate these differences with a conceptual numerical example. Consider a study with two covariates, x_1 completely observed and x_2 subject to missingness. The covariates are independent N(0,1), and failure time is exponential with hazard $\exp(x_1 + x_2)$. Censoring is uniform (1.8, 2.5), independent of failure time and covariates. The simulated data set with $n = 5,000$ was created, containing 3,167 events. A Cox model fit to the simulated data set gave estimates of $\hat{\beta}_1 = 0.99$ and $\hat{\beta}_2 = 1.03$ with $\widehat{se} = 0.02$ for each coefficient. We consider three scenarios for missingness for x_2.

1. Suppose that large values of x_2 are difficult to measure so that the probability of x_2 being missing is an increasing function of x_2. For example, x_2 may represent income and people with higher incomes are less willing to report it. We used the following function.
$$\text{logit}(1 - \pi_{1i}) = -\log(4.5) + 2.5x_2.$$
2. Suppose that the importance of x_2 was not recognized until the end of the study period. It must be ascertained retrospectively. Therefore, it may not be obtainable from subjects who have died ($\delta_i = 1$) or from those who entered the study early and thus have long followup times. We used
$$\text{logit}(1 - \pi_{2i}) = -\log(150) + 3T_i + \delta_i.$$
3. Both of the above mechanisms are operative:
$$\text{logit}(1 - \pi_{3i}) = -\log(150) + 3T_i + \delta_i + 2.5x_2.$$

We introduced missing values for x_2 via each of the three models above and then estimated $\hat{\beta}$ by complete case analysis and the Pugh method. Table 7.1 summarizes the estimates. The amount of missingness is between 31 and 32% in all three cases. The two methods can give quite different results. Unfortunately, there is no way to tell from the data set itself which missingness mechanism holds. Of course, these problems are not unique to Cox regression. Both complete case analysis and the completeness propensity score have been applied in numerous regression settings (as well as many other methods for dealing with missing covariates). In general, it is found that complete case analysis yields valid (if inefficient) inference provided that missingness depends on the predictor variables, whether missing or not, but not on the outcome; and the completeness propensity score approach is valid when the probability of being missing depends only on the values of observed data, response, or predictors, and not on the values of missing covariates [94].

8

Multiple Events per Subject

8.1 Introduction

There is increasing interest, and need, to apply survival analysis to data sets with multiple events per subject. This includes both the cases of multiple events of the same type, and events of different types. Examples of the former would be recurrent infections in AIDS patients or multiple infarcts in a coronary study. Examples of the latter are the use of both survival and recurrence information in cancer trials, or multiple sequelae (toxicity, worsening symptoms, etc.) in the management of chronic disease. With the increasing emphasis on quality of life, rehospitalization, and other secondary endpoints such analyses will become more common.

A major issue in extending proportional hazards regression models to this situation is intrasubject correlation. Other concerns are multiple time scales, discontinuous intervals of risk, stratum by covariate interactions, and the structure of the risk sets. Several approaches to such data have appeared in the literature:

- Time to first event, ignoring the multiplicity. This is simple and easy to interpret, but there is always the concern that information is being wasted.

- Random effects or *frailty* model, such as that described in Oakes [114]. The model includes a random per-subject effect; multiple outcomes are assumed to be independent conditional on the per-subject coefficient. These are examined in more detail in Chapter 9.

- A marginal models approach. This has much in common with the generalized estimating equations (GEE) approach of Zeger, et al. [163].

- A more ambitious plan is to model the subject's correlation directly within the Cox framework. Prentice and Cai [120] explore this for a sample of industrial failure data. The method is very computer intensive, however, and as pointed out by the discussant of their paper, required the estimation of 226 parameters from only 20 pairs of data.

This chapter focuses on marginal models, including three common variants of the approach due to Andersen and Gill [6] (AG), Wei, Lin, and Wiessfeld [155] (WLW) and Prentice, Williams and Petersen [122] (PWP). This is partly due to the ready availability of software for this approach in both the S-Plus and SAS packages. As well, the method affords great flexibility in the formation of strata and risk sets, manipulation of the time scale, and has a well-developed estimator of variance. In each case the analysis is based on three steps:

- Decide on a model (issues such as strata, time-dependent covariates, etc.) and structure the data set accordingly.

- Fit the data as an ordinary Cox model, ignoring the possible correlation.

- Replace the standard variance estimate with one which is corrected for the possible correlations.

In the sections below we first deal with the third issue, then the first and second, and finally a list of examples. Application of these methods to actual data sets most clearly illustrates the relevant issues in the models' practical usage.

8.2 Robust variance and computation

8.2.1 Grouped jackknife

The ordinary Cox model estimate of variance for $\hat\beta$ treats each of the observations as independent. When a given subject may contribute multiple events this assumption obviously does not hold, but an appropriate correction is available using an argument that directly follows the discussion of a robust variance in Section 7.2. Essentially, the jackknife will provide an honest estimate of variance for correlated data whenever the observation(s) left out at any step are independent of the observations left in. For data in which the correlation is restricted to disjoint groups (e.g., multiple observations per subject) the obvious choice is then a grouped jackknife estimate that leaves out one *subject* at a time rather than one *observation* at a time.

As the simplest example consider a data set with doubled observations; for example, suppose that through some programming error each line of data has been entered twice. As a specific example we use the 85 observations for time to first event from the bladder cancer data discussed in Section 8.5.4; two data sets `single` and `double` contain the correct and doubled data set, respectively. The variable `id` contains the subject identifier. We can fit the two data sets in S-Plus as the following.

```
> coxph(Surv(futime, status) ~ rx + size + number + cluster(id),
                  data=single, method='breslow')

           coef exp(coef) se(coef) robust se      z      p
    rx -0.5176      0.596   0.3158    0.3075 -1.683 0.0920
  size  0.0679      1.070   0.1012    0.0853  0.796 0.4300
number  0.2360      1.266   0.0761    0.0721  3.275 0.0011

Likelihood ratio test=9.66  on 3 df, p=0.0216  n= 85

> coxph(Surv(futime, status) ~ rx + size + number + cluster(id),
                  data=double, method='breslow')

           coef exp(coef) se(coef) robust se      z      p
    rx -0.5176      0.596   0.2233    0.3075 -1.683 0.0920
  size  0.0679      1.070   0.0716    0.0853  0.796 0.4300
number  0.2360      1.266   0.0538    0.0721  3.275 0.0011

Likelihood ratio test=19.3  on 3 df, p=0.000234  n= 170
```

The `cluster` term in the model is the key addition. It performs exactly the same operations as were needed when a subject was broken into multiple observations for artificial reasons, such as to represent a time-dependent covariate, that is, the creation of D, collapsing this to $\widetilde{D}$, followed by formation of the alternate variance $\widetilde{D}'\widetilde{D}$, and incorporation of the result into the printout.

We have purposely used the Breslow approximation in the example to avoid any correction for ties; doing this leads to identical coefficients in the two data fits and simplifies comparison of the standard errors. Comparing the `se` columns, the doubled data set has a variance of exactly half the correct value: $.2233 = .3158/\sqrt{2}$, while the robust standard error is unchanged.

A fit using SAS requires extra processing since `phreg` does not directly handle the clustering. But it is instructive since it shows how the robust estimate can be obtained using only the dfbeta residuals; the technique may be useful in other packages as well.

```
proc phreg data=double;
    model futime * status(0) = rx + size + number;
    output out=temp1 dfbeta= rx size number;
    id id;

proc sort data=temp1; by id;
proc means data=temp1 noprint;          *add up rows to get D-tilde;
    by id;
    var rx size number;
    output out=temp2 sum=rx size number;

proc iml;                                *compute matrix product;
    use temp2;
    read all var{rx size number} in dtil;
    v = dtil' * dtil;
    reset noname;
    vname = {"rx", "size", "number"};
    print, "Robust variance matrix",,
                            v[colname=vname rowname=vname];
```

The %phlev macro found in Appendix B is an extension of the above which merges the coefficients and robust variance into a single printout.

With correlated groups the sandwich estimate $\widetilde{D}'\widetilde{D}$ will often be substantially larger than the model-based variance $\mathcal{I}^{-1}$. All three of the usual tests, the Wald, score, and likelihood ratio test, will then be anticonservative. A robust Wald test is $\hat{\beta}'[\widetilde{D}'\widetilde{D}]^{-1}\hat{\beta}$, that is, replacing the usual variance with the sandwich estimate. An version of the score test that is adjusted for possible correlation can also be created. First, note that the per-subject leverage matrix can be written as $\widetilde{D}_{m\times p} = B_{m\times n}D_{n\times p}$ where B is an matrix of 0s and 1s that sums the appropriate rows, so that $\widetilde{D}'\widetilde{D} = \mathcal{I}^{-1}U'B'BU\mathcal{I}^{-1}$. The first step of the Newton–Raphson iteration is $\hat{\beta}^{(1)} = \hat{\beta}^{(0)} + U\mathcal{I}^{-1}$, where (0) refers to the initial parameter estimate (usually $\beta = 0$) and U and $\mathcal{I}$ are computed at $\beta^{(0)}$. Writing the usual score test

$$T = [1'U]\,\mathcal{I}^{-1}\,[U'1]$$

as

$$[1'U\mathcal{I}^{-1}]\,\mathcal{I}\,[\mathcal{I}^{-1}U'1]$$

(i.e., as a Wald test based on the one-step estimate of $\hat{\beta}$), insertion of the inverse of the sandwich estimate of variance for the central term, again based at the starting estimate of β, gives a robust score test

$$T_r = [1'U]\,[U'B'BU]^{-1}\,[U'1]$$

The test can also be derived directly without using an approximate Wald argument.

8.2.2 Connection to other work

Lee et al. [83] consider highly stratified data sets that arise from inter-observation correlation. As an example they use paired eye data on visual loss due to diabetic retinopathy, where photocoagulation was randomly assigned to one eye of each patient. There are $n/2 = 1,742$ clusters (patients) with two observations per cluster. Treating each pair of eyes as a cluster, they derive the modified sandwich estimate $V = \mathcal{I}^{-1}(B'B)\mathcal{I}^{-1}$, where each row of the matrix B is based on a sum of score vectors, summed over the two eyes of each individual. Some algebraic manipulation reveals that this is precisely the estimate $\widetilde{D}'\widetilde{D}$ suggested above, where each row of $\widetilde{D}'\widetilde{D}$ is obtained by summing rows of the per-observation dfbeta matrix D over each individual's pair of eyes. Wei et al. [155] consider multivariate survival times, an example being the measurement of both time to progression of disease and time to death for a group of cancer patients. They propose a sandwich estimator of variance that reduces to $\widetilde{D}'\widetilde{D}$.

For a generalized linear model with loglikelihood function $l(\beta)$, the score function is

$$U_{ij} = \frac{\partial l}{\partial \eta_i}\frac{\partial \eta_i}{\partial \beta_j},$$

where $\eta_i = \beta_0 + \beta_1 x_{i1} + \ldots$ is the linear predictor for subject i. Defining an approximate dfbeta residual as before (i.e., the product of U with the inverse information matrix for the model), it can be shown that $\widetilde{D}'\widetilde{D}$ is equal to the *working independence* estimate of variance proposed by Liang and Zeger [162] for generalized estimating equation (GEE) models. They deal with the case of longitudinal data, so the summation of each individual's contributions in going from D to $\widetilde{D}$ is over observations at multiple time points.

In the special case of a linear model this dfbeta matrix has rows

$$D_i = (y_i - X_i\beta)X(X'X)^{-1}$$

and the variance estimate $D'D$ can be written as

$$D'D = (X'X)^{-1}X'RX(X'X)^{-1},$$

where R is a diagonal matrix of the squared residuals. This is the estimator proposed by White [157, 158] for the analysis of nonhomoscedastic data. If one were to replace R by $\hat{\sigma}^2 I$, and identity matrix times the average residual, the estimator collapses to the standard linear models form.

Lipsitz et al. [92] discuss clustered survival data and propose a clustered jackknife estimator whose first approximation again turns out to be $\widetilde{D}'\widetilde{D}$. Interestingly, they make the connection to White's work [158] and to the GEE models, but do not note the relationship to the leverage measure of Cain and Lange or Reid and Crépeau [27, 124], nor to the robust variance papers of Lin and Wei or of Wei et al. [87, 155].

Self and Prentice [132] discuss estimation of $\hat\beta$ in the context of a case-cohort study, which consists of a random sample (the *cohort*) from the population of interest, augmented with all of the events for those not in the cohort, and derive an appropriate variance estimate that consists of the usual variance plus a correction term. Barlow [9] suggests as an alternative the use of $D'D$, since the Self and Prentice estimate was considered to be very hard to compute. With algebraic rearrangement, however, it can be shown that the correction term is ${D_c}'D_c$ times a constant, D_c being the subset of rows of D corresponding to the cohort subjects [145].

Widely differing notation has caused problems with recognition of cross-linkages in this area.

8.3 Selecting a model

As shown above the computation of a marginal model is very easy once a data set has been created: in S-Plus make use of the `cluster()` directive to force an approximate jackknife variance; in SAS make use of the `phlev` macro. The difficult part of the analysis is the creation of an appropriate data set, in particular, the choice between alternative models.

One aspect of multiple event data sets is that there are a number of choices to be made in setting up the model. These include the choice of strata and membership within strata, time scales within strata, constructed time-dependent covariates, stratum by covariate interactions, and data organization. For a "standard" Cox model these issues are fairly well understood.

- Stratification, if used, is based on external variables such as enrolling institution or disease subtype. These generally correspond to predictors for which we desire a flexible adjustment, but not an estimate of the covariate effect. Each subject is in exactly one stratum.

- The time scale is almost invariably time since entry to the study, although, as discussed in Section 3.7.2, alternate time scales are possible using the counting process notation.

- Time-dependent covariates usually reflect directly measured data such as repeated lab tests. Strata by covariate interactions (i.e., separate coefficients per stratum for some covariate) are infrequent.

- The counting process form may be used for a time-dependent covariate, but normally the data set will consist of one observation per subject.

In a multiple events data set there are possible extensions in each of these four areas.

The first issue is to distinguish between data sets where the multiple events have a distinct ordering and those where they do not. Two examples of correlated *unordered* events are paired survival data, such as the subjects' two eyes in the diabetic retinopathy data, and genetic studies where the correlated group is a family (there is no constraint that Aunt Millicent die before Uncle Joe, or vice versa). An example of ordered events is multiple sequential infections for a single subject. Since the issues for unordered events are simpler, we deal with them first.

8.4 Unordered outcomes

We look at correlated, but unordered, outcomes using four examples, illustrating the application to competing risks and to multiple (parallel) events per subject. A fifth example concerning familial clustering is presented in Chapter 9 on random effects (frailty) models. A common feature of all is that setup of the data is straightforward; each observation is entered into the data just as it would be were correlation not an issue. Fits are then easily accomplished with either package, using the sandwich estimate $\widetilde{D}'\widetilde{D}$ to account for the correlation structure. Often, the analysis is stratified by the type of endpoint; for example, we assume that the baseline hazard functions for time-to-death and time-to-progression may differ.

8.4.1 Long-term outcomes in MGUS patients

The plasma cell lineage comprises only a small portion of human blood cells, <3%, but is responsible for the production of immunoglobulins, an important part of the body's immune defense. Each cell creates a distinctive molecule, allowing the body to respond to a broad spectrum of threats; when the immoglobulins are assayed using protein electrophoresis one sees a roughly uniform density of molecular weights over the defined range. In the case of a plasma cell malignancy (multiple myeloma, macroglobulinemia, amyloidosis, and other related disorders) the assay will often reveal a sharp spike — in spite of its inappropriate (unbounded) growth, the malignant clone is still manufacturing its unique product.

The presence of a monoclonal peak in persons without evidence of overt disease is termed "monoclonal gammopathy of undetermined significance" (MGUS); it may often be discovered inadvertently when protein electrophoresis is performed for other diagnostic reasons. The population prevalence of MGUS increases with age from about 1% at age 50 to 3% for patients over 70 [78]. Given its connection to serious plasma cell diseases, the potential prognostic importance of MGUS is of interest: is it a precursor state to malignancy, an incidental finding of no prognostic importance, or something inbetween? Kyle [77] studied all 241 cases of MGUS identified at the

Mayo Clinic before Jan. 1, 1971, with between 20 and 35 years of total followup on each patient. This can be analyzed as a competing risks problem. The response variable is time to the first of multiple myeloma ($n = 39$), amyloidosis ($n = 8$), macroglobulinemia ($n = 7$), other lymphoproliferative disease ($n = 5$), or death ($n = 130$). Important covariates are the age at diagnosis, the size of the monoclonal spike, hemoglobin, and creatinine levels.

We use two data sets; the first data set `mgus` has one observation per subject and corresponds to the usual "time to first outcome" analysis. The second data set `mgus2` allows for a competing risks analysis. It contains one stratum for each outcome type, with all 241 subjects appearing in each stratum. For simplicity, and because of the small numbers of events, the outcomes are collapsed into "death," "multiple myeloma," and "other." The first two subjects in the study experience death without progression at 760 days and lymphoproliferative disease at 2,160 days, respectively. They generate the following six observations in the `mgus2` data set.

```
id  time status endpoint  sex age   hgb  creat mspike
1    760    1    death      2   79   1.5   1.2    2.0
1    760    0    myeloma    2   79   1.5   1.2    2.0
1    760    0    other      2   79   1.5   1.2    2.0
2   2160    0    death      2   76  13.3   1.0    1.8
2   2160    0    myeloma    2   76  13.3   1.0    1.8
2   2160    1    other      2   76  13.3   1.0    1.8
```

To fit the simple "time to first event" and "competing risks" models, the S-Plus code is as follows.

```
>  coxph(Surv(time, status) ~ sex + age + mspike + hgb +
             cluster(id), data=mgus)

          coef exp(coef) se(coef) robust se      z       p
   sex -0.3494     0.705  0.15611   0.15277 -2.287 2.2e-02
   age  0.0516     1.053  0.00732   0.00725  7.119 1.1e-12
mspike -0.0945     0.910  0.18673   0.18292 -0.517 6.1e-01
   hgb -0.1669     0.846  0.04418   0.03506 -4.759 1.9e-06

Likelihood ratio test=76.8  on 4 df, p=7.77e-16  n=238
        (3 observations deleted due to missing)

> coxph(Surv(time, status) ~ sex + age + mspike + hgb
             + cluster(id) + strata(endpoint), data=mgus2)

          coef exp(coef) se(coef) robust se      z       p
   sex -0.3493     0.705  0.15611   0.15276 -2.287 2.2e-02
   age  0.0516     1.053  0.00732   0.00725  7.121 1.1e-12
mspike -0.0947     0.910  0.18673   0.18289 -0.518 6.0e-01
   hgb -0.1669     0.846  0.04418   0.03505 -4.761 1.9e-06
```

```
Likelihood ratio test=76.8  on 4 df, p=7.77e-16  n=714
        (9 observations deleted due to missing)
```

The analyses are nearly identical! In fact, the two results would match exactly were it not for a handful of tied events, leading to a slight change in the computation of the Efron approximation (3 tied event times become untied by being separated into two strata). The robust (sandwich) estimate as a correction for multiple events is not required in the competing risks case when each subject may have at most one outcome event. This was noted empirically in Lunn and McNeil [96]. The reason for the equivalence is clear from the partial likelihood equation (3.3): it has one term for each event, said term compares the subject with the event to the other subjects who were "at risk" at the time of the event. Because of the replication of observations into each stratum, the likelihood term for any given event is the same in `fit1` and `fit2`.

The advantage of the larger data set is that it allows for easy estimation of within-event-type coefficients. For instance, one might ask if the effect of age is identical for both outcomes, while controlling for a common effect of hemoglobin. This can be investigated by coding two dummy variables.

```
> age1 <- mgus2$age * (mgus2$endpoint=='death')
> age2 <- mgus2$age * (mgus2$endpoint!='death')
>  coxph(Surv(time, status) ~ hgb + age1 + age2
           + strata(endpoint), data=mgus2)

         coef exp(coef) se(coef)      z      p
 hgb -0.14057     0.869  0.04410 -3.187 0.0014
age1  0.07873     1.082  0.00928  8.486 0.0000
age2  0.00511     1.005  0.01212  0.421 0.6700
```

The median age of the study subjects is 64 years, and it is not surprising that age is a significant predictor of the overall death rate. Age is, however, of far less import in predicting the likelihood of a plasma cell malignancy.

8.4.2 Diabetic retinopathy study

This example is used in Lee et al. [83] to motivate the robust estimate, and in Huster et al. [70] to illustrate parametric models for paired data. Diabetic retinopathy is a complication associated with diabetes mellitus, which can cause abnormalities in the microvasculature of the retina which in turn can lead to macular edema and visual loss. It is the leading cause of blindness in patients under 60 years of age in the United States. Between 1972 and 1975, 1,742 patients were enrolled in a multicenter study to evaluate the efficacy of photocoagulation treatment for proliferative diabetic retinopathy; photocoagulation was randomly assigned to one eye of each study patient, with the other eye serving as an untreated control. A major goal was to assess whether treatment significantly delayed the onset of severe visual loss. Several other potentially important covariates such as age, gender, and duration of diabetes were also recorded. We use the subset of 197 patients defined in Huster et al. [70], which is a 50% sample of the high-risk patients as defined by the study.

Since each eye is at risk for failure both before and after its companion has failed, the analysis data set consists of $2n$ observations, each at risk from enrollment (time 0) onwards. There is no obvious stratification variable (left eye vs. right eye, dominant vs. nondominant, etc.), so the analysis will have a single stratum corresponding to an overall baseline hazard or "time to failure" distribution. The risk set when a particular eye fails is all *eyes* that have not yet failed.

```
> dfit <- coxph(Surv(time, status) ~ adult + trt + cluster(id),
                  data=diabetes)
> summary(dfit)

  n= 394
          coef exp(coef) se(coef) robust se      z      p
  adult  0.0539    1.055    0.162     0.179  0.302    .76
    trt -0.7789    0.459    0.169     0.149 -5.245 <.0001

Rsquare= 0.055   (max possible= 0.988 )
Likelihood ratio test= 22.5  on 2 df,   p=1.31e-05
Wald test            = 27.9  on 2 df,   p=8.94e-07
Score (logrank) test = 22.4  on 2 df,   p=1.4e-05,
               Robust = 26.4  p=1.89e-06

(Note: the likelihood ratio and score tests assume independence of
 observations within a cluster; the Wald and robust score tests
 do not).
```

The covariate defining adult versus juvenile onset of disease is not significant, as noted by other authors. The standard error for the corresponding coefficient is underestimated by the model-based variance, as it does not account for correlation between the eyes; the approximate jackknife variance $\tilde{D}'\tilde{D}$ corrects for this. The robust variance for treatment is *smaller* than the model-based estimate, however. Because the treatment is balanced within subjects there is an improvement in the precision of the estimated treatment coefficient, analogous to that obtained with a paired t-test. Note the warning message that follows the fit, which shows that only the Wald and robust score test have been corrected for correlation. The two corrected statistics are quite similar, as are the two uncorrected values.

As shown by Lee et al. [83], the resulting estimate and its variance are much more efficient than a matched analysis, which places each pair of patients into a separate stratum.

	UDCA	Placebo
Death	6	10
Transplant	6	6
Drug toxicity	0	0
Voluntary withdrawal	11	18
Histologic progression	8	12
Development of varices	8	17
Development of ascites	1	5
Development of encephalopathy	3	1
Doubling of bilirubin	2	15
Worsening of symptoms	7	9

TABLE 8.1: *Total number of events in the UDCA trial*

```
> coxph(Surv(time, status) ~ adult + trt + strata(id), diabetes)

        coef exp(coef) se(coef)     z       p
treat -0.962     0.382    0.202 -4.77 1.8e-06

Likelihood ratio test=25.5  on 1 df, p=4.45e-07  n= 394
```

The model-based standard error is valid for a stratified analysis, but it is about 35% larger than the result of the marginal fit. There is a larger estimated treatment effect as well; we come back to this when discussing frailty models.

8.4.3 UDCA in patients with PBC

Primary biliary cirrhosis (PBC) is a chronic cholestatic liver disease characterized by slow but progressive destruction of the bile ducts. PBC frequently progresses to cirrhosis, and in turn death from liver failure. Liver transplantation is the definitive treatment for end-stage disease, but this is an extensive and costly procedure and is furthermore available only to a portion of the patients due to the shortage of donor organs. Trials have been held for several promising agents, but an effective therapy remains elusive. Although progression of the disease is inexorable the time course can be very long; many patients survive 10 or more years from their initial diagnosis before requiring a transplant.

A randomized double-blind trial of a new agent, ursodeoxycholic acid (UDCA), was conducted at the Mayo Clinic from 1988 to 1992 and enrolled 180 patients. The data are reported in Lindor et al. [89]. For this analysis, we exclude 10 patients who had incomplete followup for some of the event types (they were the last 10 enrolled in the study). The endpoints of the study were predefined and are shown in Table 8.1. Although nearly all of the comparisons favor UDCA, none are significant individually. The primary report was based on an analysis of time to the first event; 58/84 placebo and 34/86 UDCA patients have at least one event. Each of the event endpoints is unique; that is, no single patient had more than one instance of death, transplant, doubling of bilirubin, and so on.

	Number of Events					
	0	1	2	3	4	5
Placebo	39	28	9	5	1	2
UDCA	59	17	6	4	0	0

TABLE 8.2: *Number of adverse outcomes per subject in the UDCA study, after exclusion of voluntary withdrawal*

Because there was concern that voluntary withdrawal could be influenced by external factors (e.g., a patient guessing she was on placebo) the primary analysis was also done with that outcome excluded; we do so as well. For the remaining events, the number per subject is shown in Table 8.2; 45 of the placebo and 27 of the UDCA subjects have at least one event. An analysis using all events would seem to be more complete than one using first events however, since it would be based on 75 placebo and 41 UDCA events, a potential gain in "information" of 61%.

The obvious starting point for analysis, of course, is time to the first adverse outcome. Each patient is represented by a single observation and correlation is not an issue; the relevant data set `udca1` has 170 observations. The data set for the WLW method is essentially a concatenation of the 8 individual data sets that would be created for an analysis of time to death (censoring all other causes), time to transplant, time to histologic progression, and the like; this data set will have $170 * 8 = 1,360$ observations. (Because there were no instances of drug toxicity, this outcome has no impact on the computation and can be excluded.) The data set contains a code variable `etype` or "event type" which is 1 for the first block of 170 observations, 2 for the second block of 170, and so on.

The SAS and S-Plus code to fit the models is as follows.

```
data temp1; set udca1;
    lbili = log(bili);
%phlev(data=temp1, time=time, event=status,
                    xvars= treat lbili stage, id=id);
data temp2; set udca2;
    lbili = log(bili);
%phlev(data=temp2, time=time, event=status,
                    xvars= treat lbili stage, strata=etype,
                    id=id, collapse=Y);

> fit1 <- coxph(Surv(time, status) ~ treat + log(bili) + stage +
                               cluster(id), data=udca1)
> fit2 <- coxph(Surv(time, status) ~ treat + log(bili) + stage +
                          cluster(id) + strata(etype), data=udca2)
```

Results are shown in Table 8.3; the covariates in the model are treatment and two of the potential risk factors for disease progression. The second fit is stratified by event type; that is, we do not assume that the baseline hazard rates for death, development of ascites, transplant, and so on are all equal. (Table 8.1 shows that the overall rate for encephalopathy, for instance, is obviously lower than that for worsening of symptoms.)

	β	SE(β)	Robust SE
Time to first event			
Treatment	−1.03	0.26	0.26
Log(bili)	0.62	0.15	0.16
Stage	−0.07	0.29	0.31
Marginal model			
Treatment	−0.97	0.21	0.27
Bilirubin	0.66	0.12	0.17
Stage	0.03	0.24	0.33

TABLE 8.3: *Results of two models for the UDCA data*

Three consequences are immediately obvious. First, for the simple model the usual estimate $\mathcal{I}^{-1}$ and the robust sandwich estimate of variance are essentially the same, as we might expect if there were no serious violations of the model assumptions. Second, the naive variance is an underestimate in the multiple event model — accounting for the within-patient correlation is important. The last is that the variance using all the data is no smaller than that obtained using first events only; the use of multiple events has added no information to the analysis! The standard error for treatment in the marginal model is actually somewhat higher. The ratio of the model-based variances for the two fits, which do not correct for the correlation, is $(.255/.203)^2 = 1.58$, almost exactly the 61% "increase in information" predicted by the total event count.

A closer look at the data reveals the cause of the difficulty. Patients on the study returned for evaluation once a year, which is the point at which most of the outcomes were measured (excluding death and transplantation of course). One patient who had five events, for instance, has four of them recorded on July 20, 1990, followed by death on July 22. Similar outcomes are seen for many others. Figure 8.1 shows the event times for the 27 subjects with multiple adverse outcomes, with a circle marking each event. The data have been jittered slightly to avoid overlap. It appears that the use of multiple event types was useful in this study only to make the detection of "liver failure" more sensitive. Given that failure has occurred, the number of positive markers for failure was irrelevant. Multiple event analysis does not always lead to gains.

One commonly asked question is whether the different outcomes could be weighted according to severity. Assume, for instance, that the investigator believed that liver death (patient death or liver transplant) were twice as momentous as any of the other outcomes and should receive proportionately more weight. This is easily accomplished by giving each observation in the death and transplant stratum a weight of 2. The outcome is shown below; note that death and transplant are event types 1 and 2 in the data set.

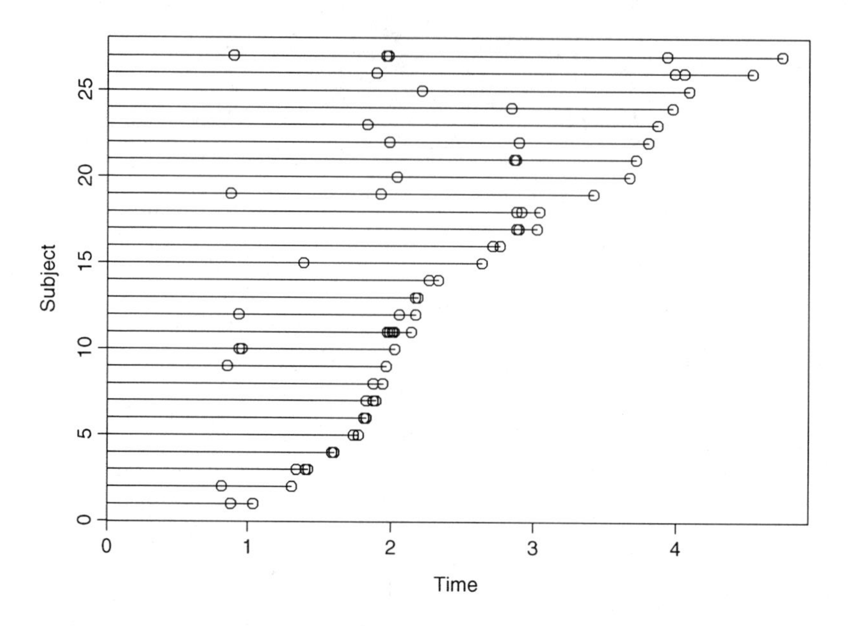

FIGURE 8.1: *Multiple failure times for the UDCA data*

```
> temp <- 1 + 1*(udca2$etype <= 2)
> coxph(Surv(time, status) ~ treat +log(bili) + stage +
                                cluster(id)+ strata(etype),
                        data=udca2, weights=temp)

               coef exp(coef) se(coef) robust se      z       p
     treat -0.9210     0.398    0.181     0.281 -3.276 1.1e-03
 log(bili)  0.7178     2.050    0.106     0.178  4.027 5.7e-05
     stage  0.0754     1.078    0.220     0.341  0.221 8.2e-01
```

The estimated treatment effect is just a little smaller, and the standard error of the treatment coefficient has increased slightly from 0.27 to 0.28. If we were to do a more extreme reweighting, say 20-fold weights for the death/transplant outcome, the standard error is substantially increased to .39 as seen below. (The robust se is corrected for an importance weight such as this; the ordinary estimate is not.) In the limit (e.g., a relative weight of 1,000) the analysis would be based essentially only on those two outcomes.

```
> temp <- 1 + 20*(udca2$etype <= 2)
> coxph(Surv(time, status) ~ treat +log(bili) + stage +
                                 cluster(id)+ strata(etype),
                    data=udca2, weights=temp)

            coef exp(coef) se(coef) robust se      z       p
     treat -0.750     0.472   0.0826     0.394 -1.904 0.05700
 log(bili)  0.892     2.441   0.0465     0.233  3.832 0.00013
     stage  0.277     1.319   0.1104     0.507  0.546 0.59000
```

8.4.4 Colon cancer data

The data set is from a study of adjuvant treatment of large bowel carcinoma conducted by the North Central Cancer Treatment Group. There were three treatment arms of observation, Levamisole (Lev), and the combination of Levamisole and 5-fluorouracil (5FU). For details of the study see Laurie et al. [81]. The data set is also used in Lin [86]; his version of the data, however, has less followup than that used here.

In this trial 315, 310, and 304 patients with stage C disease were randomized to the observation, Lev, and Lev + 5FU arms, respectively. Both time to death and time to recurrence were of interest. Since we would not expect the baseline hazards for the two event types to be the same, the analysis is stratified on event type. The data set, then, has $929 * 2 = 1,858$ observations. The first 929 encode time to recurrence information, the latter 929 time to death. As before the data set contains a covariate `etype` which is 1 for the first stratum and 2 for the second (a character variable coded as "death" or "progression" would work equally well in either package). Both events were observed for 414 of the subjects, neither event (censored at last followup) for 423, 38 had death without documented recurrence, and 54 were still alive following recurrence. Here is a simple analysis of time to recurrence, ignoring death.

```
> fitr <- coxph(Surv(time, status) ~ rx + extent+ node4,
                        data=colon, subset=(etype==1))
> print(fitr)
            coef exp(coef) se(coef)     z       p
    rxLev -0.031     0.969   0.1071 -0.29 7.7e-01
rxLev+5FU -0.518     0.596   0.1187 -4.36 1.3e-05
   extent  0.538     1.713   0.1135  4.74 2.1e-06
    node4  0.845     2.328   0.0957  8.83 0.0e+00

Likelihood ratio test=127  on 4 df, p=0  n= 929
```

In SAS the code would be as follows.

	Progression	Death	Combined
Levamisole vs. Obs	−0.031	−0.042	−0.036
Lev +5FU vs. Obs	−0.518	−0.379	−0.449
Extent of disease	0.538	0.493	0.516
$\geq$ 4 Nodes	0.845	0.915	0.880

TABLE 8.4: *Fits for the colon cancer trial*

```
data temp; set colon;
    rx_lev = 1*(rx='Lev');
    rx_lev5= 1*(rx='Lev+5FU')
    if (etype=1);

proc phreg data=temp;
    model time * status(0) = rx_lev rx_lev5 extend node4/
                ties=efron;
```

Here is SAS code and output for a combined analysis.

```
data temp; set save.colon;
    rx_lev = (rx='Lev');
    rx_lev5= (rx='Lev+5FU');

%phlev(data=temp, time=time, event=status,
        xvars= rx_lev rx_lev5 extent node4,
        id=id, collapse=Y);

             Parameter              Robust                    Robust
Variable  Estimate       SE       SE  Chi-Square Chi-Square DF        P

rx_lev       -0.0368 0.07684 0.1042       0.230        0.12         0.723
rx_lev5      -0.4447 0.08396 0.1160      28.058       14.68         0.000
extent        0.5141 0.07942 0.1080      41.912       22.65         0.000
node4         0.8653 0.06805 0.0948     161.672       83.25         0.000
Wald                                                 135.172     4 0.000
robust score                                         115.724     4 0.000
```

The most important covariates are the extent of disease (four levels) and whether there were four or more positive lymph nodes. The first coefficient of the model tests the contrast between observation and Levamisole alone, and shows that monotherapy confers no significant survival benefit. The combination treatment of Lev + 5FU, however, reduces the risk by 36%; $\exp(-.4447) = 0.64$.

The results for the marginal fit, which considers both outcomes jointly, and the individual fits by outcome type are shown in Table 8.4. The Levamisole/observation contrast is near 0 for all models. For the other, significant, covariates the combined analysis gives a solution somewhere between the two single-outcome models.

The marginal solutions shown so far, both for the colon cancer and UDCA studies, have made the assumption that the effect of each covariate is constant for all of the outcome types, that is, that higher bilirubin was associated with a uniform $\exp(.66) = 1.9$-fold increase in all eight UDCA outcomes. One important issue to consider is outcome type by covariate interactions. Do we wish to assume that "$\geq$4 nodes" has the same effect on both the death and progression risks? Assume that the node4 effects should be different and fit the appropriate model.

```
coxph(Surv(time, status) ~ rx + extent + cluster(id) +
                           node4*strata(etype), data=colon)

                coef exp(coef) se(coef) robust se      z       p
      rxLev -0.0364     0.964   0.0768    0.1056 -0.345 7.3e-01
  rxLev+5FU -0.4490     0.638   0.0840    0.1168 -3.844 1.2e-04
     extent  0.5154     1.674   0.0796    0.1097  4.700 2.6e-06
      node4  0.8460     2.330   0.0956    0.0994  8.512 0.0e+00
node4:etype  0.0688     1.071   0.1359    0.0534  1.287 2.0e-01
```

S-Plus has added a contrast variable corresponding to the interaction term; the corresponding coefficient shows that the estimated effect for node4 is .0688 units larger for the etype = 2 (death) stratum than it is for the recurrence outcome. We see that the statistical evidence for a difference in the effect size is weak, with a p-value of 0.2.

8.5 Ordered multiple events

For ordered outcomes (i.e., multiple events of the same type) several suggestions have been offered. The most common approaches are the independent increment (Andersen-Gill), marginal (WLW), or conditional (PWP) models. All three are "marginal" regression models in that $\hat{\beta}$ is determined from a fit that ignores the correlation followed by a corrected variance $\widetilde{D}'\widetilde{D}$, but differ considerably in their creation of the risk sets. All can be fit in both SAS and S-Plus.

8.5.1 The three approaches

Andersen–Gill

This method is the simplest to visualize and set up, but makes the strongest assumptions. It is closest in spirit to Poisson regression, and can in fact be accurately approximated with Poisson regression software in the same manner in which Laird and Olivier [80] approximate an ordinary single-event Cox model.

Using the counting process style of data input, each subject is represented as a series of observations (rows of data) with time intervals of (entry time, first event], (first event, second event], ..., (mth event, last followup]. A subject with zero events would have a single observation, one with one event would have one or two observations (depending on whether there was additional followup experience after the first event), and so on. Depending on the time scale, the first observation may or may not begin at zero.

When the time scale is "time since entry", the intensity process for the ith subject is

$$Y_i(t)\lambda_0(t)\exp(X_i(t)\beta).$$

Note that this is formally identical to the Cox model for survival data; compare equation (3.1). The difference lies in the definition of $Y_i(t)$; for survival data, the individual ceases to be at risk when an event occurs and Y_i goes to zero, but for The Andersen-Gill model for recurrent events, $Y_i(t)$ remains one as events occur. No extra strata or strata by covariate interaction terms are induced by the multiple events. Strata, if they are used, would be based on the same considerations as for an ordinary single-event model.

This model is ideally suited to the situation of mutual independence of the observations within a subject. This assumption is equivalent to each individual counting process possessing *idependent increments*, i.e., the numbers of events in nonoverlapping time intervals are independent, given the covariates. Such processes are typically modeled as time-varying Poisson processes, hence the Poisson connection.

One alternative time scale is the sojourn- or gap-time scale, with intervals of $(0, t_1]$, $(0, t_2 - t_1]$, ..., corresponding to "time since entry or last event". The model assumption in this case is that the gap times form a renewal process. The famed lack of memory of the exponential distribution implies that a renewal process with exponential gap times is also a counting process with independent increments; but in general counting processess cannot possess both independent increments and independent gap times.

If the model assumptions are met then the three variance estimators $\mathcal{I}^{-1}$, $D'D$, and $\widetilde{D}'\widetilde{D}$ all estimate the same quantity. This model can also be used as a marginal model when one anticipates correlations among the observations for each individual, as might be induced by unmeasured covariates. In that situation, it is wisest to use the per-subject jackknife estimate $\widetilde{D}'\widetilde{D}$.

WLW model

A marginal data model is used by Wei, Lin, and Weissfeld [155] to analyze a bladder cancer data set with multiple recurrences per subject. Further examples of this approach for ordered data are found in Lin [86]. Essentially, one treats the ordered outcome data set as though it were an unordered competing risks problem. If there is a maximum of four events, say, in the data set, then there will be four strata in the analysis. Every subject will have four observations, one in each stratum (barring deletion due to missing covariates). In most applications the analysis has been on the "time from study entry" scale; since all the time intervals start at zero the model can in this case be fit without recourse to the counting process style of input.

The intensity or hazard function for the jth event for the ith subject is:

$$Y_{ij}(t)\lambda_{0j}(t)\exp(X_i(t)\beta_j)$$

Note that, unlike the AG model, this model allows a separate underlying hazard for each event and and for strata by covariate interactions, as shown by the notation β_j. The at-risk indicator for the jth event, $Y_{ij}(t)$ is one until the occurrence of the jth event, unless, of course, some external event causes censoring. When either of those occurs, it becomes zero.

Conditional model

The conditional model was proposed in Prentice, Williams, and Peterson [122], and is sometimes labeled as the "PWP model". It assumes that a subject cannot be at risk for event 2 until event 1 occurs; in general, a subject is not at risk for the kth event until he/she has experienced event $k-1$. To accomplish this, the counting process style of input is used, as in the AG model, but each event is assigned to a separate stratum. The time scale may be either time since entry or gap time. The use of time-dependent strata means that the underlying intensity function may vary from event to event, unlike the AG model, which assumes that all events are identical. The intensity in the time since entry scale is formally identical to the WLW intensity given above, except for the definition of the at risk indicator: $Y_{ij}(t)$ is zero until the $j-1$st event and only then becomes one.

Oakes [114] argues persuasively for the conditional approach, and states that the marginal method will be inefficient.

8.5.2 *Fitting the models*

The key to fitting any of the models is creation of an appropriate data set. Assume a subject with events at times 10, 30, and 42, with no further followup after the last event. He will be represented in the data set by three observations, but the time intervals and strata differ as shown in Table 8.5. For the Andersen–Gill and conditional setups, it is also possible to use "time since last event" as the time scale. This is uncommon with the AG model, but more frequent for the conditional. In the data shown, the three intervals on this scale would be $(0, 10]$, $(0, 20]$, and $(0, 12]$; one would not need to use a counting process for the data.

Figure 8.2 shows the four models in schematic form. Possible transitions are represented by an arrow, with each distinct arrow corresponding to a separate stratum in the Cox model. Each "event" for a subject corresponds to a traversal of one of the arrows. This type of figure will prove useful in the more complicated data examples.

Another way to look at the difference is to consider the risk sets. Suppose that subject "Smith" has experienced his second event on day 32. Who are the subjects at risk when Smith has his second event?

	Interval	Stratum
AG	(0, 10]	1
	(10, 30)	1
	(30, 42)	1
WLW	(0, 10]	1
	(0, 30)	2
	(0, 42)	3
PWP	(0, 10]	1
	(10, 30)	2
	(30, 42)	3

TABLE 8.5: *Representation of a hypothetical subject for the three marginal models*

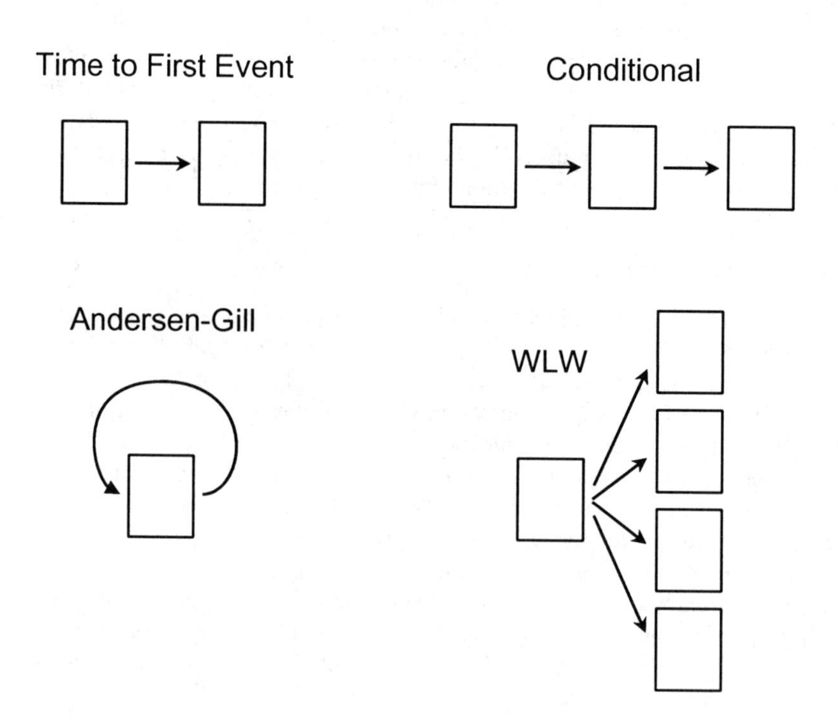

FIGURE 8.2: *Schematic form of the three models. Each arrow represents a stratum*

AG : All subjects who were under observation on day 32.

WLW: All subjects who were under observation on day 32,
and have not yet had a second event.

PWP: All subjects who were under observation on day 32,
have not yet had a second event,
and have experienced a first event.

Both the Andersen–Gill and conditional methods treat the data as time-ordered outcomes, differing only in their use of stratification (a difference that can cause major changes in the conclusions). A single (start, stop] data set can be used to fit both the Andersen–Gill and conditional models, including the gap-time version of the latter. A subject with followup to time 10 but no events would be represented by a single row with interval $(0, 10]$ in the data set, and a status of 0 (censored). One with three events at times 20, 30, and 42, with additional followup to time 81 would have four rows of data with intervals of $(0, 20]$, $(20, 30]$, $(30, 42]$, and $(42, 81]$. Only the last observation would be censored.

The data set for the WLW marginal analysis will look exactly like the data created for the UDCA trial discussed in Section 8.4.3. First event, second event, and so on are treated in the same way that survival, liver transplant, and worsening of symptoms were treated in the UDCA data set. If the largest number of events experienced by any one subject were four, say, then the data will have four strata corresponding to the four possible "types" of event. There will be n observations for stratum 1, followed by n observations for stratum 2, n for stratum 3, and n observations for stratum 4. If there are k possible events, then the data set will have nk rows.

In the examples that follow `data1` refers to the Andersen–Gill style data set, and `data2` to the WLW style data set. The second of these is usually considerably larger. In each data set, an indicator variable `enum` has been included. This variable is 1 for the first observation of any given patient, 2 for the second, and so on.

Four analysis plans are to use `data1` or `data2`, and either stratify or not stratify the Cox model by `enum`. (Any of the models might be stratified by another variable such as enrolling institution, of course.) Use of `data1` without stratifying on `enum` is an Andersen–Gill model, `data1` with stratification on `enum` is a conditional model. Use of `data2` and stratification on `enum` is the WLW model. An unstratified model based on the second data set is less common; the diabetic retinopathy data set was one example. It is difficult to conceive of a use for the unstratified `data2` analysis for ordered outcomes, however.

8.5.3 Hidden covariate data

We first illustrate the methods with a simple test case using simulated data, one which shows that each method has potential biases. Let the time to next event be exponential with rate $\exp(\beta_1 x_1 + \beta_2 x_2)$, where x_1 is a randomly assigned 0/1 treatment and x_2 is a per-patient covariate distributed uniformly between -2 and 2. The true coefficients were chosen to be $\beta_1 = -1$ and $\beta_2 = 1$, particularly easy numbers to remember when reading the output. Sequential events were independent, and the followup time for each subject was 1 year, which gave a mean number of events of 1.3. For simplicity of presentation, the few subjects with more than seven events were censored after their seventh. The sample size was 2,000, which allows us to illustrate any biases in the estimates. The number of events experienced was as follows.

	Number of Events							
	0	1	2	3	4	5	6	7
Control	367	312	174	88	39	13	5	2
Treatment	680	250	50	14	6	0	0	0

To do the AG and conditional analyses the data are set up in the counting process form. Assume that subject 10 is on treatment with a covariate value of .2, and has events on days 100 and 200, with followup to day 365. The subject is represented as three rows of data with the following variables.

Id	Start	Stop	Status	Enum	x_1	x_2
10	0	100	1	1	1	.2
10	100	200	1	2	1	.2
10	200	365	0	3	1	.2

The marginal data set is somewhat larger. Since at least one patient in the study had a seventh event, then all patients must be coded for that event type. The data rows for our hypothetical subject are the following.

Id	Time	Status	Enum	x_1	x_2
10	100	1	1	1	.2
10	200	1	2	1	.2
10	365	0	3	1	.2
10	365	0	4	1	.2
10	365	0	5	1	.2
10	365	0	6	1	.2
10	365	0	7	1	.2

The modeling statements to fit the data for the three methods are similar. S-Plus statements for the AG, conditional, and marginal models, respectively, are as follows.

```
> afit <- coxph(Surv(start, stop, status) ~ x1 + x2 + cluster(id),
                    data=data1)
```

	Fits with the Covariate		Fits without the Covariate
	β_1	β_2	β_1
Andersen–Gill			
Coefficient	−0.93	1.05	−0.92
Variance	.066, .066	.056, .056	.066, .084
WLW			
Coefficient	−1.60	1.82	−1.23
Variance	.069, .117	.063, .113	.066, .113
Conditional			
Coefficient	−0.91	1.03	−0.67
Variance	.073, .069	.065 , .064	.070, .068

TABLE 8.6: *Simple models, with both the model-based and sandwich (robust) variance estimates*

```
> cfit <- coxph(Surv(start, stop, status) ~ x1 + x2 + cluster(id)+
                                 strata(enum), data=data1)
> wfit <- coxph(Surv(time, status) ~ x1 + x2 + cluster(id) +
                                 strata(enum), data=data2)
```

Each of these tests for an overall treatment effect. Results for the three fits are shown in Table 8.6. An important point of comparison is when x_2 is *not* included in the model. This corresponds, in real data sets, to those important covariates that are unmeasured. In fact, the potentially "hidden" covariate x_2 was purposely chosen so as to have a larger overall effect on the outcome than treatment (same size coefficient, but x_2 has a larger variation than x_1); this is unfortunately the usual case in medical research, where a large number of important factors will be unmeasured or even unsuspected.

The Andersen–Gill model assumes that the data are a set of independent increments, which this data set is. When both covariates are included in the Cox fit, we are fitting a correct model, and Table 8.6 reveals that the fit is essentially unbiased as all coefficients are within 1 standard error of the true values of -1 and 1. The model-based and robust variance estimates agree. When an important covariate is omitted, we see that the model does well in its estimate of β; the standard error of the coefficient, however, is underestimated. Although the time increments between events are conditionally uncorrelated given the covariates, omission of an important covariate induces a dependence: if a subject's first event time is short, relative to the population as a whole, his second is likely to be also.

When x_2 is included then the conditional model is correctly specified as well, and the estimates are close to the true values of $(-1, 1)$. There is a slight increase in the variance of $\hat{\beta}$ with respect to the Andersen–Gill fit because of the extra stratum parameters but the effect is quite small. When x_2 is unknown the conditional model seriously underestimates the treatment effect, however. This bias is due to a loss of balance in the unmeasured covariate. The mean level of x_1 for the first stratum (event number 1) is near 0 for both treatment and control. For stratum 2, however, the mean levels

	trt1	trt2	trt3	trt4	trt5	trt6	trt7
Marginal	−0.99	−1.7	−2.1	−2.3	−4.2	−4.2	−4.2
Conditional	−0.99	−0.9	−0.6	−0.3	$-\infty$		

TABLE 8.7: *Models with interaction*

are 0.6 and 0.8, respectively, in the control and treatment arms: high-risk patients are more likely to have an event, and since treatment is effective the treated patients must be, on average, of higher risk than controls to have had one. By stratum 4, the baseline risk for an average subject on the treatment arm is 40% greater than that for an average control subject, entirely through the process of patient selection. Essentially, stratum 1 is a randomized trial but strata 2 through 7 are not.

Table 8.7 shows the estimated treatment effects within strata for the WLW and PWP (conditional) models, for fits that ignore x_2. (These can be obtained either by adding an interaction term `rx *strata(enum)` to the overall model, or by fitting each stratum separately.) For stratum 1, time to first event, the conditional model is correct and reliable, and is in fact identical to a "time to first event" analysis. The estimated treatment effect then steadily decreases for strata 2, 3, and 4. By stratum 5 there are only 6 treated patients; 0/6 of these had an event as compared to 13/39 for the control subjects. This leads to an infinite relative hazard, which is not, however, significantly different from zero by a likelihood ratio test. Strata 6 and 7 have only control subjects and a treatment effect cannot be estimated.

The WLW model on the other hand overestimates the treatment effect, and inclusion of the covariate x_2 into the model makes matters even worse. The per-stratum fits of Table 8.7 show a steady growth of the estimated coefficient, with stratum 1 again being identical to a time to first event model. The problem here is that the data for strata 2, 3, and so on no longer obey the proportional hazards model.

Consider the even simpler case of an exponential model where treatment is the only important covariate, there is no censoring, and the hazard ratio for treatment versus control is λ_1/λ_2. The time to the kth event will then follow a gamma distribution, and the hazard ratio for treatment/control in stratum k can be shown to have value $(\lambda_1/\lambda_2)^k$ at time 0, trending towards (λ_1/λ_2) over time. Figure 8.3 shows the actual hazard ratios for first, second, and third events when $\lambda_1 = 1$ and $\lambda_2 = 2$, and Figure 8.4 shows the estimated ratios for the simulated data set using the `cox.zph` function. The lack of proportional hazards for the later strata is clear.

In summary, this example suggests the following.

- The Andersen–Gill model gives a nearly unbiased estimate of the treatment effect, even when an important covariate has been omitted. The naive estimate of variance may be too small, but the robust estimate $\widetilde{D}'\widetilde{D}$ corrects for this.

- The conditional model gives seriously biased estimates when an important covariate is omitted, due to loss of balance in the later strata.

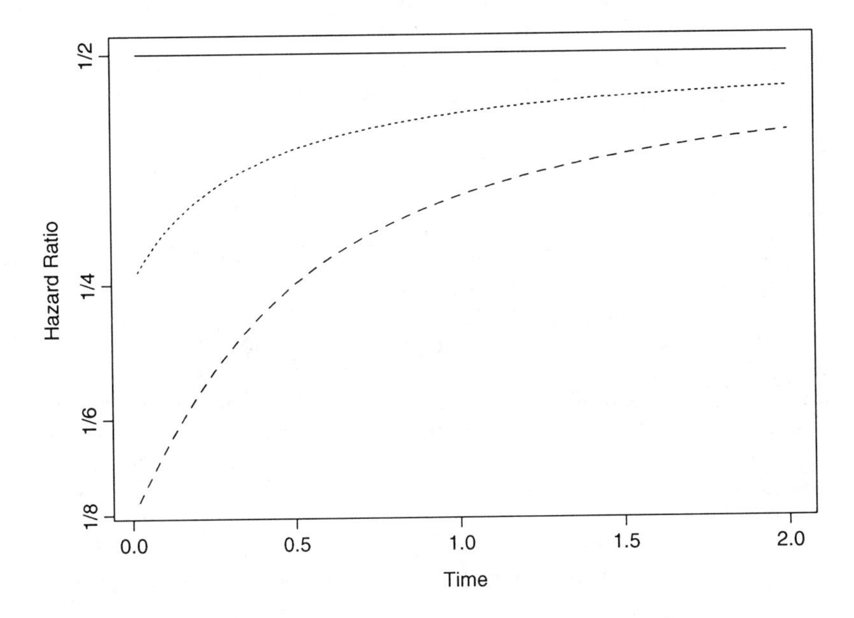

FIGURE 8.3: *Hazard ratios for the first three strata of a WLW model, applied to simple exponential data*

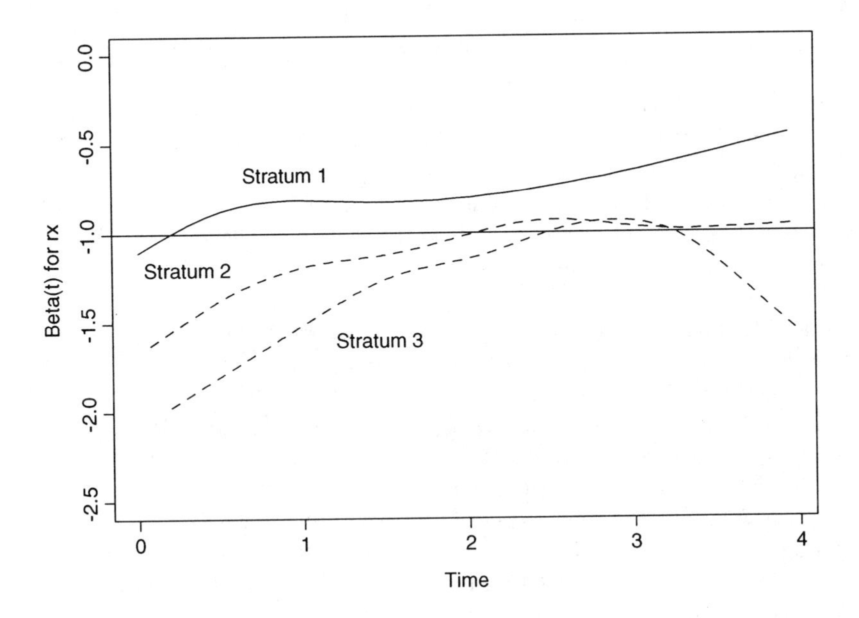

FIGURE 8.4: *Estimated hazard ratios for the first three strata of the simulation*

	Actual SE	Model-Based Standard Error	Sandwich Standard Error
With Covariate			
First	0.234	(0.223, 0.234, 0.249)	(0.214, 0.230, 0.252)
AG	0.132	(0.126, 0.132, 0.141)	(0.116, 0.129, 0.146)
Cond	0.143	(0.135, 0.145, 0.157)	(0.122, 0.139, 0.160)
WLW	0.246	(0.132, 0.141, 0.153)	(0.214, 0.235, 0.263)
Without Covariate			
First	0.223	(0.217, 0.225, 0.235)	(0.214, 0.225, 0.239)
AG	0.159	(0.124, 0.131, 0.139)	(0.146, 0.161, 0.177)
Cond	0.143	(0.130, 0.139, 0.152)	(0.127, 0.142, 0.164)
WLW	0.229	(0.125, 0.133, 0.143)	(0.220, 0.232, 0.246)

TABLE 8.8: *Actual standard error for each case of the simulation, as computed from the 1,000 realizations of $\hat{\beta}$, compared to the estimated values from the fits. The model-based and sandwich columns show the 10th, 50th, and 90th percentiles of the 1,000 respective variance estimators*

- The competing risks (WLW) model may violate the proportional hazards assumption, even when the overall data set does not.

One critique of the above is that it is based on a single realization of the simulation. Perhaps the outcomes we have shown are atypical. Figure 8.5 shows the results of a larger simulation that had 1,000 replicates. Each of the replicates is for a sample of size 100 with a somewhat smaller covariate effect than before — uniform(−1,1) — and a maximum of six events for any subject. This matches more closely some of the actual data sets that we encounter in later examples.

When both of the important variables are included in the fit the figure shows that the WLW model is biased towards large values. The Andersen–Gill and conditional models, as well as the simple analysis of time to first event, are essentially unbiased. There is an advantage in efficiency for the Andersen–Gill over the conditional model but it is very slight: the two densities nearly overlay one another. Both are more efficient than time to first event.

When an important covariate is omitted the WLW model is still biased towards too large an effect, although not as greatly as it was before. The conditional model underestimates the treatment effect by about 23%. The Andersen–Gill also underestimates slightly, about 9%, but is the most accurate of the methods. Time to first event, which is a completely standard Cox model, has a bias intermediate between the two. Omori and Johnson [115] work out this bias explicitly for a single-event Cox model with a missing covariate, and show that the rate at which the bias is accrued is proportional to the variance of the missing covariate. Henderson and Oman [64] derive similar results in the context of frailty models.

Table 8.8 displays the behavior of the variance estimates from the simulation. Given its large bias, the variance of the WLW estimate is of secondary concern; nevertheless, we notice that the correction for correlated data, as provided by the robust sandwich estimator, is essential. For the

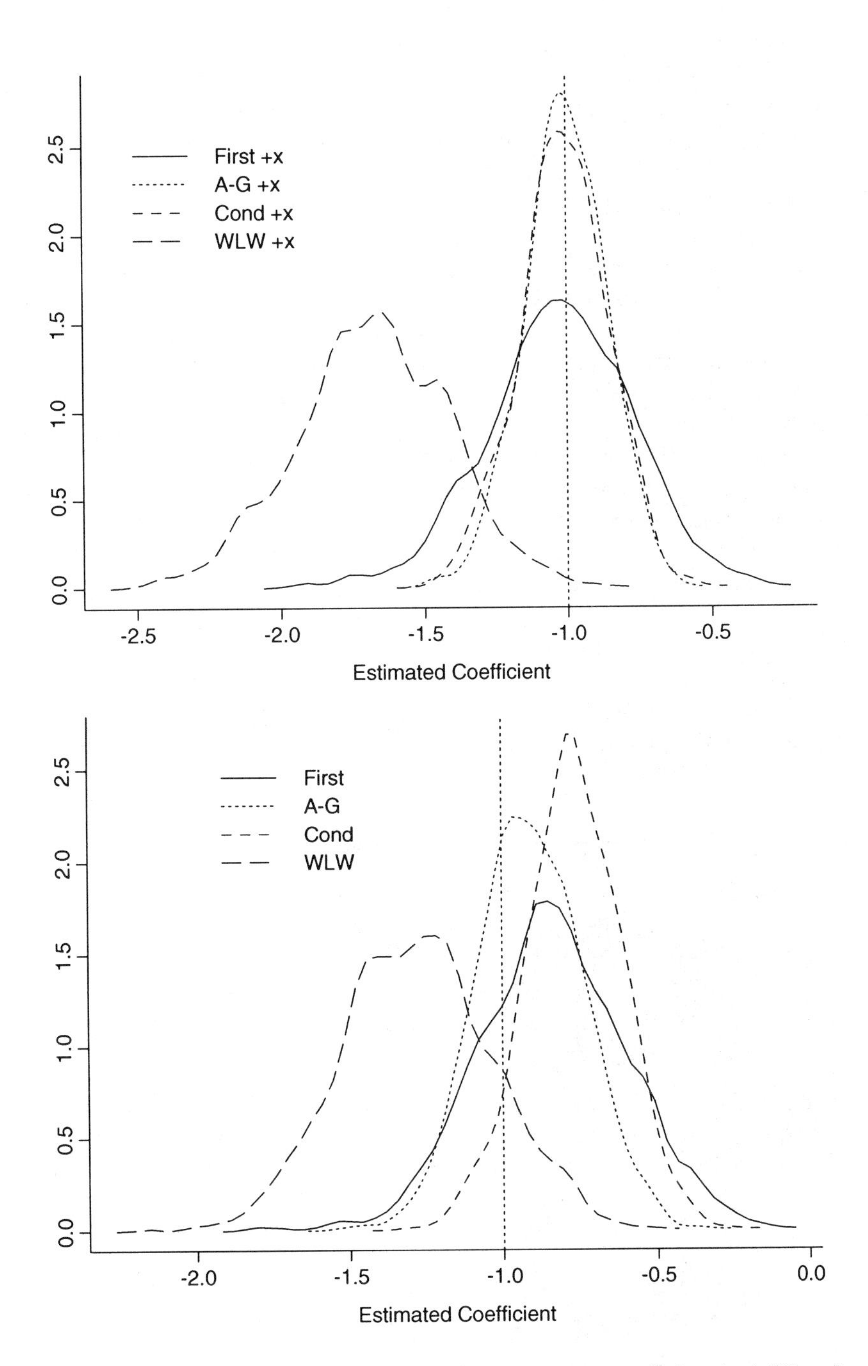

FIGURE 8.5: *Observed distribution of the estimated treatment coefficient in 1,000 replications, for models with and without the covariate x*

three "correct" models, which are the first three listed in the table, we see that both the model-based and sandwich variance estimates are of the correct size. The robust estimator is itself much more variable though; for example, for the AG model the range between the 10th and 90th percentiles is $.141 - .126 = .15$ for the model based variance, or about $\pm 10\%$ of the average value, as compared to .30 for the robust estimator. An Andersen–Gill model that does not include the second covariate underestimates the standard error by nearly 20% when independent events are assumed (i.e., the usual inverse information matrix estimate); the sandwich estimator has the right average. For the conditional estimate, the ordinary variance based on $\mathcal{I}^{-1}$ does not display this bias. This is perhaps due to the fact that *within* strata the observations are independent, but this is an area that merits further research.

Use of a per-stratum treatment coefficient within an AG model has essentially the same biases, as an estimator of per-stratum treatment effects, as the conditional model with per-stratum coefficients. The table below shows the result of two fits for one of the realizations of the simulation. Define `rx1 <- rx *(enum==1)` (S-Plus) or `rx1 = rx *(enum=1)` (SAS) and similarly for the variables `rx2`, `rx3` and `rx4`. Because only subjects with > 2 events contribute to the estimation of `rx3`, the bias due to imbalance in the hidden covariate accrues to both models, and the pattern of the coefficients is nearly identical. The AG model has somewhat smaller variances, but this is small comfort in the face of bias.

	AG Model		Conditional	
	$\hat{\beta}$	se	$\hat{\beta}$	se
rx1	−1.03	0.19	−0.85	0.23
rx2	−0.60	0.23	−0.58	0.27
rx3	−0.53	0.35	−0.42	0.40
rx4	−0.72	0.51	−1.05	0.55

8.5.4 Bladder cancer

The bladder cancer data are listed in Wei et al. [155], and used as a primary example for their method. The data record up to four recurrence times (in months) for 86 subjects. There may be followup beyond the last recurrence.

	Number of Recurrences				
	0	1	2	3	4
Number of Subjects	39	18	7	8	14
Followup After Last Event	38	17	5	6	12

One of the subjects (the one with no followup after his or her 0th recurrence) has no events and 0 months of followup. For simplicity, this subject will be removed from the data sets since he or she adds nothing to the likelihood. The covariates are initial size, initial number, and treatment group.

Data set `bladder1` is constructed in the AG style. In place of the `futime` variable there is a pair of variables `time1, time2` that define the time interval of risk. Subjects with no recurrences will have one observation, those with one recurrence have 1 or 2 observations (depending on whether there is additional followup after the recurrence), and so on. Bladder1 has 190 observations. Below is a fraction of the input data, the resultant data set, and the SAS code used to create the data set.

id	rx	futime	number	size	recurrences
0	1	0	1	1	
1	1	1	1	3	
2	1	4	2	1	
3	1	7	1	1	
4	1	10	5	1	
5	1	10	4	1	6
6	1	14	1	1	
7	1	18	1	1	
8	1	18	1	3	5
9	1	18	1	1	12, 16

id	time1	time2	status	rx	number	size	enum
1	0	1	0	1	1	3	1
2	0	4	0	1	2	1	1
3	0	7	0	1	1	1	1
4	0	10	0	1	5	1	1
5	0	6	1	1	4	1	1
5	6	10	0	1	4	1	2
6	0	14	0	1	1	1	1
7	0	18	0	1	1	1	1
8	0	5	1	1	1	3	1
8	5	18	0	1	1	3	2
9	0	12	1	1	1	1	1
9	12	16	1	1	1	1	2
9	16	18	0	1	1	1	3

```
data temp;
    infile 'data.bladder' missover;
    retain id 0;

    input rx  futime number size  r1-r4;
    if (futime =0) then delete;
    id = id +1;

data bladder1;
    set temp;
    drop futime r1-r4;
```

```
time1 =0;
enum  =0;

if (r1 ne .) then do;
    time2 = r1; status = 1; enum = 1;
    output;
    time1 = r1;
    end;

if (r2 ne .) then do;
    time2 = r2; status = 1; enum = 2;
    output;
    time1 = r2;
    end;

if (r3 ne .) then do;
    time2 = r3; status = 1; enum = 3;
    output;
    time1 = r3;
    end;

if (r4 ne .) then do;
    time2 = r4; status = 1; enum = 4;
    output;
    time1 = r4;
    end;

if (futime > time1) then do;
    time2 = futime;
    status= 0;
    enum  = enum +1;
    output;
    end;
```

The code illustrates the basic computing principle for most of these data sets: setup is tedious but straightforward. (SAS experts can certainly shorten the above layout through use of a loop, but the basic principle remains.)

The WLW style data set `bladder2` contains four lines for each subject, since that is the maximum number of events recorded for any one of the enrollees. The covariates are

`id`	subject id, 1 to 85;
`futime`	followup or recurrence time;
`status`	1 = recurrence, 0 = censoring;
`number`	initial number;
`size`	initial size;
`rx`	treatment code, 1 = placebo, 2 = thiotepa;
`enum`	event number.

The data set will have $85 * 4 = 340$ observations. The output data set for three particular subjects, ids 1, 5, and 9 is as follows.

```
id  time status  rx  number size  enum
 1    1    0      1   1      3     1
 1    1    0      1   1      3     2
 1    1    0      1   1      3     3
 1    1    0      1   1      3     4

 5    6    1      1   4      1     1
 5   10    0      1   4      1     2
 5   10    0      1   4      1     3
 5   10    0      1   4      1     4

 9   12    1      1   1      1     1
 9   16    1      1   1      1     2
 9   18    0      1   1      1     3
 9   18    0      1   1      1     4
```

The SAS data code that generated the data is below. Take special note of the last two extremely important lines: always print out all or some portion of the created data sets. Errors in coding the data set will *not* result in errors from the `phreg` or `coxph` call, and the results can then correspond to a truly inexplicable model.

```
data temp3;
    set bladder1;
    by id;
    drop temp time1 time2;

    futime = time2;
    if (enum <5) then output;
    if (last.id =1) then do;
        temp = enum +1;
        do enum = temp to 4;
            status =0;
            output;
            end;
        end;

data save.bladder2; set temp3;
    rx1 = rx * (enum=1);   *special indicator variables for later;
    rx2 = rx * (enum=2);
    rx3 = rx * (enum=3);
    rx4 = rx * (enum=4);

proc print;
    var id futime status rx rx1 rx2 rx3 rx4 size number enum;
```

Interestingly enough, the **bladder1** data set created above has a significant error. The problem shows up if we fit a model that treats **enum** as a categorical variable, that is, a **factor** in the S-Plus terminology. The model is not one that we recommend, and the error was tripped over by accident after several years of using the data set in examples and presentations.

```
> coxph(Surv(time1, time2, status) ~ rx + size +
                     number + factor(enum), data=bladder1)

                    coef exp(coef) se(coef)        z       p
              rx -0.27994  7.56e-01   0.2058 -1.3605 1.7e-01
            size -0.00375  9.96e-01   0.0703 -0.0533 9.6e-01
          number  0.14034  1.15e+00   0.0514  2.7293 6.3e-03
  factor(enum)2  0.58926  1.80e+00   0.2568  2.2948 2.2e-02
  factor(enum)3  1.68045  5.37e+00   0.3024  5.5578 2.7e-08
  factor(enum)4  1.33765  3.81e+00   0.3510  3.8108 1.4e-04
  factor(enum)5 -12.26606  4.71e-06 239.3184 -0.0513 9.6e-01

Likelihood ratio test=61.7  on 7 df, p=6.98e-11  n= 190
Warning messages:
      Loglik converged before variable  7; beta may be infinite.
```

Notice the estimated risks associated with **enum**. The reference group for the coefficient is those observations with **enum=1**, or no prior events. Subjects with one prior recurrence (enum $= 2$) have an approximately 1.8-fold recurrence rate as compared to those with no prior events, those with two prior recurrences a 5.4-fold risk, those with three prior recurrences a 3.8-fold risk, and those with four prior recurrences a 1/21,000-fold risk. The risk of another event rises for those with prior tumors, but only until a subject has had four, at which time he becomes risk-free! This is an artifact of the way the data were coded. Although several subjects have in reality more than four tumors, a maximum of four are listed in the data set as shown in the WLW manuscript. Thus, by construction, a subject who has had four recurrences cannot have another, and becomes immortal in the eyes of the model. There are 14 such subjects as shown in the initial table, 12 of which show fictitious followup after the fourth event; fictitious because the subject is not actually at risk for another *recorded* event during the extra time.

Because none of these 12 have another event the maximum likelihood estimate for the **enum5** coefficient is negative infinity. S-Plus stopped iterating with a value of -12 because the likelihood had ceased to change much at that point. SAS (code not shown) stops with a value of -16; due to a tighter default convergence criterion it does one more interation than the S-Plus code. All other coefficients agree to four significant digits.

The data set **bladder3** is a copy of **bladder1** with these 12 superfluous observations removed. Because the subjects involved had four recurrences we would expect them to be at high risk, and have high-risk values of their covariates. We might expect, then, that the inclusion of the 12 invalid observations would bias the coefficients of an overall model towards zero, by crediting each of the high-risk subjects with a block of risk-free time. This is indeed correct.

```
> coxph(Surv(time1, time2, status) ~ rx + size + number,
                        data=bladder1)$coef
     rx   size number
 -0.412 -0.041  0.164

> coxph(Surv(time1, time2, status) ~ rx + size + number,
                        data=bladder3)$coef
     rx   size number
 -0.465 -0.044  0.175
```

The incorrect data set `bladder1` is not used in further analyses. We point out again how important it is to seriously examine the data sets one creates for these analyses, particularly with respect to structural limitations such as this.

Finally, then, here are the fits to the three additive models.

```
> # Andersen-Gill
> coxph(Surv(time1, time2, status) ~ rx + size + number
                         + cluster(id), data=bladder3)
          coef exp(coef) se(coef) robust se      z      p
    rx -0.4647     0.628   0.1997    0.2656 -1.750 0.0800
  size -0.0437     0.957   0.0691    0.0776 -0.563 0.5700
number  0.1750     1.191   0.0471    0.0630  2.775 0.0055

> # Marginal risk sets or WLW
> coxph(Surv(futime, status) ~ rx + size + number +
           strata(enum) + cluster(id), data=bladder2)

          coef exp(coef) se(coef) robust se      z      p
    rx -0.5848     0.557   0.2011    0.3079 -1.899 0.0580
  size -0.0516     0.950   0.0697    0.0946 -0.546 0.5900
number  0.2103     1.234   0.0468    0.0666  3.156 0.0016

> # Conditional risk sets or PWP
> coxph(Surv(time1, time2, status) ~ rx + size + number +
           cluster(id) + strata(enum), data=bladder3)

           coef exp(coef) se(coef) robust se      z    p
    rx -0.33349     0.716   0.2162    0.2048 -1.628 0.10
  size -0.00849     0.992   0.0728    0.0616 -0.138 0.89
number  0.11962     1.127   0.0533    0.0514  2.328 0.02
```

The coefficent inflation/deflation ordering found in the hidden covariate data set is repeated, with the WLW model showing a stronger effect than

	Strata			
	1	2	3	4
Conditional	−0.418	−0.452	−0.067	0.204
WLW	−0.486	−0.662	−0.716	−0.554

TABLE 8.9: *Coefficents by strata for the bladder data*

the AG, which is in turn stronger than the conditional. The amount of difference between the models is, however, not nearly as strong as was found in that example. The robust variance is important for both the AG and WLW fits.

If we fit separate treatment coefficients to each stratum, either by including an interaction term in the model statement or by separate fits to each stratum, we see a trend for the WLW coefficients to increase in the later strata and for the conditional model's coefficients to decrease in value. (The solutions for stratum 1 are not identical because of the inclusion of the other two covariates, each as a single coefficient across strata.) The final coefficient for the conditional model actually changes sign! Table 8.9 shows the results for strata 1 to 4, and is obtained from the following fits.

```
> coxph(Surv(time1, time2, status)~ rx1 + rx2 + rx3 +rx4
        + size + number + strata(enum), data=bladder3)
> coxph(Surv(futime, status)~ rx1 + rx2 + rx3 +rx4
        + size + number + strata(enum), data=bladder2)
```

How much did the multiple events analysis gain? An approximate answer is to compare the first event and AG fits at a common value of β.

```
> fit1 <- coxph(Surv(time2, status) ~ rx + number + cluster(id),
                  data=bladder3, subset=(enum==1)) #First event
> print(fit1)
          coef exp(coef) se(coef) robust se     z      p
    rx  -0.512     0.599   0.3130    0.3116 -1.64 0.1000
number   0.231     1.260   0.0754    0.0708  3.26 0.0011

> fita <- coxph(Surv(time1, time2, status) ~ rx + number +
                                                cluster(id),
                   data=bladder3, init=fit1$coef, iter=0)
> print(fita)
          coef exp(coef) se(coef) robust se     z       p
    rx  -0.512     0.599   0.2010    0.2787 -1.84 0.06600
number   0.231     1.260   0.0431    0.0654  3.53 0.00042
```

There are 47 first recurrences and 112 total recurrences. This suggests that if the observations were independent, the standard error of treatment using all events would decrease to $\sqrt{47/112}\,(.313) = .203$, which is almost exactly the uncorrected standard error for the multiple event model. The actual reduction was to a standard error of .279, however, which is approximately equal to $\sqrt{47/59.3}\,(.313)$. There was a potential gain of $(112 - 47) = 65$ new events but a realized gain of only $(59.3 - 47) = 12.3$ "independent" observations; each recurrence was worth about 1/5 of a new subject.

And last, here is the SAS and S-Plus code to fit the all-interactions WLW model.

```
data temp; set bladder2;
    rx1 = rx *(enum=1);          rx2=rx*(enum=2);
    rx3 = rx *(enum=3);          rx4=rx*(enum=4);
    number1 = number*(enum=1);  number2=number*(enum=2);
    number3 = number*(enum=3);  number4=number*(enum=4);
    size1= size*(enum=1);       size2 = size*(enum=2);
    size3= size*(enum=3);       size4 = size*(enum=4);
%phlev(data=temp3, time=futime, status=status,
      xvars= rx1 rx2 rx3 rx4 size1 size2 size3 size4
             number1 number2 number3 number4,
      strata=enum, id=id, collapse=Y, ties='breslow');

------
> afit <- coxph(Surv(futime, status) ~ rx1 + rx2 + rx3 + rx4 +
                     (size +number)*strata(enum),
                 data=bladder2, method='breslow')
```

The S-Plus example utilizes user-defined dummy variables for the treatment variable (equivalent to the SAS code), and program-defined contrasts for the other two variables. The `breslow` option for ties causes the output to match the printed results in Wei, et al. [155]. The output of the SAS macro comprises several pages; it concludes with the following table, which has been compressed to fit on this page.

Variable	Parameter Estimate	SE	Robust SE	Robust Chi-Square	P
rx1	-0.51762	0.31576	0.30750	2.834	0.0923
rx2	-0.61944	0.39318	0.36391	2.897	0.0887
rx3	-0.69988	0.45994	0.41516	2.842	0.0918
rx4	-0.65079	0.57744	0.48971	1.766	0.1839
number1	0.06789	0.10125	0.08529	0.634	0.4260
number2	-0.07612	0.13406	0.11812	0.415	0.5193
number3	-0.21131	0.18240	0.17198	1.510	0.2192
number4	-0.20317	0.23018	0.19106	1.131	0.2876
size1	0.23599	0.07608	0.07208	10.720	0.0011
size2	0.13756	0.09190	0.08690	2.506	0.1134
size3	0.16984	0.10521	0.10356	2.690	0.1010
size4	0.32880	0.12528	0.11382	8.345	0.0039

Computational note

In their paper proposing the variance estimator, Wei et al. [88] fit each stratum separately, using multiple distinct runs of the proportional hazards program. They then combined the estimates and computed a unified variance. For this data set, the overall coefficient vector and variance matrix are

$$\hat\beta = (\hat\beta_1, \hat\beta_2, \hat\beta_3, \hat\beta_4)$$

$$V = \begin{bmatrix} D_1'D_1 & D_1'D_2 & D_1'D_3 & D_1'D_4 \\ D_2'D_1 & D_2'D_2 & D_2'D_3 & D_2'D_4 \\ D_3'D_1 & D_3'D_2 & D_3'D_3 & D_3'D_4 \\ D_4'D_1 & D_4'D_2 & D_4'D_3 & D_4'D_4 \end{bmatrix},$$

where $\hat\beta_1$, D_1 are the coefficients and dfbeta matrix from the first fit, $\hat\beta_2$, D_2 the coefficients and dfbeta matrix from the second, and so on. It is a simple (but tedious) algebraic exercise to show that the coefficients and variance resulting from this approach will be identical to those from a single fit using the $85 * 4 = 340$ observation combined data set. For example, the variance matrix below is exactly the upper 4×4corner of V^{-1}; `afit` was defined above.

```
> round(afit$var[1:4,1:4], digits=3)
      1     2     3     4
1 0.095 0.060 0.057 0.044
2 0.060 0.132 0.130 0.116
3 0.057 0.130 0.172 0.159
4 0.044 0.116 0.159 0.240
```

After the fit, WLW compute an overall estimate of treatment effect as a weighted average of the estimated coefficient vector, $k'\hat\beta$ where the vector of weights k, the average treatment effect, its standard error, and an overall test for treatment can be computed as

```
> k <- solve(afit$var[1:4,1:4], c(1,1,1,1))
> k <- k / sum(k)
> round(k, digits=3)
     1     2      3     4
 0.677 0.257 -0.076 0.142

> sum(k * afit$coef[1:4])  #Average treatment effect
[1] -0.5487979

> sqrt(k %*% afit$var[1:4,1:4] %*% k)  # Its standard error
[1,] 0.2852717

> # 4 df Wald test for treatment
> fit$coef[1:4] %*% solve(fit$var[1:4,1:4]) %*% fit$coef[1:4]
        [,1]
[1,] 3.96616
```

The last number would be compared to a chi-square distribution on four degrees of freedom, and is not significant. The `test` statement of the `phreg` procedure would be particularly useful here. Unfortunately, it cannot be applied since we need to use the robust variance matrix, which is computed in the `%phlev` macro from results of the `phreg` computations.

The WLW estimate of an overall treatment effect is equivalent to an approximate backwards-stepwise regression step from four coefficients to one coefficient, based on the score statistics of the full model fit; see Bartolucci and Fraser [11] for details of the procedure. This gives an approximation, usually a good one, to what the true overall coefficient will be in a model omitting the interaction. It is easier to simply refit the model using a single treatment effect, however.

```
> coxph(Surv(futime, status) ~ rx + (size + number)*strata(enum)
                + cluster(id), bladder2,  method='breslow')

              coef exp(coef) se(coef) robust se      z       p
       rx -0.5976     0.550   0.2031    0.3029 -1.973 0.04800
     size  0.0695     1.072   0.1009    0.0847  0.821 0.41000
        ...
```

In this case the approximation −0.545 is just a little less than the iterated estimate of −0.598 (about 1/6 of a standard error).

8.5.5 rIFN-g in patients with chronic granulomatous disease

Chronic granulomatous disease (CGD) is a heterogeneous group of uncommon inherited disorders characterized by recurrent pyogenic infections that usually begin early in life and may lead to death in childhood. Interferon gamma is a principal macrophage-activating factor shown to partially correct the metabolic defect in phagocytes, and for this reason it was hypothesized that it would reduce the frequency of serious infections in patients with CGD. In 1986, Genentech, Inc. conducted a randomized, double-blind, placebo-controlled trial in 128 CGD patients who received Genentech's humanized interferon gamma (rIFN-g) or placebo three times daily for a year. The primary endpoint of the study was the time to the first serious infection. However, data were collected on all serious infections until cessation of followup, which occurred near day 400 for most patients. Thirty of the 65 patients in the placebo group and 14 of the 63 patients in the rIFN-g group had at least one serious infection. The total number of infections was 56 and 20 in the placebo and treatment groups, respectively. A natural question is whether a multiple events regression would be useful.

A copy of the data set can be found in Appendix D of Fleming and Harrington [50], and was used in several examples there. A version with more covariates is used here. Covariates include the enrolling hospital and randomization date, age, height, weight, sex, use of antibiotics or corticosteroids at the time of enrollment, and the pattern of inheritance. This latter was a stratification factor for the study. Below is a listing of the input data for the first six subjects, along with rows for the first four subjects in the dervived counting process data set `cgd1`.

S

```
                                  I t
     C    R           H       W   n e  Fu
     e    a   T       e       e   h r
     n    n   r       i       i   e o  t
     t    d   e S  A  g       g   r i  i
I    e    o   a e  g  h       h   i d  m
D    r    m   t x  e  t       t   t s  e  ---- Infections ----------

1 204 082888 1 2 12 147.0 62.0 2 2 414 219 373
2 204 082888 0 1 15 159.0 47.5 2 2 439   8  26 152 241 249 322 350
3 204 082988 1 1 19 171.0 72.7 1 2 382
4 204 091388 1 1 12 142.0 34.0 1 2 388
5 238 092888 0 1 17 162.5 52.7 1 2 383 246 253
6 245 093088 1 2 44 153.3 45.0 2 2 364

---------------------------------------------
```

id	center	tstart	tstop	status	enum	trt	age
1	204	0	219	1	1	1	12
1	204	219	373	1	2	1	12
1	204	373	414	0	3	1	12
2	204	0	8	1	1	0	15
2	204	8	26	1	2	0	15
2	204	26	152	1	3	0	15
2	204	152	241	1	4	0	15
2	204	241	249	1	5	0	15
2	204	249	322	1	6	0	15
2	204	322	350	1	7	0	15
2	204	350	439	0	8	0	15
3	204	0	382	0	1	1	19
4	204	0	388	0	1	1	12

Here is the SAS job that created the data set; the repetitive code for events 2 through 6 has been suppressed from the listing.

```
data gamma;
    infile 'cgd.data' missover;
    input id 1-3 center 5-7 +1 random mmddyy6. trt 2.
          sex 2. age 3. height 6.1  weight 6.1
          inherit 2.    steroids 2. propylac 2.
          hos_cat 2.    futime 4.  (event1-event7) (7*4.);


data cgd1; set gamma;
    drop event1-event7 futime;

    tstart = 0;
    enum   = 1;
```

```
    if (event1 NE .) then do;
        tstop = event1;
        status = 1;
        output;
        tstart = tstop;
        enum = enum +1;
        end;
    .
    .
    .

    if (event7 NE .) then do;
        tstop = event7;
        status =1;
        output;
        tstart = tstop;
        enum = enum +1;
        end;

    if (futime > tstart) then do;
        tstop = futime;
        status =0;
        output;
        end;

proc print;
```

The cgd1 data set has 203 observations on 128 subjects. The second or WLW style data set cgd2 is not shown. There is one patient in the study with 7 recurrent infections, therefore the cgd2 data set has 7 strata and $128 * 7 = 896$ observations; each patient appears once in each stratum.

In choosing a model for the time to recurrent infections, the analyst should consider the biological processes of the disease. For instance, it is possible that after experiencing the first infection, the risk of the next infection may increase. This could happen if each infection permanently compromised the ability of the immune system to respond to subsequent attacks. From practical experience, clinical scientists conducting the trial suggested that the risk of recurrent infection remained constant regardless of the number of previous infections. This suggests use of an AG model.

The results for the four basic models are shown in Table 8.10. In the first model, time to first infection, the ordinary and robust variance estimates agree closely; a major disagreement would be evidence that some assumptions of the Cox model were violated. The Andersen–Gill model gives nearly an identical coefficient. A refit of the conditional model using "time since last event" or gap time as the time scale rather than "time since entry" differs by only $\pm.02$ in either the coefficient or standard error estimates.

There are 44 first events and 76 total events in the data set. If repeated infections contributed independent information to the model then we would expect that the standard error of the treatment effect could be reduced from 0.34 to $0.34 * \sqrt{44/76} = .26$, a reduction of 24%, which turns out to be exactly the uncorrected variance estimate. Using the robust estimate, the

	β	se(β)	Robust se
Time to first event	−1.09	0.34	0.34
AG	−1.10	0.26	0.31
Conditional	−0.86	0.28	0.29
Cond (gap time)	−0.88	0.28	0.28
WLW	−1.34	0.27	0.36

TABLE 8.10: *Fits for the CGD data*

actual gain was .31/.34 or 7%, which is approximately equal to $\sqrt{44/53}$. We thought to gain $76 - 44 = 32$ extra "units" of information and instead gained $53 - 44 = 9$; that is, each extra event was worth about $9/32 \approx 1/4$ of an original event in terms of added precision.

The pattern of results for the marginal and conditional approaches is remarkably similar to the simulated example presented earlier. If separate coefficients are fit to the first three strata, the results for the marginal model are −1.10, −1.25, and −2.74, increasing across strata, and for the conditional model they are −1.10, 0.11, and −1.28, with only five observations present in the stratum 3 treatment group.

Because of this similarity, we might expect that the Andersen–Gill and conditional models would give closer results if the model were to include significant covariates. The two most important factors, other than treatment, are age and use of steroids.

```
> # Time to first event
> fit2 <- coxph(Surv(tstop, status) ~ rx + age + inherit +
                                 steroids + cluster(id),
                          data=cgd1, subset=(enum==1))

> # Andersen-Gill
> fita2 <- coxph(Surv(tstart, tstop, status) ~ rx + age +
                          inherit +steroids + cluster(id),
                     data=cgd1)

> # Conditional
> fitc2 <- coxph(Surv(tstart, tstop, status) ~ rx + age +
                    inherit + steroids + cluster(id) + strata(enum),
                          data=cgd1)

> # Wei-Lin-Weissfeld
> fitw2 <- coxph(Surv(time, status) ~ rx + age + inherit +
                          steroids + cluster(id) + strata(enum),
                     data=cgd2)
```

Table 8.11 shows the results for the treatment effect in these models. The coefficient for the Andersen–Gill model has changed slightly, the conditional result has moved significantly in the direction of the AG solution, and the marginal model has become more extreme. If center is entered as

	β	se(β)	Robust se
Time to first event	−1.25	0.35	0.35
AG	−1.16	0.26	0.30
Conditional	−1.00	0.29	0.29
Marginal	−1.51	0.28	0.37

TABLE 8.11: *Fits for the CGD data, controlling for age, inheritance, and steroid use*

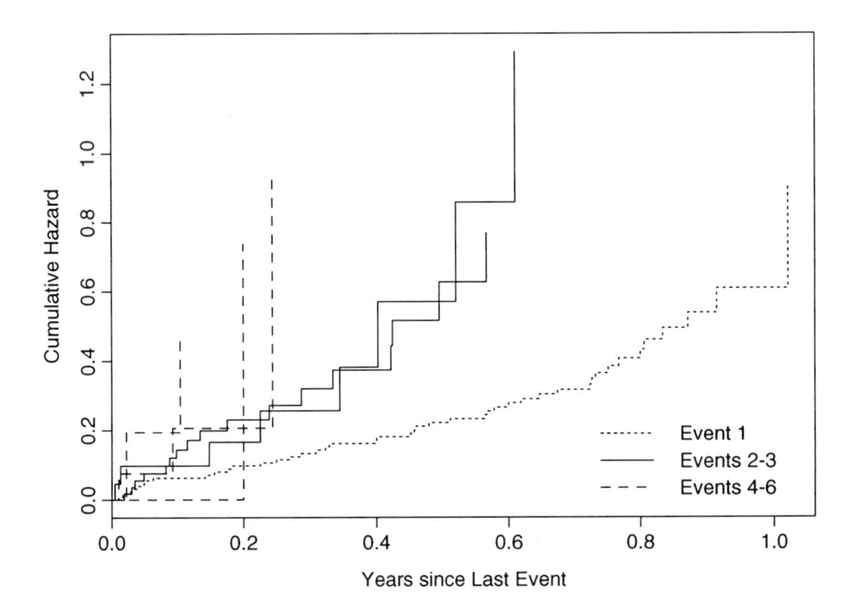

FIGURE 8.6: *Baseline cumulative hazards for each event number*

a stratification variable the results come even closer, with coefficients of −1.22, −1.26, and −1.20, respectively, for the first event, AG and conditional models. The result is similar if center is added as a factor (class) variable rather than a stratum.

It is worth looking at the cumulative hazard functions that correspond to these fits, as they will reveal one more interesting feature of the data set. By using the "time since last event" scale, all of the curves will cover a similar plotting range. Strata 7 and 8 are omitted from the plot since each contains only one event.

```
> gapfit <- coxph(Surv(tstop-tstart, status)~ rx + steroids +
                age + strata(enum), cgd1, subset=(enum<7))
> surv <- survfit(gapfit)
> plot(surv, fun='cumhaz', lty=c(2,1,1,3,3))
```

The resultant plot, shown in Figure 8.6, shows that the time to first event is much longer than the other gap times. There are at least two possible reasons for this: entry into the second stratum (i.e., experiencing a first infection on study) self-selects for the patients with a higher event rate, or that entry into a research study is itself a selection process. The eligibility

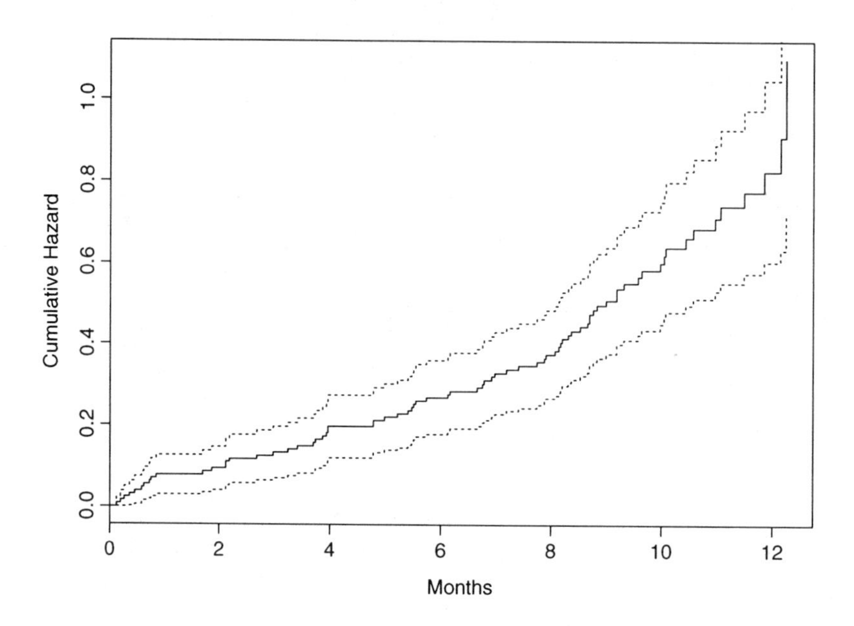

FIGURE 8.7: *Cumulative hazard for the CGD data*

criteria of clinical protocols often contain phrases like "expected survival of at least six months" or "no current serious complications." For a disease that waxes and wanes, this will serve to select patients for entry during quiescent periods. Alternatively, a study of a chronic disease such as arthritis, conducted at a tertiary care institution, may suffer from referral bias: patients are at the tertiary care center because of a flare-up or the onset of a second condition such as heart disease, and the early postenrollment period reflects sicker-than-average subjects.

A plot of the cumulative hazard curve for the multiple event data can be obtained using a null Cox model, and is shown in Figure 8.7. There is no evidence in the curve for either a higher- or lower-than-average rate of events in the first few months of the study. This argues against the hypothesis that patients enter the study during a quiescent period.

```
> dfit <- coxph(Surv(tstart, tstop, status) ~ 1, data=cgd1)
> surv <- survfit(dfit)
> plot(surv, fun='cumhaz')
```

As the S-Plus function for Kaplan–Meier curves, `survfit`, has not yet been extended to handle (start, stop] data, use of the `coxph` function is a useful "trick" to obtain them. Use of ~ `strata(rx)` as the right-hand side of the equation would have produced separate curves for each treatment arm. A slightly more subtle version of the trick works in SAS, which requires at least one covariate to be present in order to produce survival output.

```
data temp; set cgd1;
    dummy=0;
```

```
proc phreg data=temp noprint;
        model (tstart, tstop) *status(0)= dummy /ties=efron;
        strata rx;
        output out=temp2 logsurv=lsurv;

data temp3; set temp2;
    cumhaz = -lsurv;
proc plot;
    plot cumhaz * tstop;
```

(Caveat: the above statement that "`survfit` does not handle (start, stop] data" and the example of how to "fool" SAS are almost certainly version-dependent and may quickly become out of date. Both packages may soon support these features directly.)

8.5.6 rhDNase in patients with cystic fibrosis

In patients with cystic fibrosis, extracellular DNA is released by leukocytes that accumulate in the airways in response to chronic bacterial infection. This excess DNA thickens the mucus, which then cannot be cleared from the lung by the cilia. The accumulation leads to exacerbations of respiratory symptoms and progressive deterioration of lung function. More than 90% of cystic fibrosis patients eventually die of lung disease.

Deoxyribonuclease I (DNase I) is a human enzyme normally present in the mucus of human lungs that digests extracellular DNA. Genentech, Inc. has cloned a highly purified recombinant DNase (rhDNase, or Pulmozyme©) which when delivered to the lungs in an aerosolized form cuts extracellular DNA, reducing the viscoelasticity of airway secretions and improving clearance. In 1992 the company conducted a randomized double-blind trial comparing Pulmozyme to placebo. Patients were then monitored for pulmonary exacerbations, along with measures of lung volume and flow. The primary endpoint was the time until first pulmonary exacerbation; however, data on all exacerbations were collected for 169 days.

Table 8.12 shows the results on the number of exacerbations. Overall, 139/324 (43%) of the placebo and 104/321 (32%) of the rhDNase patients experienced an exacerbation during the followup period. A Cox proportional hazards model using the time to first exacerbations yields a hazard ratio of 0.69, with a 95% confidence interval of (.54, .89); strong evidence that rhDNase reduces the number of pulmonary events.

The data for second exacerbations, however, seem to point in the other direction: 42/139 (30%) of the placebo and 39/104 (38%) of the treated patients who had a first exacerbation went on to experience a second. A multiple-event Cox model can be used to clarify and understand this result.

Since pulmonary exacerbations cause scar tissue to develop which reduces lung function, it is reasonable to assume that the baseline hazard of each subsequent exacerbation was different. This suggests the use of either a stratified model, either the WLW or conditional, or an Andersen–Gill model with a time-dependent covariate for event number. Arguing against this, however, is the fact that patients are entered into the study at various

	Number of Exacerbations					
	0	1	2	3	4	5
Placebo	185	97	23	14	4	1
rhDNase	217	65	30	6	3	0

TABLE 8.12: *Frequencies of exacerbations in the rhDNase trial*

stages of disease. To attempt to control for x_1 ="number of events while on study" when x_2 ="number of events prior to study entry" is unknown is not likely to be fruitful in the AG model, especially when x_2 has both a larger mean and a larger variance than x_1.

Setting up the data sets for these models was more complicated than usual because of discontinuous intervals of risk. During an exacerbation, patients recieved IV antibiotics. While on antibiotics and for 6 exacerbation-free days beyond the end of IV therapy, a patient could not incur a new infection; it would be considered a continuation of the current exacerbation incident. Patients are thus *by definition* not at risk during this IV antibiotic + 6 day interval; that is, they are not at risk for having an event entered into the analysis data set for the study.

Consider a single treated patient who had exacerbations at days 50 and 100 with durations of 10, and 15 days, respectively, and a final followup at day 180. In the counting process data set `dnase1`, this patient would appear as follows.

```
time1   time2   status  trt     enum
  0       50       1     1       1
 66      100       1     1       2
121      180       0     1       3
```

For the marginal analysis, they would appear as 12 observations. (Since 1 person has 5 events, all subjects appear in 5 strata.)

```
time1   time2   status  trt     enum
  0       50       1     1       1

  0       50       0     1       2
 66      100       1     1       2

  0       50       0     1       3
 66      100       0     1       3
121      180       0     1       3

  0       50       0     1       4
 66      100       0     1       4
121      180       0     1       4

  0       50       0     1       5
 66      100       0     1       5
121      180       0     1       5
```

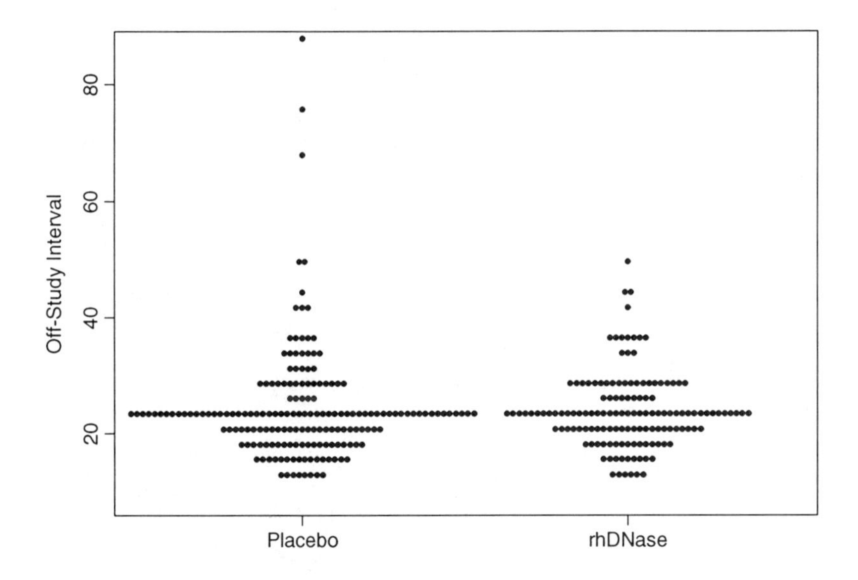

FIGURE 8.8: *Time off study due to infection for patients in the rhDNase study*

Figure 8.8 shows a plot of off-study intervals versus treatment. There is no overall difference in length of exacerbations, other than three placebo intervals of > 2 months, but the treated group has fewer events and thus slightly more total exposure time during the study.

A further consideration is the small number of events in strata 4 and 5. We have several possibilities for dealing with this. The first is to treat them exactly like the other strata, accepting the fact that the within-stratum hazard estimates will be very unstable, perhaps even useless. This is particularly true for the conditional model, which has a very small sample size in this region. A second possibility is to truncate the data set after the third event. The third approach is to amalgamate the final three strata, which is easily done by creation of a limited variable `enum3= min(enum, 3)`. The corresponding hybrid conditional/AG model corresponds to Figure 8.9. All

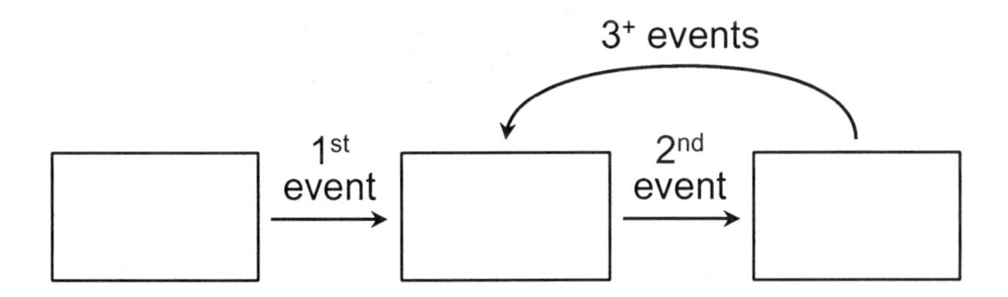

FIGURE 8.9: *Schematic for the modified conditional model*

	FEV			Treatment		
	β	se(β)	Robust	β	se(β)	Robust
First event	−0.21	0.028	0.027	−0.38	0.13	0.13
Andersen–Gill	−0.18	0.023	0.030	−0.30	0.11	0.13
Conditional	−0.15	0.023	0.027	−0.21	0.11	0.11
Conditional/3	−0.15	0.023	0.028	−0.22	0.11	0.11
WLW	−0.20	0.023	0.033	−0.35	0.11	0.15
WLW/3	−0.20	0.023	0.033	−0.35	0.11	0.15

TABLE 8.13: *Fits to the rhDNase data. The suffix /3 refers to models with strata 3, 4, and 5 combined*

of the models include FEV (forced expiratory volume in one second) as a covariate.

```
> # Time to first event, A-G, conditional, and WLW models
> fit1 <- coxph(Surv(time1, time2, status) ~ trt + fev,
                          data=dnase1, subset=(enum==1))
> fita <- coxph(Surv(time1, time2, status) ~ trt + fev +
                               cluster(id), data=dnase1)
> fitc <- coxph(Surv(time1, time2, status) ~ trt + fev +
                   cluster(id) + strata(enum), data=dnase1)
> fitw <- coxph(Surv(time1, time2, status) ~ trt + fev +
                   cluster(id) + strata(enum), data=dnase2)
> print(fita)
      coef exp(coef) se(coef) robust se     z       p
trt -0.295     0.74    0.1063    0.1312  -2.25  2.4e-02
fev -0.018     0.98    0.0023    0.0030  -5.97  2.4e-09

> # Conditional and WLW models, with fewer strata
> fitc2 <- coxph(Surv(time1, time2, status) ~ trt + fev +
                 strata(enum3) + cluster(id), data=dnase1)
> fitw2 <- coxph(Surv(time1, time2, status) ~ trt + fev +
                 strata(enum3) + cluster(id), data=dnase2)
> # Per stratum effects
> fita3 <- coxph(Surv(time1, time2, status) ~ trt1 + trt2 + trt3 +
                     fev1 + fev2 + fev3 + cluster(id),
                          data=dnase1)
> fitc3 <- coxph(Surv(time1, time2, status) ~ trt1 + trt2 + trt3 +
                     fev1 + fev2 + fev3 + cluster(id) +
                     strata(enum3), data=dnase1)
> fitw3 <- coxph(Surv(time1, time2, status) ~ trt1 + trt2 + trt3 +
                     fev1 + fev2 + fev3 + cluster(id) +
                     strata(enum3), data=dnase2)
```

The variables `trt1`, `trt2`, and `trt3` above are defined as `trt*(enum=1)`, `trt*(enum=2)`, and `trt*(enum>=3)`, respectively, and similarly for `fev`.

Table 8.13 shows the result of simple fits to the rhDNase data. Comparing the Andersen–Gill result to the first event model, we see that there is an apparent lessening of treatment effect after the first event. The overall estimates of effect based on the conditional and WLW models are smaller and larger, respectively, than the AG model, as we have seen before. Combining

	FEV			Treatment		
	β	se	robust se	β	se	robust se
Conditional						
1st event	–0.21	0.028	0.027	–0.38	0.13	0.13
2nd event	0.00	0.054	0.055	0.30	0.22	0.21
$\geq$3	–0.01	0.073	0.090	–0.28	0.36	0.35
WLW						
1st event	–0.21	0.028	0.027	–0.38	0.13	0.13
2nd event	–0.19	0.048	0.049	–0.10	0.22	0.23
$\geq$3	–0.16	0.070	0.104	–0.73	0.35	0.43

TABLE 8.14: *Per event fits to the rhDNase data*

events 3 to 5 in a single stratum has no impact on the overall estimate of effect. Table 8.14 contains the coefficients for models with a per-stratum coefficient. Here combination of the final three strata may be useful; it has sidestepped the infinite and/or missing estimates of treatment effect we have seen before for the final stratum, while still making use of the data therein. The conditional model shows an actual reversal of treatment effect for the second stratum. More importantly, the effect of FEV appears to have been diminished to zero in the second stratum, a result which on medical grounds is quite suspect — remember that the action of the drug is to help clear the lungs and it is not expected to make any change in underlying physiology. If the functional form of FEV were nonlinear, for example no differential effect for values less than the median but a sharp risk decrease thereafter, then the selection effect of having a first event could explain some of the change, but a plot examining the functional form of FEV shows its effect to be nearly linear over the observed range. The results for an Andersen–Gill model with per-event coefficients shows that it is not the stratification by event, per se, that is the issue. By its construction, the coefficient for variable `trt2` will be based on the data set intervals with `enum=2`; the coefficient is attempting to estimate the effect of treatment, conditional on having had a first event. This is a difficult quantity to estimate in this study design.

The results of the WLW fit suggest far less diminishment of the effect, and the test for nonproportional hazards is not significant as shown below. It may be the most satisfactory estimator for individual periods.

```
> print(cox.zph(fitw2))
            rho    chisq     p
  trt1 0.049376 1.304969 0.253
  trt2 0.061302 2.463456 0.117
  trt3 0.028336 0.566960 0.451
  fev1 0.015927 0.132423 0.716
  fev2 0.001115 0.000915 0.976
  fev3 0.000357 0.000134 0.991
GLOBAL       NA 2.760642 0.838
```

It is not possible to completely resolve the issues given the data at hand, in particular whether the treatment advantage actually does diminish after the first recurrence. However, the long-term effect of rhDNase was independently estimable from data collected during a postdouble-blind observational period. At the end of the 169-day trial, the treatment was determined to be efficacious based on the initial results, and all participating patients were offered enrollment in an open-label followup trial of rhDNase. All subjects received the active compound with a planned followup of 18 months. Approximately 9% of the patients dropped out during the extended followup period. However, they did not differ in either age or lung function from those who completed the trial.

The majority of the followup for the patients in the double-blind trial occurred during a six-month period beginning in February 1992, and there is a definite wet and dry season in the geographic area where the trial was conducted which could modify the "baseline" rate of exacerbation. Therneau and Hamilton [144] compared the event rates from months 7 to 12 of the second study, the calendar time period felt to best match the initial double-blind trial, to the event rate for placebo patients on the initial trial. If the effect of rhDNase were decreasing, as suggested by the conditional model, one would expect it to be apparent in this later period. The results were much closer to the marginal fit; there was a sustained 28% decrease in the overall event rate, and the effect was similar for subjects with 0, 1, or >1 prior exacerbations. Based on this analysis, rhDNase was felt to have produced a significant and sustained reduction in the risk of pulmonary exacerbations in patients with cystic fibrosis.

8.6 Multistate models

Perhaps surprisingly, the tools we have introduced can be used to investigate fairly complex multistate models. They are not a final word, certainly, but can give useful insight with only a modest amount of effort. We illustrate the idea with some examples, the first more of a "thought experiment" to illustrate the process, and the second an actual data set from our medical work.

8.6.1 Modeling the homeless

This example is actually the result of a conversation with Sally Morton (at the Rand Corporation) about potential approaches to a governmental study. Imagine that we can assign a group of homeless subjects into one of three states: living on the street (outdoors), living in a shelter or other temporary charitable housing, or jail. Over the course of the study some of the subjects will move from one state to another, possibly multiple times. A schematic is shown in Figure 8.11

In the computer model of the data, there will be six strata, one for each possible transition (arrow on the graph). Assume a subject "Jones" enters our study on day 29 at a shelter, moves out of the shelter on day 40, reenters the shelter on day 58, is jailed on day 60, and lost to our followup on day

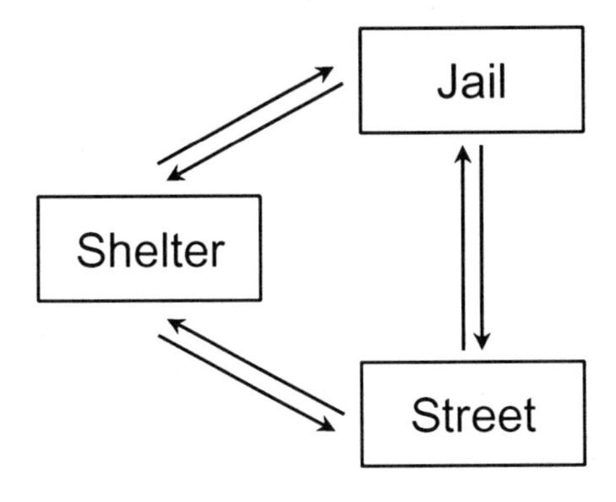

FIGURE 8.10: *Schematic for the modified conditional model*

FIGURE 8.11: *Hypothetical three-state model*

80. The data set would be as follows.

Start	Stop	Status	Stratum	Covariates
29	40	1	Shelter ⇒ Street	...
29	40	0	Shelter ⇒ Jail	
40	58	0	Street ⇒ Jail	
40	58	1	Street ⇒ Shelter	
58	60	0	Shelter ⇒ Street	
58	60	1	Shelter ⇒ Jail	
60	80	0	Jail ⇒ Shelter	
60	80	0	Jail ⇒ Street	

One important part of the setup is deciding which variables should have strata by covariate interactions, and which should not. For instance: the effect of age might well be different for shelter to street and shelter to jail transitions, reflecting local governmental policies. One may be forced to assume fewer interactions than are logically present, however, in order to limit the total number of coefficients in a model to a feasible number.

8.6.2 Crohn's disease

Our second example involves a long-term study of patients who are afflicted with Crohn's disease. This is a recurrent inflammatory disease of the gut, of uncertain origin but possibly immune-related. It frequently leads to intestinal obstruction and abcess formation, and has a high rate of recurrence.

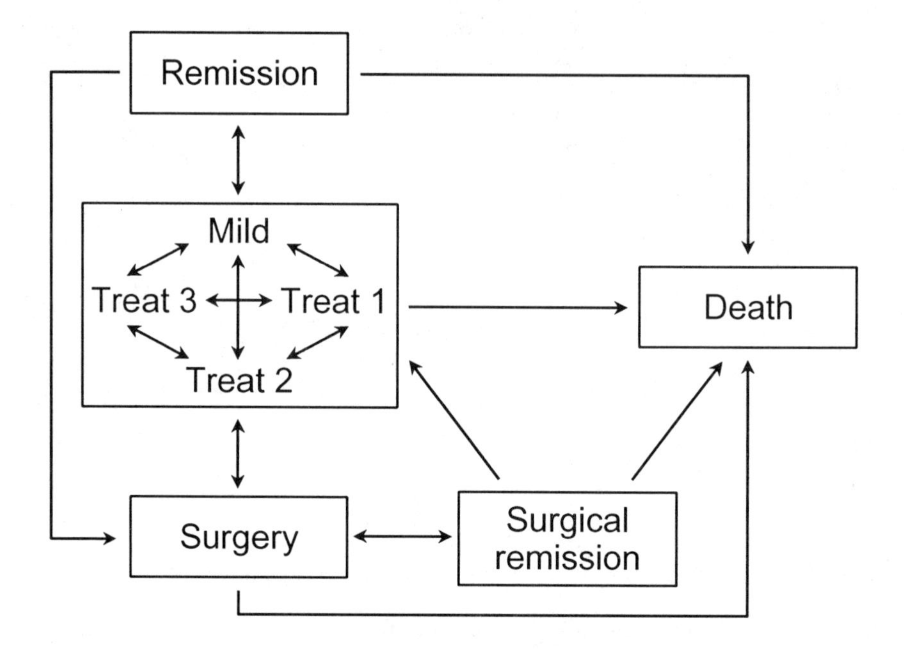

FIGURE 8.12: *States and transitions plot for the Crohn's disease data. All transitions are possible among the four states in the center box*

Flare-ups are treated with strong anti-inflammatory regimens (steroids, immunosuppression) but often lead to surgical removal of the inflamed section of the bowel followed by a quiescent period. The waxing and waning nature of Crohn's disease can make it difficult to describe long-term outcomes.

The study consists of the cohort of 174 Olmsted County, Minnesota, residents with a diagnosis of Crohn's disease from January 1, 1970, through December 31, 1993. At the time of analysis there were between two months and 24 years of completed followup on the subjects, with a mean followup of 7.3 years. Silverstein et al. [134] describe the data set in detail and fit a Markov model in order to examine long-term costs of care. Over their time course, subjects were classified into one of nine possible states.

- Pre-study. A placeholder representing the time prior to enrollment.
- Remission. Quiescent disease, no medication.
- Mild disease. Moderate medications such as antibiotic, sulfasalazine, or topical corticosteroids.
- Severe disease. Patients are being treated with oral corticosteroids or immunosuppressive therapy. There are three subcategories of drug-responsive, drug-dependent, and drug-refractory; in what follows, these three states are labeled as "Treat1," "Treat2," and "Treat3."
- Surgery. Inpatient surgical procedures.

State	No. Patients Ever in State	Entries to State					
		1	2	3	4–5	6–9	10+
Remission	146	40	49	28	16	10	3
Mild	138	50	32	20	23	11	2
Severe							
Drug-responsive	64	44	12	2	4	2	0
Drug-dependent	42	29	5	6	2	0	0
Drug-refractory	45	29	13	1	2	0	0
Surgery	100	64	20	7	7	1	1
Postsurgery remission	85	55	22	6	1	1	0

TABLE 8.15: *State changes for the Crohn's disease study. Of the 146 subjects who ever entered remission, 40 entered that state once, 49 entered it twice, etc.*

- Surgical remission. A quiescent phase following surgical intervention, no medication or treatment.
- Death from any cause.

Figure 8.12 shows the states and the possible transitions from state to state in the data. Transitions are possible between any of the four treatment states; to simplify the figure these are shown as a single box. There are from 1 to 33 state changes in the data set for each subject, the first being from "entry" to one of the observed states. The total number of subjects who ever enter a state along with the distribution of entries is shown in Table 8.15.

Creation of the analysis data set is actually fairly simple. The starting data set has one observation for each transition, containing the prior state, current state, next state, time to transition, and covariates. Consider a subject who is first diagnosed on 1Mar78 and initially categorized as mild disease, treatment escalates on 28Mar78, remission is achieved on 16May78, and the patient is then followed forward to 28Sept78. The data would look like the following.

```
 id  sex    date     age pstate current nstate   time
167    0  1Mar78     27    -1       1      2       27
167    0 28Mar78     27     1       2      0       49
167    0 16May78     27     2       0      .      136
```

Internally, the state codes for the data set are -1 = Prestudy, 0 = Remission, 1–4 = Treatment, 5 = Surgery, 6 = Surgical remission, and 7 = Dead. If the final observation does not end in a transition (e.g., a subject enters the "mild" state midway through observation and is still in it at the last followup) then the `nstate` variable is equal to missing on the last line. There are 1,314 observations in the starting data set.

Looking at the state diagram, we see that there are six possible transitions from each disease state, and of course none from the death state, so the final data set will have $7 * 6 = 42$ possible strata. All 42 appear in the final data set, with "13" as the label for a state 1 to state 3 transition and so on. The following code creates the larger analysis data set containing all of the strata and transitions.

```
data crohn2; set crohn1;
    if (0<= current <= 5) then do;
        do i = 0 to 7;
            if (nstate =i) then status =1;
                              else status =0;
            stratum = current*10 + i;
            if (i ne current and i ne 6) then output;
            end;
        end;

    else do;
        do i = 1 to 7;
            if (nstate =i) then status =1;
                              else status =0;
            stratum = current*10 + i;
            if (i ne current) then output;
            end;
        end;
```

Similar to the homeless example, if a subject moves from state 4 to state 2 after a duration of 48 days, the second data set has one observation in each of the six strata $4 \rightarrow 0$, $4 \rightarrow 1$, $4 \rightarrow 2$, $4 \rightarrow 3$, $4 \rightarrow 5$; and $4 \rightarrow 7$ corresponding to a possible transition, with a status of 1 in the "42" stratum (transition observed) and a status of 0 in the others. We have chosen to use "time since entry to the state" as the time scale, so that (start, stop] notation is not necessary. For at least some of the states, "total duration of disease" would also be medically justifiable as a time scale, but this is not pursued. One other variable in the data set, not shown in the above code, is the time spent in the prior state `prev_dur`; it is set to zero for the first observation of each subject.

A first question we might want to investigate is whether the process is Markov. That is, do the outcome and risk for a subject depend only on the current state? We fit an initial model with sex, age, duration in the previous state, and the previous state as covariates. The last variable is categorical, and needs to be entered as a set of dummy variables. We can either create our own or let the package create them, that is, the `class` statement in SAS or `factor` in S-Plus. To start, we create a factor variable with preenrollment as the first, or reference, level.

```
> pst <- factor(crohn2$pstate, levels=(-1):6,
             labels=c("PreStudy", "Remission", "Mild", "Treat1",
                      "Treat2" ,  "Treat3", "Surgery",  "Sx Rem"))

> fit1 <- coxph(Surv(time, status) ~ male + age + prev.dur + pst +
                 strata(stratum) + cluster(id), data=crohn2)
```

```
> print(fit1)
                    coef exp(coef) se(coef) robust se      z       p
        male -2.12e-01     0.809 6.16e-02  6.53e-02 -3.250 1.2e-03
         age -1.07e-04     1.000 2.02e-03  2.45e-03 -0.043 9.7e-01
    prev.dur -3.47e-05     1.000 5.06e-05  4.96e-05 -0.699 4.8e-01
pstRemission -4.65e-01     0.628 1.09e-01  1.33e-01 -3.490 4.8e-04
     pstMild -6.53e-01     0.521 1.04e-01  1.29e-01 -5.064 4.1e-07
   pstTreat1 -5.86e-01     0.557 1.35e-01  1.44e-01 -4.065 4.8e-05
   pstTreat2 -5.59e-01     0.572 1.72e-01  2.04e-01 -2.744 6.1e-03
   pstTreat3 -4.61e-01     0.631 1.61e-01  1.72e-01 -2.678 7.4e-03
  pstSurgery -8.74e-01     0.417 2.14e-01  2.15e-01 -4.057 5.0e-05
   pstSx Rem -4.96e-01     0.609 1.55e-01  1.90e-01 -2.606 9.1e-03

> waldtest(fit, 4:10)
    chisq df       p
 33.02411  7 2.6e-05
```

We see that gender is quite important, with males having a "rate" of state changes that is approximately 80% of the female rate. (One hypothesis is that this is more sociological than physiological, with the female patients being more prompt in seeking attention for medical problems.) Age and the duration of time spent in a prior state are not significant. The overall Wald test for the seven indicator variables is highly significant, however: the disease state the patient came from influences residency time in the current state. But notice that the coefficients, which are each a contrast with the prior state of "New patient," are all about the same size. Let us recode the factor so that "Remission" becomes the reference group, a change that makes certain interpretive sense as well since that is the desired state medically.

```
> pst <- factor(crohn2$pstate, levels=c(0,-1,1:6),
            labels=c("Remission", "Pre-Study", "Mild", "Treat1",
                    "Treat2", "Treat3", "Surgery", "Sx Rem"))
> fit3 <- coxph(Surv(time, status) ~ male + age + prev.dur + pst
            + strata(stratum) + cluster(id), data=crohn2)
> print(fit3)
                  coef exp(coef) se(coef) robust se       z      p
      male -2.12e-01     0.809 6.16e-02  6.53e-02 -3.2508 0.0012
       age -1.07e-04     1.000 2.02e-03  2.45e-03 -0.0435 0.9700
  prev.dur -3.47e-05     1.000 5.06e-05  4.96e-05 -0.6995 0.4800
  pstEntry  4.65e-01     1.592 1.09e-01  1.33e-01  3.4900 0.0005
   pstMild -1.88e-01     0.829 1.07e-01  1.37e-01 -1.3711 0.1700
 pstTreat1 -1.21e-01     0.886 1.31e-01  1.31e-01 -0.9251 0.3500
 pstTreat2 -9.44e-02     0.910 1.70e-01  1.75e-01 -0.5402 0.5900
 pstTreat3  4.26e-03     1.004 1.55e-01  1.62e-01  0.0264 0.9800
pstSurgery -4.09e-01     0.664 2.03e-01  1.88e-01 -2.1747 0.0300
 pstSx Rem -3.16e-02     0.969 1.37e-01  1.76e-01 -0.1801 0.8600
```

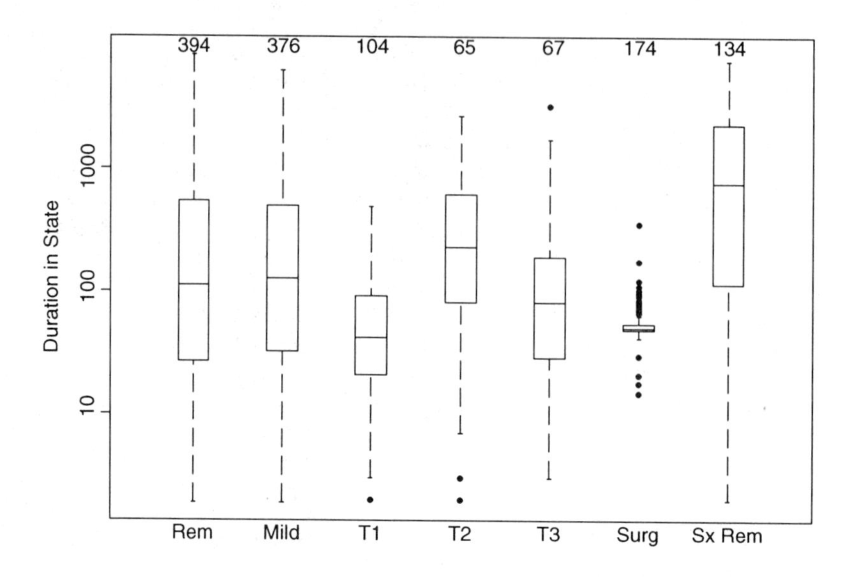

FIGURE 8.13: *Number of visits to each state, with the duration of each*

If a subject is new, he/she has a 1.6-fold higher rate of transition; that is, the initially assigned state doesn't "endure" as long. Perhaps, lacking a history of working with the patient, the initial treatment decision is less accurate, or perhaps patients are more likely to come during a period of disease transition. None of the other prior states is significantly different than remission in regard to effect on the current state's duration, with the exception of surgery. If a subject is coming off surgery, the current state is likely to persist longer.

Figure 8.13 shows the average duration in each state, and immediately reveals a flaw in the prior two models. The total time a patient spends in the surgery state is severely prescribed, it is essentially the hospital recovery time, and as such is unlikely to be related at all to age, sex, or prior duration. Secondly, the longer duration of the "Surgery Remission" state might have made surgery look better in general, since surgery is the only way to enter that state. We can easily verify that age, gender, and duration in prior state are unrelated to the recovery time.

```
data temp; set save.crohn2;
   if (current=5);    * only retain surgery state observations;

%phlev(data=temp, time=time, event=status, strata= stratum,
        xvars= age male prev_dur, id=id, collapse=Y);
```

```
          Parameter              Robust                        Robust
Variable  Estimate      SE         SE     Chi-Square Chi-Square DF      P
age       -0.006001 0.00491 0.00414      1.494       2.104          0.147
male       0.028570 0.16138 0.14491      0.031       0.039          0.844
prev_dur  -0.000041 0.00012 0.00009      0.118       0.184          0.668
```

```
wald                                          2.205    3  0.531
robust score                                  1.367    3  0.713
```

A second fit (not shown) shows that the time is also not significantly related to which state preceded surgery. The outlier in the surgery time period (361 days) is at first worrisome, but an examination of the dfbeta residuals (not shown) reveals that it actually does not have a major effect on the estimates, helped by the fact that a Cox model is essentially based on the ranks of the exit times.

Because it involves transitions from only a single state, the above result can also be obtained from the unexpanded data set `crohn1`. If using the Breslow approximation, the approach gives precisely the same coefficients; for others the parameter solution changes slightly because stratification induces some artifical separation of tied event times. This is the same issue as was discussed in the competing risks framework, see Section 8.4.1.

```
data temp; set save.crohn1;
   if (current=5);
%phlev(data=temp, time=time, event=status,
       xvars= age male prev_dur, id=id, collapse=Y);
```

Based on what has been discovered thus far, we fit a summary model. We first create two new covariates: `entry`, which is 1 if this is a subject's first state after entry into the study, and `priorsx` which is 1 for the first state after a surgery. The surgery state strata (i.e., transitions from surgery to another state) are left out of the model, since time in that state is clearly not related to the covariates or to the prior state. (This is, in one sense, a particular state by covariate interaction.)

```
> entry   <- 1*(crohn2$previous == -1)
> priorsx <- 1*(crohn2$previous ==  5)

> fit4 <- coxph(Surv(time, status) ~ entry + priorsx + male +
                         strata(stratum) + cluster(id),
                   data=crohn2, subset=(current != 5))
> print(fit4)
          coef exp(coef) se(coef) robust se     z       p
  entry  0.588     1.801   0.0963    0.1231  4.78 1.8e-06
priorsx -0.324     0.723   0.1969    0.1762 -1.84 6.6e-02
   male -0.267     0.766   0.0671    0.0757 -3.53 4.2e-04

Likelihood ratio test=53.3  on 3 df, p=1.55e-11  n= 6840
```

The coefficient for being in a prior surgical state is not significant in the reduced model. Overall, then, we see that the first state after entry has a reduced duration (1.8-fold increased rate of departure from the state), but beyond that first transition a Markov model might be entertained as neither the prior state nor the duration in that state has significant predictive power. We have not looked at more complicated possible dependencies, such as the pattern formed by the prior two states, prior three states, and the like, but this could be explored by creation of the proper interaction variables (given sufficient sample size).

The analysis so far has only looked for a covariate's overall effect on "time in state," not distinguishing the states. Does gender, for instance, affect some transition times more than others? Does "new patient" status imply shortening for *each* of the possible follow-on states? We first look at the second question, by adding an interaction term to the model.

```
> cst <- factor(crohn2$current, levels=c(0:6),
           labels=c("Remission", "Mild", "Treat1",
                    "Treat2",    "Treat3", "Surgery", "Sx Rem"))
> fit5 <- coxph(Surv(time, status) ~ male + entry + entry:cst +
           + strata(stratum) + cluster(id),
           data=crohn2, subset=(current!=5))

> print(fit5)
                    coef exp(coef) se(coef) robust se      z      p
           male -0.281     0.755    0.067    0.0759 -3.697  .0002
          entry  0.882     2.416    0.123    0.1699  5.193  .0000
  entrycst:Mild -0.742     0.476    0.224    0.2849 -2.604  .0092
entrycst:Treat1 -0.247     0.781    0.421    0.2938 -0.839  .40
entrycst:Treat2     NA        NA    0.000    0.0000
entrycst:Treat3 -1.072     0.342    0.733    0.4517 -2.372  .018
entrycst:Surgery    NA        NA    0.000    0.0000
entrycst:Sx Rem     NA        NA    0.000    0.0000
```

Although "automatically" generated dummy variables are nice, such automatic generation does not always work as well as we'd like. Here S-Plus has generated three unnecessary indicator variables, all of which end up as NA in the printout: one for subjects whose first state is postsurgery (impossible by the definition of states), one for those whose first state is surgery (removed in this analysis), and the last for those whose first state is `Treat2` (no actual occurrences in the data). The reference level for the covariate is "first entry into remission," and we see that there are significant differences between this and first entry into either the `Mild` or `Treat3` state.

As an alternative, we can code our own dummy variables.

```
data temp; set save.crohn2;
   if (current = 5) then delete;
   ent_rem  = 1*(pstate= -1 and current=0);
   ent_mild = 1*(pstate= -1 and current=1);
   ent_trt1 = 1*(pstate= -1 and current=2);
   ent_trt3 = 1*(pstate= -1 and current=4);

%phlev(data=temp, time=time, event=status, strata=stratum,
       xvars= male ent_rem ent_mild ent_trt1 ent_trt3,
       id=id, collapse=Y)
```

```
           Parameter            Robust                  Robust
Variable    Estimate      SE       SE   Chi-Square Chi-Square DF       P

male        -0.28007 0.0670 0.07576     17.464     13.668        0.0002
ent_rem      0.87823 0.1229 0.16922     51.063     26.935        0.0000
ent_mild     0.14065 0.1869 0.22158      0.566      0.403        0.5256
ent_trt1     0.63145 0.4024 0.23967      2.462      6.941        0.0084
ent_trt3    -0.18763 0.7221 0.42489      0.068      0.195        0.6588
wald                                               45.275      5 0.0000
robust score                                       43.492      5 0.0000
```

The difference between coefficients 2 and 3 above, .878 − .141, is the treatment contrast printed in the S-Plus code. Initial entries into the remission or `Treat1` state tend to have a shorter duration in those states, than when remission is entered at a later time. (The `test` statement of SAS `phreg` would be useful in many instances such as these, for example, to test equality of the `ent_rec` and `ent_trt1` coefficients, but is not available when using the `%phlev` macro to get a correct variance.)

We can also look at the gender by state interaction.

```
> male0 <- crohn2$male * (crohn2$current==0) # remission
> male1 <- crohn2$male * (crohn2$current==1) # mild
> male2 <- crohn2$male * (crohn2$current==2) # treat1
> male3 <- crohn2$male * (crohn2$current==3) # treat2
> male4 <- crohn2$male * (crohn2$current==4) # treat3
> male6 <- crohn2$male * (crohn2$current==6) # post-surgery rem

> fit6 <- coxph(Surv(time, status) ~ male0 + male1 + male2 +
                                    male3 +male4 + male6 + entry +
                                    strata(stratum) + cluster(id),
                         data=crohn2, subset=(current!=5))
> print(fit6)
        coef exp(coef) se(coef) robust se      z       p
male0 -0.186     0.830   0.1130     0.120 -1.551 1.2e-01
male1 -0.251     0.778   0.1133     0.130 -1.935 5.3e-02
male2 -0.729     0.482   0.2307     0.203 -3.598 3.2e-04
male3 -0.403     0.668   0.3009     0.320 -1.258 2.1e-01
male4 -0.103     0.902   0.2600     0.291 -0.354 7.2e-01
male6 -0.281     0.755   0.2155     0.253 -1.112 2.7e-01
entry  0.599     1.820   0.0963     0.123  4.866 1.1e-06
```

The gender effect is weakest with respect to duration of the remission and `Treat3` states, and strongest in the more severe treatment states. Although not persuasive for either side, it does invite discussion about the relative importance of biologic and patient advocacy factors in the gender difference. All of the coefficients are negative, and we can perform an overall Wald test for whether they differ by fitting an interaction model.

```
> fit6a <- coxph(Surv(time, status) ~ male + male:cst + entry +
                                   strata(stratum) + cluster(id),
                      data=crohn2, subset=(current!=5))
> round(fit6a$coef,3)
   male entry malecstPre-Study malecstMild malecstTreat1
 -0.186 0.599               NA      -0.065        -0.543
 malecstTreat2 malecstTreat3 malecstSurgery malecstSx Rem
         -0.21         0.083             NA        -0.095
> waldtest(fit6a, 3:10)
  chi     p df
 5.94 0.312  5
```

The printout of the coefficients shows that S-Plus will list the main effects first, even if an interaction precedes it in the equation. The overall Wald test has a p of 0.3, indicating that the gender by state interaction, although interesting, is not proven.

Last, it is interesting to look at the hazard functions that correspond to each of the transitions. We use the unstratified data set to look at the transition rate out of each state, after adjusting (partially) for gender and study entry. Use of the smaller data set `crohn1` leads to a single cumulative hazard for departing "remission," say, where use of `crohn2` would lead to one for "departing remission to mild," "departing remission to `treat 1`,"and so on. Assume that the necessary variables `ent.rem` and `ent.trt1` have been added to the data set. Stratum 5 is left in for contrast, although it properly does not belong in the fit of these covariates. The resulting cumulative hazard curves are shown in Figure (8.14).

```
> crohn1$status <- !(is.na(crohn1$nstate))
> fit7 <- coxph(Surv(time, status) ~ male + ent.rem + ent.trt1 +
                                   strata(current), data=crohn1)
> tdata <- data.frame(male=1, ent.rem=0, ent.trt1=0)
> fsurv <- survfit(fit7, newdata=tdata)

> fsurv$time <- sqrt(fsurv$time/30.5)
> plot(fsurv, fun='cumhaz', lty=1, xaxt='n',
        xlab='Months', ylab='Cumulative Hazard')
> temp <- c(0,1, 10, 50, 100, 200)
> axis(1, sqrt(temp), as.character(temp))

> print(fsurv)
              n events mean se(mean) median 0.95LCL 0.95UCL
current=0 394    339 5.17   0.3554   2.85    2.43    3.77
current=1 376    340 3.65   0.2063   2.41    2.06    2.89
current=2 103    100 1.43   0.0806   1.36    1.16    1.59
current=3  64     55 3.50   0.2655   2.91    2.73    4.32
current=4  67     63 2.48   0.3726   1.83    1.53    2.31
current=5 173    170 1.40   0.0345   1.31    1.29    1.32
current=6 134     90 7.73   0.5468   6.44    5.14    9.51
```

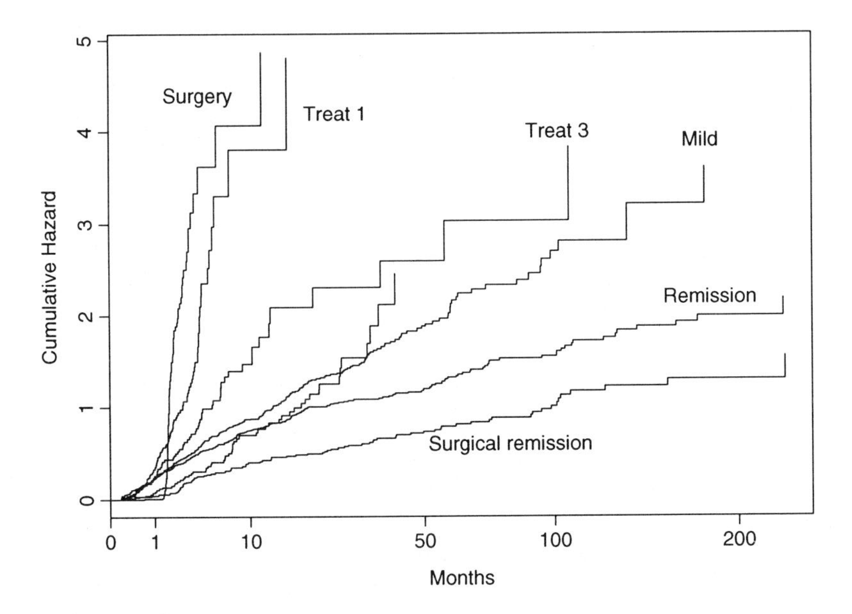

FIGURE 8.14: *Cumulative hazard curves for duration remaining in each state of the Crohn's disease data. The unlabeled curve is "Treat 2"*

Survival curves following a Cox model are discussed in Chapter 10; we are using them here to get group curves *adjusted* for possible differences in gender and prior state. The `tdata` object is a data set of one observation, and defines the reference set for the plot: these are curves for a hypothetical male subject, with neither remission nor `Treat1` as his prior state. A bit of trickery was used to get the plot on a square root scale while still using the prepackaged `plot` function; normally the four lines below the `survfit` call could be replaced with a single call to `plot(fsurv)`. It happens that square-root scale most easily separates the plots for labeling. The unusual pattern of the surgery curve — a horizontal start followed by a sharp upwards turn — reflects the tight clustering of the surgery state durations around a central value. Surgical remission is the longest lasting state, followed by remission and then mild treatment. The fact that so many of the curves are nearly linear on this scale suggests that a Weibull model with scale = .5 would also be a reasonable choice.

This look at the data is far from complete, but does show how some fairly important questions can be addressed very quickly with a multiple-state Cox model approach.

8.7 Combination models

The multistate model of the last section does not fit neatly into any of our three standards: like the WLW model, patients have a "competing risks" set of new states that they can enter when leaving a particular state; like the Andersen–Gill, subjects can reenter the same state multiple times; and like the conditional model, they may traverse a series of disjoint states

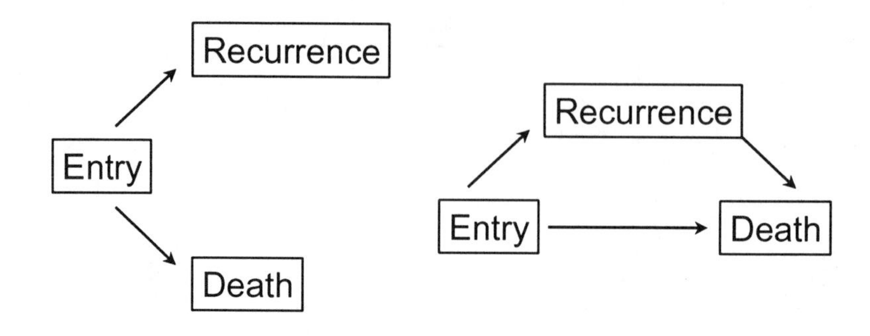

FIGURE 8.15: *Alternate analysis plans for the colon cancer data*

using a "time since entry" time scale. Likewise, a combination model can be used for some of the earlier simpler problems.

Figure 8.15 shows two alternate state diagrams for the colon cancer data discussed earlier in Section 8.4.4. The left diagram corresponds to the WLW analysis that was carried out in the discussion there. The right-hand figure corresponds to an alternate view that patients who have experienced a recurrence are no longer at the same risk of death as those who have not, and should at the point of recurrence be assigned to a separate stratum. The most natural time scale for the R→D stratum is, by the same reasoning, the time since recurrence.

Consider patient 1 of the data set, who has a recurrence on day 968 and death on day 1,521. Under the WLW formulation, he is coded as two rows of data, the first in stratum "entry-recurrence" with time = 986 and status = 1, and the second in stratum "entry-death" with time = 1,521 and status = 1. For the new analysis, the subject is encoded as three observations. The first, in the "entry-recurrence" stratum, is just as before. The second, for the "entry-death" stratum, has time = 986 and status = 0; with respect to the "death without recurrence" hazard function the patient has become censored. A third observation in the "recurrence-death" stratum has time = 553 and status = 1. There are 461 observations in the third stratum, one for each recurrence subject who has followup beyond the date of progression (five subjects have death/recurrence on the same day). A similar analysis of mortality in patients with liver cirrhosis, with variceal bleeding as the intermediate state, is presented in Andersen et al. [5].

Table 8.16 shows the coefficients for the two analyses side by side. There is not much difference in their realizations. The more important value of the alternate formulation is for coding treatment by stratum interactions. For instance, one could examine the hypothesis that extent of disease, after controlling for nodes and treatment, has an impact on time to progression but not on the duration of postrecurrence survival. There is, of course, also the philosophical argument with respect to the WLW formulation of

	WLW	Alternate
Levamisole vs. Obs	–0.036	–0.059
Lev +5FU vs. Obs	–0.449	–0.470
Extent of disease	0.516	0.528
>4 Nodes	0.880	0.829

TABLE 8.16: *Fits to the colon cancer data set under a WLW and an alternative model*

whether two patients at some time t, one with and one without recurrence, really should be considered to have a common baseline hazard of death at that point.

8.8 Summary

The examples have shown, hopefully, the tremendous flexibility available with marginal survival models. For multiple unordered events, the appropriate setup is usually obvious and the gains, as shown by the diabetic retinopathy data, can be substantial. The UDCA data set, however, stands as a cautionary note that supposedly "different" outcome events can be highly correlated, leading to essentially no gain for the extra analysis work.

For multiple recurrent events within a given subject the gain in power was modest; in the bladder cancer and CGD studies each secondary event appeared to be worth between 1/5 and 1/3 of a new patient. This gain is not guaranteed, and should not be counted on when planning sample sizes for a trial. Nevertheless, it is sizeable enough to make multiple-event models worthwhile in the analysis.

The Andersen–Gill model is efficient, and gives the most reliable estimate of the overall effect of treatment. Use of the robust variance for the AG model is not necessary *in theory*, but in practice is the wiser choice. Two basic assumptions of the model are that the events do not change the subject (no change in baseline hazard), and that an *overall* estimate of effect is of interest.

The WLW approach allows for changes in the model effects over time by using stratum by covariate interaction terms. The data set for the model can get quite large. The interpretation of the model is less clear, however, since the assumption that a subject is "at risk" for a kth event before event $k-1$ has occurred is uncomfortable. As well, the model may badly violate the proportional hazards assumption.

The conditional model has the most natural interpretation, and is easy to set up. However, the existence of unmodeled risk factors can badly bias the coefficients. The risk sets for the later event numbers will also get quite small, making estimates of per-stratum risk unstable.

What are the practical conclusions for real data sets? It is well to remember the dictum of G. E. P. Box that "All models are wrong, but some are useful." These models are certainly imperfect, but still provide us with important information.

9

Frailty Models

9.1 Background

In the last several years there has been significant and active research concerning the addition of random effects to survival models. In this setting, a random effect is a continuous variable that describes excess risk or *frailty* for distinct categories, such as individuals or families. The idea is that individuals have different frailties, and that those who are most frail will die earlier than the others. Aalen [1] provides theoretical and practical motivation for frailty models by discussing the impact of heterogeneity on analyses, and by illustrating how random effects can deal with it. He states

> It is a basic observation of medical statistics that individuals are dissimilar. ... Still, there is a tendency to regard this variation as a nuisance, and not as something to be considered seriously in its own right. Statisticians are often accused of being more interested in averages, and there is some truth to this.

Aalen shows that with a sufficiently important frailty the population relative risk can go from r to $1/r$ over time, even though the true relative risk stays at r.

As an example of the possiblity of reversing risks, assume that we have a treatment for multiple recurrent infections. Unknown to us, the population is stratified as follows.

Proportion	Rate	Drug Effect
.4	1/year	.5
.4	2/year	.5
.2	10/year	.2

The drug is very effective for the majority of patients, reducing the rate of infections by half. There is a subset of relatively intractable patients with severe disease, however, for which it is less effective but still quite worthwhile, reducing the infection rate by 20%. A study is planned with one year of followup per patient, 1,000 subjects per arm. Assuming that infections follow a simple Poisson process with the above rates, we can compute the expected number of subjects who will finish the year with 0, 1, ... events directly.

	Number of Infections					
	0	1	2	3	4	5+
Placebo	201	256	182	98	46	217
Treatment	390	269	106	35	18	182

For a patient with two infections already, what is the chance of a third? In the placebo arm it is $361/543 = 66\%$ and for the treatment arm the chance of another infection within the year is $235/341 = 69\%$, higher than the placebo group! Among those with four events, 68% of the placebo and 91% of the treated group have a fifth. This reflects an important medical question for the treating physician — if a patient continues to fail on treatment, should treatment be stopped? The above data would seem to indicate yes, even though we know the contrary to be true; this drug helps every patient. The problem is that the treatment arm's "2 events or more" group is dominated by the severe disease patients, 58%, while the placebo group is 37% severe disease patients at that point. Methods that can account for this unmeasured heterogeneity would be very useful.

9.2 Computation

Computationally, frailties are usually viewed as an unobserved covariate. This has led to the use of the EM algorithm as an estimation tool; see, for example, Klein [76], Nielsen et al. [113], Guo and Rodríguez [57], Hougaard [67], and several others. However, the algorithm is slow, proper variance estimates require further computation, and no implementation has appeared in any of the more widely available packages. Section 9.6 shows that the computation can be approached instead as a penalized Cox model; the general framework for penalized survival models in S-Plus along with its application to smoothing splines was discussed in Section 5.5. Penalized models are not yet an option in `phreg`.

A simple random effects scenario, and the main one currently supported in S-Plus, is the shared frailty model. Assume that each subject i, $i = 1, \ldots, n$ is a member of a single group j, $j = 1, \ldots, q$, for example, a set of family members from q pedigrees. Write the proportional hazards model as

$$\lambda_i(t) = \lambda_0(t) e^{X_i\beta + Z_i\omega},$$

(cf equation (5.11)), where X_i and Z_i are the ith rows of covariate matrices $X_{n\times p}$ and $Z_{n\times p}$ respectively. X and β correspond to p fixed effects in the model (covariates such as age, gender, etc.), ω is a vector containing the q unknown random effects or frailties, and Z is a design matrix — Z_{ij} equals 1 if subject i is a member of family j, 0 otherwise. Z has the same form as the design matrix in a one-way analysis of variance. Then

- a penalized Cox model with penalty function $p(\omega) = (1/\theta)\sum[\omega_i - \exp(\omega_i)]$ is equivalent to the gamma frailty model discussed in Klein [76] and in Nielsen et al. [113]. The ω_is are distributed as the logs of iid gamma random variables and the tuning parameter θ is their variance. For this frailty distribution, the correlation of subjects within groups (Kendall's tau) is $\theta/(2+\theta)$;

- a penalized Cox model with penalty function $p(\omega) = (1/2\theta)\sum\omega_i^2$ is equivalent to the Gaussian random effects model of McGilchrist and Aisbett [102], where again the tuning parameter θ of the penalty function is the variance of the ω_is.

The exact connection between gamma frailty and a penalized model holds only for the shared frailty case, but the Gaussian correspondence holds for general Z. The fact that both penalties are the loglikelihood for a random sample of $\omega_1, \ldots, \omega_q$ from the appropriate distribution raises the question of whether other frailty distributions can be accommodated within the penalized framework.

From the viewpoint of the penalized fitting procedure θ is a nuisance or "tuning" parameter of the computation. The `coxph` function supports several options for selecting the variance.

- The variance can be a fixed parameter set by the user, either set directly, or chosen indirectly by specifying the degrees of freedom for the random effects term. Since the random effect is a penalized version of a factor variable, the degrees of freedom range from 0 for a variance of $\theta = 0$ (infinite penalty) to q, the number of random effects, when the variance is infinite (no penalty). The df is computed as the trace of the appropriate matrix, just as for a smoothing spline. Hodges and Sargent [66] investigate this relationship between degrees of freedom and the variance of random effects for a linear mixed model.

- The program can seek an overall best variance by minimizing Akiake's Information Criterion (AIC) or a corrected AIC [69]. The corrected AIC uses a much larger penalty as the number of parameters approaches the sample size n, leading to somewhat smaller models and avoiding pathological AIC solutions that can arise when the sample size is small. In the `coxph` program the total number of events in the data set is used for n in the corrected AIC formula, making it

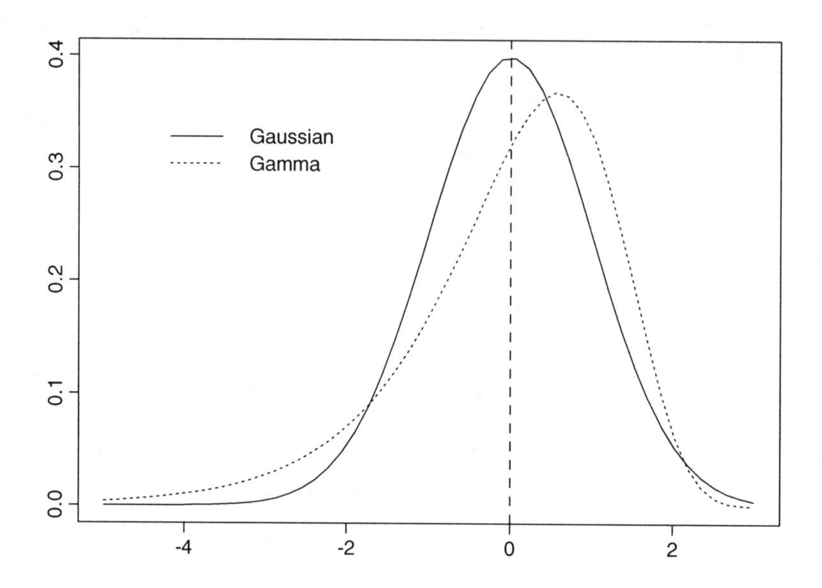

FIGURE 9.1: *Assumed density of the random effect, gamma and Gaussian distributions*

invariant to the particulars of how a data set is divided into observations.

- For the gamma frailty, the profile likelihood for θ can be used. This gives a global solution that is identical to the EM algorithm for a shared gamma frailty model. It is the default when a gamma distribution is chosen for the frailty term.
- When a Gaussian distribution of the frailty is chosen, the variance θ of the random effect can be chosen based on an approximate REML equation. This is the default choice for Gaussian frailties.

The assumed random effect density for the log of a gamma and Gaussian distributions is shown in Figure 9.1, with both densities scaled to have mean zero and variance one. The horizontal axis is ω, the loghazard scale. Unlike the Gaussian, the gamma distribution is asymmetric on this scale, implying that although most of the population has frailty near 0, there is a portion with large negative values (i.e., families with exceptionally low risk). This may or may not be plausible; for instance, in a study of a genetic disease we might presume a few families with outlying high risk corresponding to a rare but high-risk allele, but be less willing to assume genetic immortality.

To illustrate the computations we consider a data set of litter-matched rats. The data are presented in Mantel et al. [99], and are used to illustrate the frailty computation in Nielsen et al. [113]. There are 50 litters of 3 rats each, one of which received a potentially tumorgenic treatment; 40/150 rats developed a tumor during followup. The near balance of the data set makes the estimate of treatment effect nearly invariant to the value chosen for θ; making random effects models rather unexciting. Below are the marginal model and gamma frailty fits.

```
> fitw <- coxph(Surv(time, status) ~ rx + cluster(litter),
                  data=rats)
> print(fitw)

    coef exp(coef) se(coef) robust se    z      p
rx 0.905      2.47    0.318     0.303 2.99 0.0028

Likelihood ratio test=7.98  on 1 df, p=0.00474  n= 150
> print(fitw$loglik)
[1] -185.6556 -181.6677

> fitf <- coxph(Surv(time, status) ~ rx + frailty(litter),
                  data=rats)
> print(fitf)
                 coef se(coef)   se2 Chisq   DF      p
              rx 0.914 0.323    0.319  8.01  1.0 0.0046
frailty(litter)                       17.69 14.4 0.2400

Iterations: 6 outer, 19 Newton-Raphson
     Variance of random effect= 0.499   I-likelihood = -180.8
Degrees of freedom for terms=  1.0 14.4
Likelihood ratio test=37.6  on 15.38 df, p=0.00124  n= 150

> print(fitf$loglik)
[1] -185.6556 -166.8325
```

The first fit treats each litter as a cluster, and is directly comparable to the analysis of paired eyes used for the diabetic retinopathy data; see Section 8.4.2. The LR test statistic of 7.98 is twice the difference between the log partial-likelihood of the model with $\hat{\beta} = 0$ (-185.66) and that for the final fit (-181.67). The second fit, a gamma frailty fit, gives essentially the same treatment coefficient and standard error as the marginal model. The variance of the random effect is estimated to be 0.499, corresponding to 14.4 degrees of freedom. (To exactly match the results of Nielsen, redo the fit using the Breslow approximation for ties.) Kendall's tau for the the within-litter correlation would be estimated as $\theta/(\theta + 2) = .2$. In general, the treatment coefficients are not be expected to be the same in the marginal and frailty models, as they are estimating different quantities unless the within-litter correlation is zero. The marginal model estimates the population averaged relative risk due to treatment; that is, the risk of a random sample of treated rats relative to a random sample of untreated, and the frailty model estimates the relative risk within litters.

The program required 6 "outer loop" estimates of θ, with an average of 3 Newton–Raphson iterations per θ for the inner Newton–Raphson loop, which solves for the treatment and litter coefficients given θ. The EM algorithm for this data set requires on the order of 150 iterations.

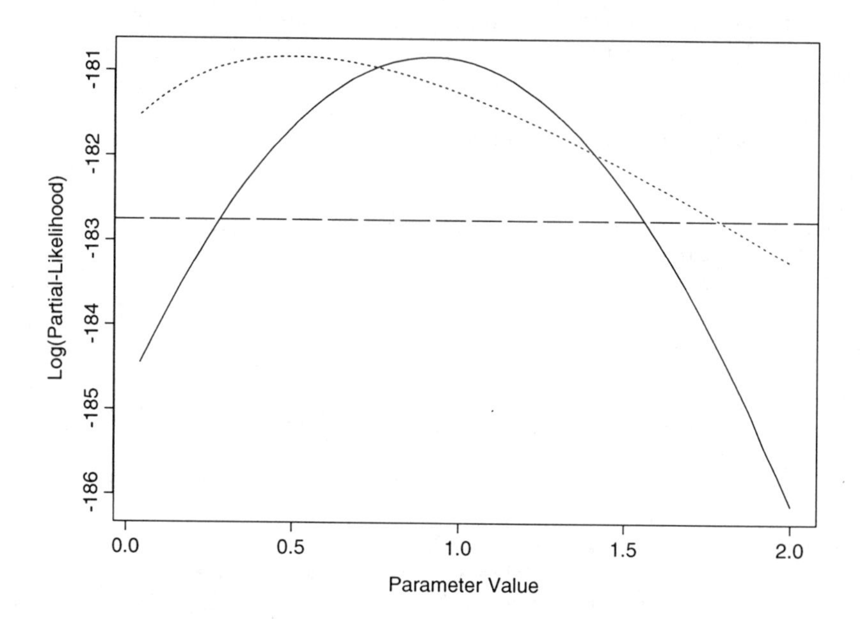

FIGURE 9.2: *Profile likelihoods for the treatment parameter β (solid line) and for the random effect variance θ (dashed line)*

An approximate Wald test for the frailty is 17.7 on 14.4 degrees of freedom. It is $\omega' V_{22} \omega$, where V_{22} is the lower right $q \times q$ portion of the variance matrix H^{-1}, and H is minus the Hessian of the penalized Cox partial log-likelihood, equation (5.13). (It is assumed that the user does not want to have all 50 per-litter ω coefficients printed out by default.) A likelihood ratio test for the frailty is twice the difference between the log partial-likelihood with the frailty terms integrated out, shown as "I-likelihood" in the printout, and the loglikelihood of a no-frailty model, or $2(181.7 - 180.8) = 1.8$. It has one degree of freedom and p-value $= 0.18$, similar to the Wald test. Formal justification for the approximate Wald test of the frailty term is lacking: it can be derived by the same arguments used for penalized splines in Section 5.8.1, although they assume fixed θ, rather than an estimated θ, as here. Nonetheless it seems to do fairly well as a general guide; the likelihood ratio test is preferred for formal assessment of θ.

The printed "LR test" for the model as a whole is the difference between the (unpenalized) log partial-likelihoods at the final and initial values of the full set of $p+q$ parameters. The likelihood at the initial values of $\beta = 0$, $\omega = 0$ is obviously the same as that for a nonfrailty model at $\beta = 0$. As shown in Gray [56], the actual distribution of this test is a weighted sum of chi-squares; the p-value based on a single chi-square with 15.38 degrees of freedom is somewhat conservative.

Figure 9.2 shows the profile likelihoods for the treatment parameter β and for the frailty parameter θ on a common scale. Each is the result of 50 separate fits to the data; those for computing the treatment profile treat β as an offset term ranging from .04 to 2 and maximize over θ, those for the θ profile treat the frailty variance as fixed and maximize over the treatment parameter β; as follows.

```
> for (i in 1:50) {
    a <- .04 *i
    fit1 <- coxph(Surv(time, status) ~ offset(rx *a) +
                              frailty(litter), rats)
    fit2 <- coxph(Surv(time, status) ~ rx +
                              frailty(litter, theta=a),  rats)
    }
```

The figure includes a horizontal line 3.84/2 units below the maximum value of the curves; the intersection of the profile likelihood with this curve is a 95% confidence interval for the parameter.

- The 95% confidence interval for the treatment effect is (0.28, 1.56), almost identical to the confidence interval of $0.914 \pm 1.96(.323) = (.28, 1.55)$ given by the usual printout. This will not always be the case; the standard error for treatment in the model `fitf` is computed assuming that the tuning parameter of the penalty function (i.e., θ), is fixed when in fact it is a parameter to be estimated. However, the balanced design of the rat data makes the estimate of β nearly orthogonal to that of θ. The value at $\theta = 0$ is $\hat\beta = .91$ and at $\theta = 1.8$ is $\hat\beta = .95$.
- The 95% confidence interval for θ is (0, 1.8); there is no clear evidence for a frailty effect. The LR test for a significant frailty involves the boundary of the parameter space, but Neilson et al. [113] have shown that the one degree of freedom chi-square approximation is valid. The profile loglikelihood for a transformed parameter, either $\sqrt{\theta}$ or $\rho = \theta/(\theta + 2)$ would be more quadratic in shape, and should lead to faster convergence of the computing algorithm. The asymmetry also shows that $\hat\theta \pm 1.96\,\mathrm{se}(\hat\theta)$ will not be an accurate 95% confidence interval.
- The treatment parameter β can be estimated more precisely than the frailty parameter. A frailty variance of 2 is a very large biological effect; using $\sqrt{\mathcal{E}(\omega_i - \omega_j)^2}$ as the "average" distance between two subjects randomly chosen from different litters, this implies an average $\exp(2) = 7.4$-fold difference in risk between random selections. Treating 0–2 as the a priori plausible range for θ, the confidence interval from the rat litter data set is able to exclude only a fraction of the values.

A Gaussian random effect can be fit as

```
> coxph(Surv(time, status) ~ rx +frailty(litter, dist='gaussian'),
                      data=rats)

                          coef se(coef)   se2 Chisq   DF      p
                       rx 0.913 0.323   0.319  8.01  1.0 0.0046
frailty(litter, dist = "g                      15.57 11.9 0.2100
```

```
Iterations: 6 outer, 16 Newton-Raphson
     Variance of random effect= 0.412
Degrees of freedom for terms=  1.0 11.9
Likelihood ratio test=35.3  on 12.87 df, p=0.000712  n= 150

> coxph(Surv(time, status) ~ rx +
                 frailty(litter, dist='gauss', method='aic'),
                                  data=rats)

                           coef se(coef)   se2 Chisq   DF      p
                        rx 0.924 0.326   0.321  8.02  1.0 0.0046
frailty(litter, dist = "g                       23.40 17.2 0.1400

Iterations: 4 outer, 13 Newton-Raphson
     Variance of random effect= 0.711
Degrees of freedom for terms=  1.0 17.2
Likelihood ratio test=46.0  on 18.13 df, p=0.000323  n= 150
```

The first fit chooses the value of $\hat{\theta}$ using a REML criterion. The second fit uses Akaike's information criterion to choose the variance of the random effect, that is, it maximizes the value of (LR test − df), two quantities that are printed on the last line. The AIC method has given a larger estimated frailty variance, but given the uncertainty in $\hat{\theta}$ with this small data set, no meaningful interpretation can be given to the difference in the solutions. The integrated likelihood is not (yet) printed for Gaussian frailties; it can be computed by equation (9.13).

Which frailty distribution/variance selection combination is best for everyday work is not yet clear.

9.3 Examples

9.3.1 Random institutional effect

The data set `lung` contains survival times for advanced lung cancer patients enrolled in trials within the North Central Cancer Treatment Group. Because the enrolling institutions range from community practices to a large tertiary care center, differences in the baseline risk of enrollees might be a concern. There are 18 separate institutions that enrolled at least one subject in the trials.

```
> table(lung$inst)
  1 2  3 4 5  6 7 10 11 12 13 15 16 21 22 26 32 33 NA
 36 5 19 4 9 14 8  4 18 23 20  6 16 13 17  6  7  2  1
```

Can we do a restricted adjustment for institution?

```
> coxph(Surv(time, status) ~ sex + ph.karno + pat.karno,
                           data=lung)

                coef exp(coef) se(coef)      z      p
       sex -0.51178     0.599  0.16927 -3.023 0.0025
  ph.karno -0.00616     0.994  0.00682 -0.903 0.3700
 pat.karno -0.01702     0.983  0.00653 -2.605 0.0092

Likelihood ratio test=22.9  on 3 df, p=4.21e-05

> coxph(Surv(time, status) ~ sex + ph.karno + pat.karno
                  + factor(inst), data=lung)

                    coef exp(coef) se(coef)      z      p
           sex -0.5197    0.5947  0.17635 -2.947 0.0032
      ph.karno -0.0108    0.9892  0.00726 -1.494 0.1400
     pat.karno -0.0190    0.9812  0.00686 -2.770 0.0056
 factor(inst)2  0.5159    1.6752  0.54269  0.951 0.3400
 factor(inst)3 -0.4168    0.6592  0.33146 -1.257 0.2100
    ...
Likelihood ratio test=42.4  on 20 df, p=0.00244

> coxph(Surv(time, status) ~ sex + ph.karno + pat.karno +
                 frailty(inst, df=9), data=lung)

                            coef se(coef)     se2 Chisq   DF      p
                  sex -0.50823 0.17187  0.17051  8.74 1.00 0.0031
             ph.karno -0.00867 0.00706  0.00688  1.51 1.00 0.2200
            pat.karno -0.01822 0.00670  0.00661  7.39 1.00 0.0066
frailty(inst, df = 9)                           10.62 8.94 0.3000

Iterations: 3 outer, 10 Newton-Raphson
     Variance of random effect= 0.163    I likelihood = -714.1
Degrees of freedom for terms= 1.0 1.0 1.0 8.9
Likelihood ratio test=37.3  on 11.85 df, p=0.000179
```

The model with institution as a factor or "class" variable has 17 degrees of freedom for the 18 enrolling clinics, and the first model has none. The random effects model was chosen to be intermediate between the two of them with 9 df for institution. In this particular data example the gain in df is not very compelling, however; some large trials may have over 100 enrolling centers in which case the limitation to fewer degrees of freedom is desirable.

The standard errors of the coefficients for the frailty model are based on the assumption that the variance of the frailty is fixed. Because of the one to one relationship between degrees of freedom and the frailty variance, for any given data set, choosing the degrees of freedom also fixes the variance. Thus, the standard error estimates for the other coefficients such as `sex` are justified. The relationship between df and θ is not available in closed form, however. For any given value of θ, the penalized problem is solved and then the degrees of freedom can be computed post hoc from a matrix trace; the program may need to attempt several values of θ before matching the specified df, but this is only a computational issue (in this case, three attempts before getting "close enough" with 8.9 df).

9.4 Unordered events

9.4.1 Diabetic retinopathy data

The four models below are a marginal, stratified, gamma frailty, and Gaussian frailty model for the diabetic retinopathy data set.

```
> coxph(Surv(time, status) ~ trt + adult + cluster(id), diabetes)
          coef exp(coef) se(coef) robust se      z       p
  trt -0.7789      0.459    0.169     0.149 -5.245 1.6e-07
adult  0.0539      1.055    0.162     0.179  0.302 7.6e-01

Likelihood ratio test=22.5  on 2 df, p=1.31e-05  n= 394

> coxph(Surv(time, status) ~ trt +adult + strata(id), diabetes)
        coef exp(coef) se(coef)     z       p
  trt -0.962     0.382    0.202 -4.77 1.8e-06
adult     NA        NA    0.000    NA      NA

Likelihood ratio test=25.5  on 1 df, p=4.45e-07  n= 394

> coxph(Surv(time, status) ~ trt +  adult + frailty(id),
                        data=diabetes)

              coef se(coef)    se2  Chisq DF       p
         trt -0.911 0.174    0.171  27.31  1 1.7e-07
       adult  0.041 0.221    0.166   0.03  1 8.5e-01
frailty(id)                        113.79 84 1.7e-02

Iterations: 6 outer, 24 Newton-Raphson
     Variance of random effect= 0.851   I-likelihood = -850.8
Degrees of freedom for terms=  1.0  0.6 84.0
Likelihood ratio test=201  on 85.56 df, p=2.77e-11  n= 394

> coxph(Surv(time, status) ~ trt +  adult +
                        frailty(id, dist='Gauss'), data=diabetes)
```

```
               coef se(coef)   se2  Chisq   DF        p
       trt -0.8991 0.174    0.171  26.65  1.0 2.4e-07
     adult  0.0602 0.209    0.163   0.08  1.0 7.7e-01
frailty(id)                        109.02 71.5 2.8e-03

Iterations: 6 outer, 19 Newton-Raphson
     Variance of random effect= 0.774
Degrees of freedom for terms=  1.0  0.6 71.5
Likelihood ratio test=197  on 73.03 df, p=2.9e-13  n= 394
```

The Gaussian and gamma frailty models both estimate a substantial random effect for subject, of size 0.77 and 0.85, respectively. The estimated size of the treatment coefficient increases with the variance of the random effect, as is expected theoretically [64], but only by a small amount. The stratified model, which treats each adult as a separate stratum, is the most aggressive correction for possible correlation, and has the largest treatment effect but also the largest variance. The adult/juvenile covariate is not estimable in the stratified model, since the covariate value is constant within a given stratum.

The UDCA dataset is another case where data already known about the study would lead us to anticipate a large variance for the random effect, and in fact this is so. For a gamma frailty model $\hat{\theta} = 1.54$.

9.4.2 Familial aggregation of breast cancer

The aggregation of breast cancer within families has been the focus of investigation for at least a century [25]. There is clear evidence that both genetic and environmental factors are important, but despite literally hundreds of studies, it is estimated that less than 50% of the cancer cases can be accounted for by known risk factors. The Minnesota Breast Cancer Family Resource is a unique collection of 426 families, first identified by V. Elving Anderson and colleagues at the Dight Institute for Human Genetics as a consecutive series of patients seen between 1944 and 1952 [8]. Baseline information on probands, relatives (parents, aunts and uncles, sisters and brothers, sons and daughters) was obtained by interviews, followup letters, and telephone calls. Sellers et al. [133] have recently extended the followup of all pedigrees through 1995 as part of an ongoing research program, 98.2% of the families agreed to further participation. There are currently 6,663 relatives and 5,185 marry-ins in the cohort, with over 350,000 person-years of followup. A total of 1,053 breast and 161 ovarian cancers have been observed.

Age is the natural time scale for the baseline risk. Figure 9.3 shows breast cancer incidence as a function of age, based on the Iowa SEER registry for 1973 to 1977 [142]. The followup for most of the familial members starts at age 18, that for marry-ins to the families begins at the age that they married into the family tree.

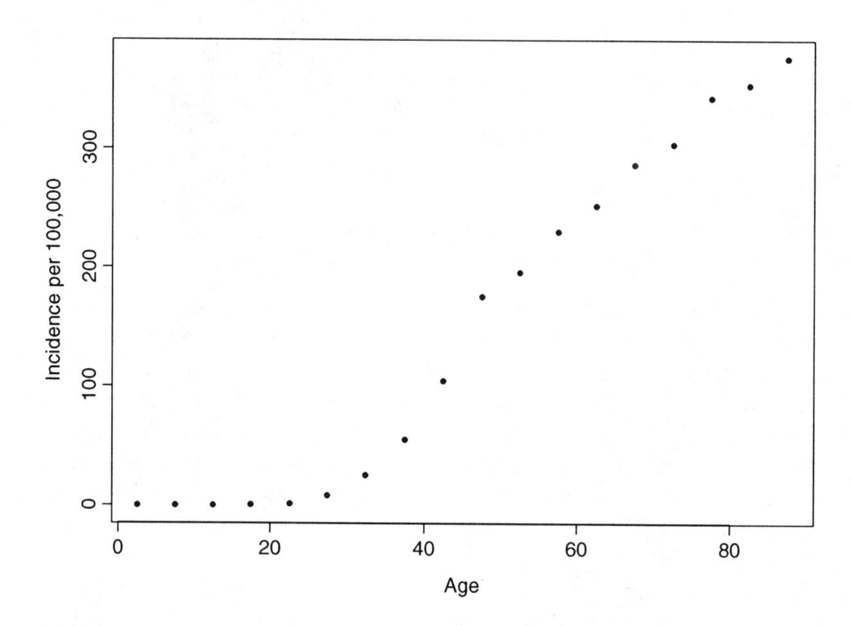

FIGURE 9.3: *Breast cancer incidence rates*

For efficiency, many of the proposed screening studies focus first on the highest risk subjects and/or families. One selection criterion is to use those families with the largest number of breast and/or ovarian cancers. However, this does not take into account family size, the age-intervals of followup, or the ages at which cancers occurred. An alternative which does take those factors into account is to fit a random effects model with one "frailty" per family, and then rank the families by the size of the estimated frailty coefficient. This has the further advantage that it allows the model to control for other important but non-genetic factors such as parity (number of children). Those who have married into the pedigrees are each treated as a separate family of size 1; the mean frailty coefficient for these subjects is taken as the "population" value to which the realized familial coefficients can be compared. In the code below, this is done by creating a variable `id2` which is equal to the family id (a unique three digit number assigned to each pedigree) for the descendants and to 1,000 + subject id for the marry-ins. Some subjects are deleted due to a missing value for parity; this leaves 422 families and 3,961 marry-ins.

```
> table(is.na(cohort$parity), cohort$relation)

      daughter granddaughter marry in niece sister
FALSE      553          1519     3961  2394    552
 TRUE        5             2       39    24     24
```

```
> id2 <- ifelse(cohort$relation=='marry in', 1000 + cohort$id,
                                             cohort$famid)
> ffit <- coxph(Surv(startage, endage, bcancer) ~ parity +
                     frailty(id2, dist='Gaussian'), data=cohort)
> ffit
                  coef se(coef)   se2  Chisq  DF      p
     parity -0.333 0.123     0.121   7.31   1 0.0069
frailty(id2)                        224.00 173 0.0053

Iterations: 5 outer, 18 Newton-Raphson
     Variance of random effect= 0.385
Degrees of freedom for terms=   1 173
Likelihood ratio test=395  on 173.79 df, p=0
  n=8979 (94 observations deleted due to missing)

> length(ffit$frail)
  4383
>> jitplot(ncancer, exp(ffit$frail[1:422]))
```

The parity variable is 1 for those women with 1 or more offspring and 0 for nulliparous women. It is a powerful effect, reducing risk by nearly a third. (A more complete analysis would also consider the age at first birth and the total number of children.) The per-family risks after adjusting for parity are given in Figure 9.4, showing a plot of the random effects, $\hat{\omega}$s, using the frailty scale (e^{ω}) as the y-axis label since that is easily interpretable as relative risk and is familiar to physicians. The random effects under a Gaussian model are constrained to have mean 0; the average value for the marry-in cases was -0.005. Two of the points are labeled by their family identifier. There have been five identified breast/ovarian cancers in family 115 among 33 blood relatives (not counting the initial index case), but the overall risk estimate for the family is below the average of the marry-in subjects. A simple count of breast/ovarian cancers would have placed this family in the high risk group. Family 574 is estimated to have high risk; there are two breast cancers and only three blood relatives, and one of the cancers occured before the age of 35.

A marginal fit gives a very similar estimate of the parity effect with about the same standard error.

```
> coxph(formula = Surv(startage, endage, bcancer) ~ parity +
                  cluster(famid), data=cohort)


         coef exp(coef) se(coef) robust se     z      p
parity -0.343      0.71     0.12     0.122 -2.80 0.0066
```

9.5 Ordered events

9.5.1 *Hidden covariate data*

The hidden covariate data set is a simulation introduced in Section 8.5.3 to investigate the performance of marginal models under a particular kind of model misspecification. The test data sets were in effect simulations from

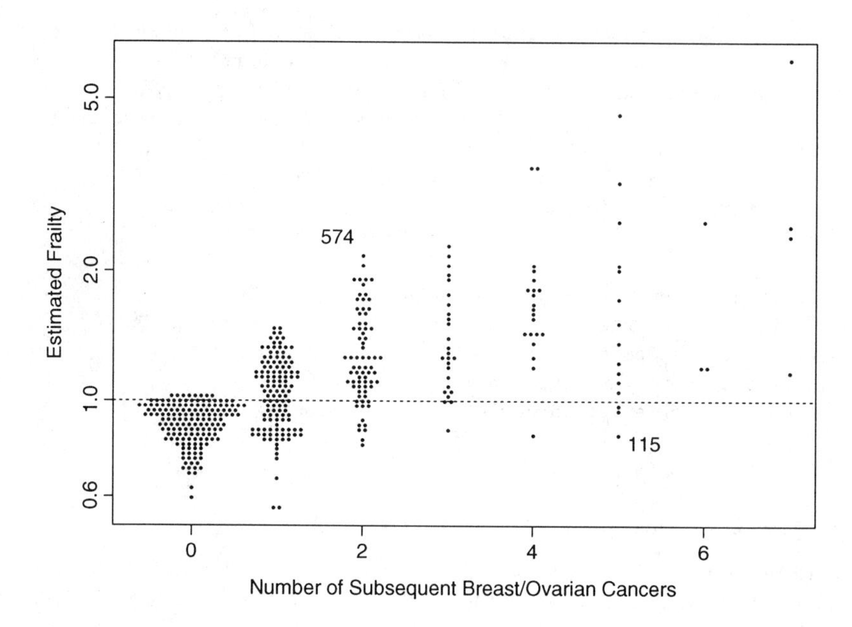

FIGURE 9.4: *Estimated excess risk for each of 422 families*

a frailty model, where the random effect or "hidden covariate" is from a uniform(−1,1) distribution, which is mean 0 with a variance of 4/12.

Figure 9.5 shows the result of 1,000 simulated data sets, fitting an AG model, an AG model with gamma frailty, and an AG model with gamma frailty and known θ, as follows.

```
> fita <- coxph(Surv(start, stop, status) ~ x1 + cluster(id))
> fitb <- coxph(Surv(start, stop, status) ~ x1 + frailty(id))
> fitc <- coxph(Surv(start, stop, status) ~ x1 +
                                 frailty(id, theta=.33))
```

The simulations used the same random number seed as Figure 8.5 and so are directly comparable. The two solid curves on the plot are the results shown earlier in Section 8.5.3; the AG model with the hidden covariate x_2 known, "AG + x" in the plot, is the gold-standard for the simulation: all the information is known and incorporated properly into the model. The second solid curve is for the AG model without knowlege of x_2; the density of $\hat{\beta}$ is biased towards the right and has a larger variance. The two densities corresponding to the fit of a gamma frailty with an estimated variance and with a known variance of 4/12 are nearly identical. The addition of a frailty term has almost completely rectified the bias, at the price of some increase in variance over the AG fit. The estimated MSE for the treatment coefficient in the four fits are .020, .036, .037, and .034, respectively. The performance of the random effects model is exciting. Figure 9.6 shows the concordance between the actual value of x_i for one of the simulated data sets and the "reconstructed" value ω_i for a given subject. The realization has 306 events for 100 subjects; 8, 20, 19, 13, 11, 9, and 20 subjects have 0, 1, ..., 6 events, respectively. The frailty model has reconstructed the

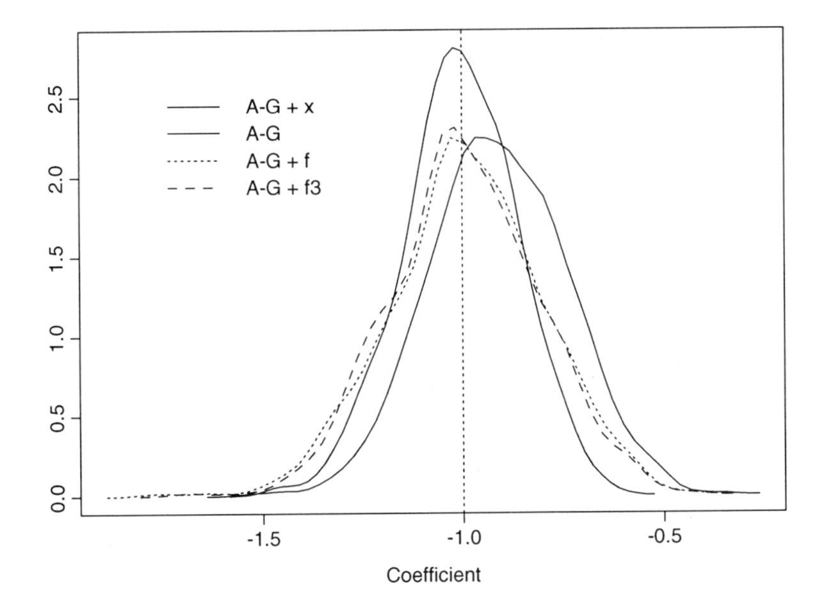

FIGURE 9.5: *Andersen–Gill models fit to the hidden covariate data*

missing covariate sufficiently well to remove bias, but with far from perfect accuracy.

Figure 9.7 shows the corresponding curves for the conditional model. The fit with x known is, as noted before, almost identical to the AG fit with x known. It is essentially unbiased, while the density for a conditional fit without x is seriously shifted to the right. Addition of a frailty term with known variance of 1/3 again almost completely removes the bias. Addition of a frailty term with unknown variance is not very successful, it removes some of the bias, but with substantially larger variance than the other methods. Table 9.1 reveals that the conditional fit estimated a no-frailty model 92% of the time, with the remainder of the estimates scattered from .05 to .65. The frailty variance estimated from an Andersen–Gill model, however, is much more tightly clustered about the true value of 1/3.

9.5.2 *Survival of kidney catheters*

The following data set is presented in McGilchrist and Aisbett [102], and has been used by several authors to illustrate frailty. Each observation is the time to infection, at the point of insertion of the catheter, for kidney patients using portable dialysis equipment. Catheters may be removed for reasons other than infection, in which case the observation is censored. There are 38 patients, each with exactly two observations. Variables are the subject id, age, sex (1 = male, 2 = female), disease type (glomerulo nephritis, acute nephritis, polycystic kidney disease, and other), and the time to infection or censoring for each insertion. We first fit two ordinary Cox models, followed by a gamma frailty fit.

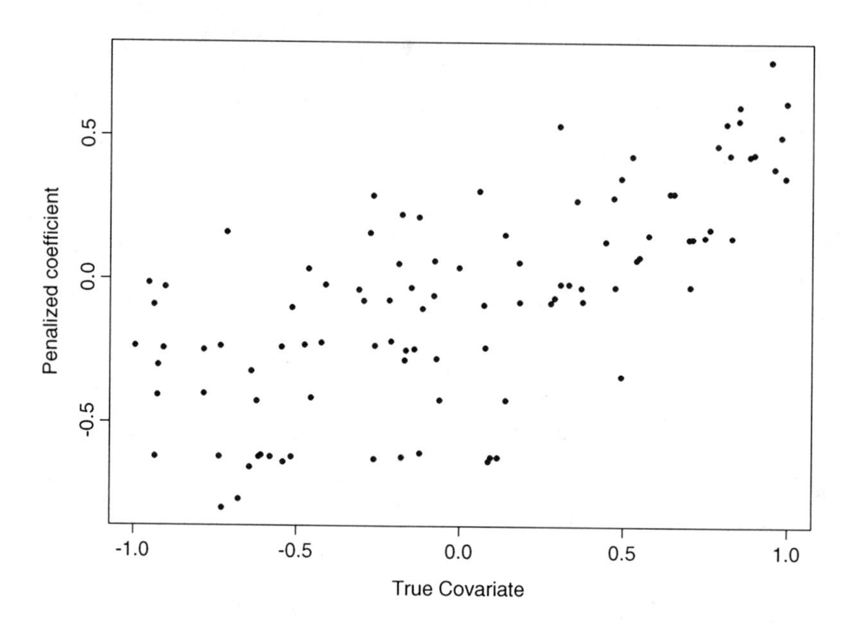

FIGURE 9.6: *Correlation between the actual and "reconstructed" covariates*

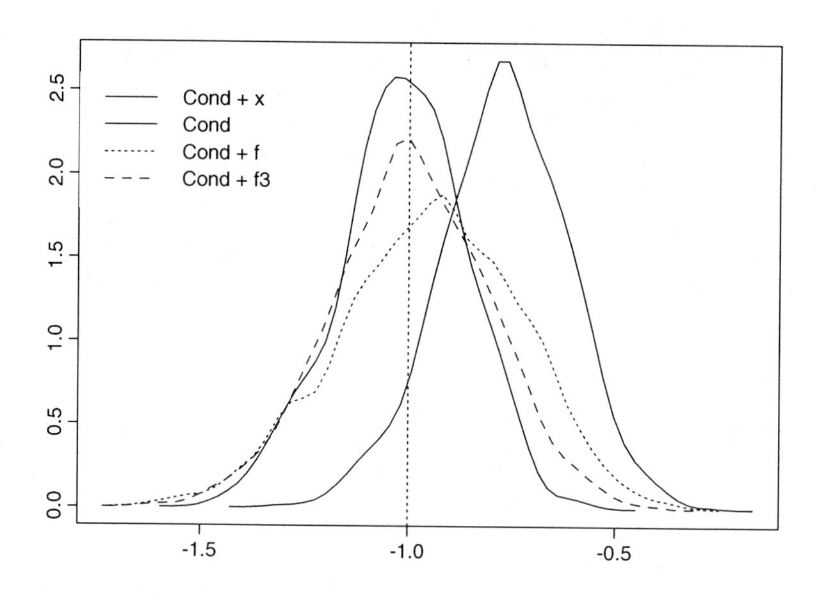

FIGURE 9.7: *Conditional models fit to the hidden covariate data*

	Andersen–Gill	Conditional
0–.1	9	921
.1–.2	106	14
.2–.25	125	5
.25–.3	190	7
.3–.35	197	10
.35–.4	152	5
.4–.5	160	8
.5–.6	42	11
.6+	9	18

TABLE 9.1: *Distribution of the estimated frailty variance θ in 1,000 simulations*

```
> kfit1 <- coxph(Surv(time, status) ~ age + sex, data=kidney)
> kfit2 <- coxph(Surv(time, status) ~ age + sex + disease,
                data=kidney)
> kfit3 <-  coxph(Surv(time, status) ~ age + sex + disease +
                                         frailty(id), data=kidney)
> kfit3
                 coef se(coef)    se2 Chisq DF       p
        age  0.00318 0.0111   0.0111  0.08 1  7.8e-01
        sex -1.48314 0.3582   0.3582 17.14 1  3.5e-05
  diseaseGN  0.08796 0.4064   0.4064  0.05 1  8.3e-01
  diseaseAN  0.35079 0.3997   0.3997  0.77 1  3.8e-01
diseasePKD -1.43111 0.6311   0.6311  5.14 1  2.3e-02
frailty(id)                           0.00 0  9.5e-01

Iterations: 6 outer, 29 Newton-Raphson
Penalized terms:
     Variance of random effect= 1.47e-07   I-likelihood = -179.1
Degrees of freedom for terms= 1 1 3 0
Likelihood ratio test=17.6  on 5 df, p=0.00342  n= 76
```

The partial likelihood values for first two models are -184.3 and -179.1, with two and five degrees of freedom, respectively. Hence, the disease variable is a significant addition. In the third fit, the program provided an estimate of the MLE of θ, the variance of the random effect, that is, essentially 0.

When the disease variable is left out of the random effects model, however, we get a quite different result.

```
> kfit4 <- coxph(Surv(time, status) ~ age + sex + frailty(id),
        data=kidney)
> kfit4
                 coef se(coef)    se2 Chisq   DF       p
        age  0.00522 0.0119   0.0088  0.19  1.0 0.66000
        sex -1.58335 0.4594   0.3515 11.88  1.0 0.00057
frailty(id)                          22.97 12.9 0.04100

Iterations: 7 outer, 49 Newton-Raphson
     Variance of random effect= 0.408   I-likelihood = -181.6
Degrees of freedom for terms=  0.6  0.6 12.9
Likelihood ratio test=46.6  on 14.06 df, p=2.36e-05  n= 76
```

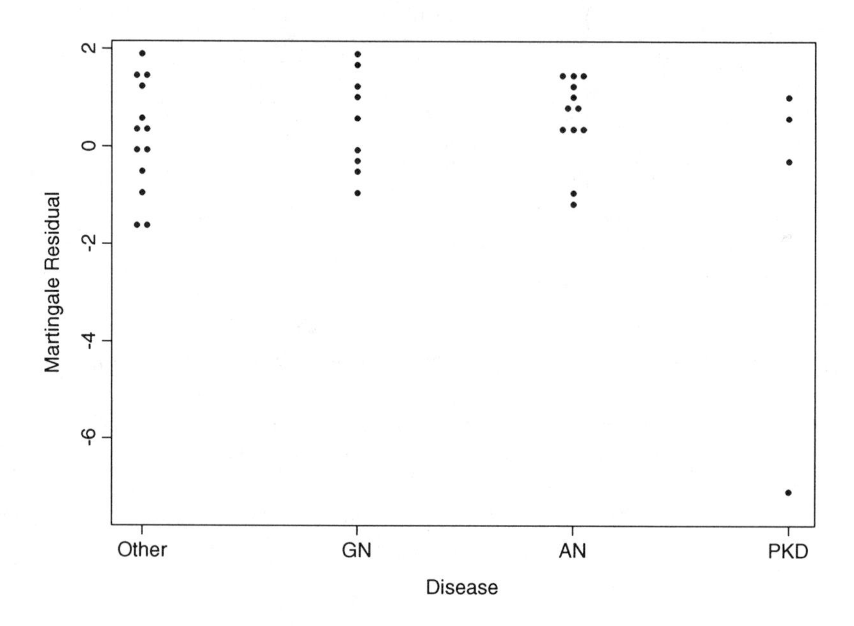

FIGURE 9.8: *Residuals for the kidney data, from model 1*

```
> kfit1$loglik
[1] -187.9028 -184.3446
```

The likelihood ratio test for significance of the frailty is −184.3 vs. −181.6, which gives a chi-square statistic of 5.4 on one degree of freedom for a p-value of 0.02. In this case, both the approximate Wald test and the likelihood ratio test indicate that the variance of the random effect is greater than zero.

Figure 9.8 shows the reason for the between the fits with and without disease type. The graph shows the martingale residuals for each subject (the sum of the residuals from the two observations), based on the simplest model, `kfit1`. Note the outlier in the lower right. The subject, number 21, is a 46-year-old male, whose age is quite close to the median for the study (45.5 years). There were 10 males and most had early failures: 2 observations were censored at 4 and 8 days, respectively, and the remaining 16 male kidneys had a median time to infection of 19 days. Subject 21, however, had failures at 154 and 562 days. With this subject removed, neither the disease (p=0.53) nor the frailty (p>0.9) is important. With this subject in the model, it is a toss-up whether the disease or the frailty term will be credited with "significance." Using a Gaussian frailty with REML gives partial importance to each.

```
> mfit1 <- coxph(Surv(time, status) ~ age + sex + disease +
                 frailty(id, dist='Gauss'), data=kidney)
```

```
> mfit1
                 coef se(coef)     se2 Chisq   DF       p
        age   0.00489 0.015    0.0106  0.11  1.0 0.74000
        sex  -1.69727 0.461    0.3617 13.56  1.0 0.00023
  diseaseGN   0.17985 0.545    0.3927  0.11  1.0 0.74000
  diseaseAN   0.39294 0.545    0.3982  0.52  1.0 0.47000
 diseasePKD  -1.13633 0.825    0.6173  1.90  1.0 0.17000
frailty(id)                           17.89 12.1 0.12000

Iterations: 8 outer, 32 Newton-Raphson
Penalized terms:
     Variance of random effect= 0.493
Degrees of freedom for terms=  0.5  0.6  1.7 12.1
Likelihood ratio test=47.5  on 14.9 df, p=2.83e-05  n= 76
```

The standard error estimates reported by a penalized `coxph` model in S-Plus are computed under the assumption of θ fixed. For some models, such as a smoothing spline with user-specified degrees of freedom, this assumption is correct. For the above frailty models it clearly is not and the standard errors are an underestimate. A more correct estimate may be obtained using the bootstrap.

```
> nboot <- 100
> cmat  <- matrix(0, nboot, 5)  #coefs
> frail <- double(nboot)        #frailties

> temp <- matrix(1:76, nrow=2)
> id2  <- kidney$id
> for (i in 1:nboot) {
     # Make data set
     idlist <- sample(1:38, 38, replace=T)
     irows  <- as.vector(temp[, idlist])

     fit <- coxph(Surv(time, status) ~ age + sex + disease +
                    frailty(id2), data=kidney, subset=irows)
     cmat[i,] <- fit$coef
     frail[i] <- fit$history[[1]]$theta
     }
> quantile(frail)
   0%  25%  50%  75% 100%
    0  0.2 0.41 0.54 1.26

> round(sqrt(apply(cmat,2,var2)),3)  # bootstrap se estimate
[1] 0.012 0.642 0.481 0.406 1.206
```

The results are interesting. The estimate of frailty itself is quite variable. Comparing the standard errors of the coefficients to those based on a fixed frailty variance of 0.49 (`mfit1`), the uncertainty for `age` is virtually unchanged. This is perhaps not too surprising since subject 21 is near the center of the age distribution. The standard errors for `sex` and `PKD` are both approximately doubled, reflecting the interdependence of these coefficients with the estimated frailty effect for subject 21.

The S-Plus code above is more complex than most we have shown, and deserves some comment. At each of the `nboot=100` iterations, the code first chooses 38 subjects, with replacement, from the 38 persons in the study and stores their ids in the vector `idlist`. The row numbers of for the data corresponding to these resampled subjects are then placed in the `irows` vector, making implicit use of the fact that rows 1–2 are subject 1, rows 3–4 of the data set are subject 2's observations, and so on. Since this bootstrap resample is intended to represent, logically, a hypothetical *new* set of experimental data, the `id` variable for the fit needs to be (1,1,2,2,3,3,...,38,38), found in variable `id2`. The coefficents of the 100 fits are stored in the `cmat` matrix, and the frailty variances in the `frail` vector. The `history` component of a penalized model contains information specific to the iteration history of the outer loop of the optimization, element `[[1]]` for the first penalized term, element `[[2]]` for the second, etc.

The results of these fits differ slightly from McGilchrist's [101] results. That paper presents formulae that are completely valid only for untied data, and this data set has five tied pairs and one quadruple. This is a small proportion of the data, and in a standard Cox model the ties would barely perturb the answers. Unfortunately, the REML solution for θ can be very sensitive to small changes in the data.

9.5.3 *Chronic granulotamous disease*

In the CGD analysis presented earlier in Section 8.5.5 it was found that controlling for important covariates lessened the apparent difference between an Andersen-Gill and conditional analysis. It is of some interest to see whether a random effects model can provide a similar effect.

```
> coxph(Surv(tstart, tstop, status) ~ rx + frailty(id), cgd1)

              coef se(coef)   se2 Chisq   DF        p
         rx  -1.05 0.308    0.264 11.8   1.0 0.00061
frailty(id)                       57.1  37.9 0.02300

Iterations: 5 outer, 18 Newton-Raphson
Variance of random effect= 0.827
Degrees of freedom for terms=  0.7 37.9
Likelihood ratio test=98.8  on 38.67 df, p=3.67e-07  n= 203


> coxph(Surv(tstart, tstop, status) ~ rx + strata(enum) +
                frailty(id, theta=.827), cgd1)
```

```
              coef se(coef)    se2 Chisq   DF      p
          rx -1.05 0.329     0.283 10.3   1.0 0.0013
frailty(id)                        50.8  36.4 0.0560

Iterations: 1 outer, 5 Newton-Raphson
Variance of random effect= 0.827
Degrees of freedom for terms=  0.7 36.4
Likelihood ratio test=75.8  on 37.12 df, p=0.000181  n= 203
```

To retain comparability, the stratified fit has been constrained to use the frailty variance of .827 from the AG model fit. Under this restriction, the random effects term seems to have "reconstructed" the hidden covariates sufficiently well to synchronize the two solutions.

9.6 Formal derivations

9.6.1 *Penalized solution for shared frailty*

Assume that the data for subject i, who is a member of the jth family, follows a proportional hazards shared frailty model. In the literature, this is usually written as

$$\lambda_{i(j)}(t) = \lambda_0(t)\varpi_j e^{X_i\beta},$$

where ϖ_j is the frailty for family j. This can easily be rewritten in the form of equation (5.11), with i ranging over all subjects, $\varpi_j = \exp(\omega_j)$, and Z a matrix of indicator variables such that $Z_{ij} = 1$ iff subject i is a member of family j and 0 otherwise. In this model, each individual can belong to only one family.

Suppose that θ were known. The log penalized partial-likelihood function is $PPL(\beta, \omega, \theta) = \ell(\beta, \omega) - g(\omega, \theta)$ where

$$\begin{aligned} \ell(\beta,\omega) &= \textstyle\sum_{i=1}^n \int_0^\infty [Y_i(t)(X_i\beta + Z_i\omega) - \\ &\qquad \log\{\sum Y_k(t)\exp(X_k\beta + Z_k\omega)\}]\, dN_i(t) \end{aligned}$$

To estimate ω_j, one solves the score equation

$$\begin{aligned} \frac{\partial PPL}{\partial \omega_j} &= \frac{\partial \ell}{\partial \omega_j} - \frac{\partial g(\omega;\theta)}{\partial \omega_j} \\ &= 0. \end{aligned}$$

Let

$$\bar{z}_j(t) = \bar{z}_j(\beta,\omega,t) = \frac{\sum Z_{ij} Y_i(s)\exp[X_i\beta + Z_i\omega]}{\sum Y_i(s)\exp[X_i\beta + Z_i\omega]}. \tag{9.1}$$

Then

$$\frac{\partial \ell}{\partial \omega_j} = \sum_{i=1}^n \int_0^\infty (Z_{ij} - \bar{z}_j(t))dN_i(t).$$

To exhibit the tie-in with the EM approach, we rewrite this, assuming time-fixed covariates for notational simplicity. Note that for given β and ω,

$$d\hat{\Lambda}_0(t;\beta,\omega) = \sum dN_i(t) / \sum Y_i(t)\exp(X_i\beta + Z_i\omega)$$

[117]. Let $\hat{\lambda}_i = \hat{\lambda}_i(\beta,\omega) = \int_0^\infty Y_i(s)d\hat{\Lambda}_0(t;\beta,\omega)$. Simple algebra gives

$$\frac{\partial PPL}{\partial \omega_j} = \sum_{i=1}^n \left[Z_{ij}\delta_i - Z_{ij}\hat{\lambda}_i e^{X_i\beta + Z_i\omega} \right] - \frac{\partial g(\omega;\theta)}{\partial \omega_j} = 0. \tag{9.2}$$

The above equation can be extended to time-dependent covariates by writing the first portion as an integral with respect to $dN_i(s)$. Because of the structure of the matrix Z, equation (9.2) simplifies to

$$\frac{\partial PPL}{\partial \omega_j} = \left[d_j - \hat{A}_j e^{\omega_j} \right] - \frac{\partial g(\omega;\theta)}{\partial \omega_j} = 0, \tag{9.3}$$

where d_j represents the number of events occurring in family j, and $\hat{A}_j$ is the sum of $\hat{\lambda}_i \exp(X_i\beta)$ over all the individuals in the family.

The score equations for β, on the other hand, are identical to those for an ordinary Cox model treating $Z\omega$ as a fixed or *offset* term because β does not enter into the penalty function.

9.6.2 EM solution for shared frailty

If we think of ϖ as missing data, the problem can be approached using the EM algorithm. Parner [117] lays out a general framework which starts with a full likelihood involving λ_0 rather than with the partial-likelihood of Cox regression which is, in fact, a profile likelihood with λ_0 profiled out (see Johansen [72]). If we knew the ω_js, but not θ, the loglikelihood would be

$$\begin{aligned} \textstyle\sum_i \quad & \left[\int_0^\infty Y_i(t)[\log(\lambda_0(t)) + X_i\beta + Z_i\omega]\, dN_i(t) \right. \\ & \left. - \int_0^\infty Y_i(t)\exp[X_i\beta + Z_i\omega]\lambda_0(t)dt \right] + \log p(\omega;\theta), \end{aligned}$$

where $p(\omega;\theta)$ is the density of ω. The loglikelihood of the observed data is found by integrating over the distribution of ω. Let $\phi(s) = \phi(s,\theta)$ be the Laplace transform of the distribution of ϖ, and let $\phi^{(n)}(s)$ be its nth derivative with respect to s. Let $A_j = A_j(\beta,\lambda_0) = \sum \int_0^\infty Y_i(s)\exp(X_i\beta)d\Lambda_0(s)$, where the sum is over the members of family j and let d_j be the number of events in the jth family, as above. Parner shows that the observed data loglikelihood for shared frailty is

$$L_m(\beta,\lambda_0;\theta) = \sum_{i=1}^n \delta_i \log\left(\int_0^\infty Y_i(t)e^{X_i\beta}\lambda_0(t) \right)$$

$$+\sum_{j=1}^{q} \log[(-1)^{d_j} \phi^{(d_j)}(A_j)]. \tag{9.4}$$

For any fixed value of θ, he suggests maximizing this likelihood for β and λ_0 by the EM algorithm. It alternates between the following steps.

1. M-step. Treat the current estimate of ω as a fixed value or *offset*, and update β and λ_0 as in usual Cox regression;

2. E-step. Compute ϖ as the expected value given the current values β and λ_0 and the data.

Parner [117] shows that, for the shared frailty model, the E step is

$$e^{\omega_j} = -\frac{\phi^{(d_j+1)}(\hat{A}_j)}{\phi^{(d_j)}(\hat{A}_j)}, \tag{9.5}$$

where $\hat{A}_j = A_j(\beta, \hat{\lambda}_0(\beta, \omega))$, the same as $\hat{A}_j$ defined below equation (9.3). Equations (9.4) and (9.5) require the shared frailty model and unfortunately do not hold for more complex frailties, such as nested or crossed frailty parameters.

The estimates depend on θ and can be denoted $\hat{\beta}(\theta)$ and $\hat{\lambda}_0(\theta)$. As a side benefit, one also gets an estimate of ω, $\hat{\omega}(\theta)$. Parner suggests that estimation of θ be done by maximizing the profile loglikelihood

$$L_m(\theta) = L_m(\hat{\beta}(\theta), \hat{\lambda}_0(\theta), \theta). \tag{9.6}$$

9.6.3 Gamma frailty

Details of the EM approach for the shared gamma frailty model can be found in Nielsen et al. [113] and Klein [76]. Equations (9.5) and (9.4) can be used to rederive their results, and help make the connection to penalized methods. Let the frailty have a gamma distribution with mean 1 and variance $\theta = 1/\nu$. The log of the density function of ϖ can be written as

$$\log[f(\varpi;\nu)] = (\nu-1)\log(\varpi) - \nu\varpi + \nu\log(\nu) - \log\Gamma(\nu),$$

and the density has a Laplace transform of $\phi(s) = (1+s/\nu)^{-\nu}$. The derivatives of $\phi(s)$ are

$$\phi^{(d)}(s) = \left(-\frac{1}{\nu}\right)^d \left(1+\frac{s}{\nu}\right)^{-(\nu+d)} \prod_{i=0}^{d-1} (\nu+i),$$

and equation (9.5) reduces to

$$e^{\omega_j} = \frac{d_j+\nu}{\hat{A}_j+\nu}. \tag{9.7}$$

Note that the log of the density of ω is $[\omega - \exp(\omega)]/\theta$ plus a function of θ and

$$PPL = \ell - (1/\theta)\sum_{j=1}^{q}[\omega_j - \exp(\omega_j)]. \tag{9.8}$$

The use of a log–density as the penalty function will appear again when discussing Gaussian frailty.

Lemma: The solution to the penalized partial likelihood model with penalty function
$g(\omega;\theta) = -1/\theta\sum_{j=1}^{q}[\omega_j - \exp(\omega_j)]$ coincides with the EM solution for equation (9.4) with gamma frailty for any fixed value of θ.

Proof: For β, the EM and penalized methods have the same update equation, which includes $Z\omega$ as a fixed offset. Thus if the solutions for ω are the same, those for β will be also. Let $(\hat\beta, \hat\omega) = (\hat\beta(\theta), \hat\omega(\theta))$ be a solution from the the EM algorithm. Then $\hat\omega$ must satisfy equation (9.7) *exactly.* Rearranging that equation gives $\hat A_j = \exp(-\hat\omega_j)(d_j + \nu) - \nu$. Substituting this into the penalized score equation, equation (9.2), noting that $\nu = 1/\theta$, and using the fact that $\partial g(\omega;\theta)/\partial\omega_j = 1 - e^{\omega_j}$ we see that, evaluated at $(\hat\beta, \hat\omega)$,

$$\begin{aligned}\frac{\partial PPL}{\partial \omega_j} &= \left[d_j - e^{-\hat\omega_j}\left(d_j + \tfrac{1}{\theta} - \tfrac{1}{\theta}e^{\hat\omega_j}\right)e^{\hat\omega_j}\right] + \tfrac{1}{\theta}(1 - e^{\hat\omega_j}) \\ &= 0\end{aligned}$$

for all j. This shows that the solution to the EM algorithm is also a solution to the penalized score equations. Therefore, for any fixed θ, the penalized loglikelihood and the observed-data loglikelihood in equation (9.4) have the same solution, although these two equations are *not* equal to one another.

Furthermore, we can write the profile loglikelihood for θ, equation (9.6), as the profile PPL plus a correction that only involves ν and the d_js. Using the fact that each row of Z has exactly one 1 and $q-1$ 0s, we see that the Cox partial loglikelihood for $(\hat\beta, \hat\omega)$ must be the same as that for $(\hat\beta, \hat\omega + c)$ for any constant c. Simple algebra shows that the value c which minimizes the penalty function must satisfy

$$\sum_{i=1}^{q} e^{\omega_j} = q. \tag{9.9}$$

Let $PPL(\theta) = PPL(\hat\beta(\theta), \hat\omega(\theta), \theta)$, the log profile penalized partial-likelihood. Using the identities in equations (9.7) and (9.9), we show in Section 9.6.5 that

$$L_m(\theta) = PPL(\theta) + \sum_{j=1}^{q} \nu - (\nu + d_j)\log(\nu + d_j) + \nu\log\nu + \log\left(\frac{\Gamma(\nu + d_j)}{\Gamma(\nu)}\right). \tag{9.10}$$

It is useful to consider $L_m(\theta) + \sum_{j=1}^{q} d_j$, rather than $L_m(\theta)$ because the profile loglikelihood converges to $\ell(\hat{\beta}) - \sum d_j$ as the variance of the random effect goes to zero. This modification makes the maximized likelihood from a frailty model with small θ comparable to a nonfrailty model.

The fitting program for a shared gamma frailty consists of an inner and outer loop. For any fixed θ, Newton–Raphson iteration is used to solve the penalized model in a few (usually three to five) steps, and return the corresponding value of the PPL. The outer loop chooses θ to maximize the profile likelihood in equation (9.10), which is easily done as it is a unimodal function of one parameter.

9.6.4 Gaussian frailty

McGilchrist and Aisbett [102, 101], suggest a Gaussian density for the random effects in a shared frailty model. This leads to the penalized partial likelihood

$$PPL = \ell - (1/2\theta)\sum_{j=1}^{q} \omega_j^2 \,, \tag{9.11}$$

where θ is the variance of the random effect.

The authors do not provide an exact connection to the marginal likelihood that can be used to choose the variance or "shrinkage" parameter θ. Instead, they note the similarity of the Cox model's Newton–Raphson step to an iteratively reweighted least-squares calculation. Using this observation, they propose using standard estimators from Gaussian problems. This leads to choosing θ such that it satisfies

$$\theta = \frac{\sum_{j=1}^{q} \omega_j^2 + r}{q}. \tag{9.12}$$

The value of the parameter r varies, depending on the estimation technique used. For the BLUP estimate of θ r is 0, for the ML estimate of θ $r =$ trace$[(H_{22})^{-1}]$ and for the REML estimate $r =$ trace$[(H^{-1})_{22}]$, where, as before, H is minus the Hessian of the penalized partial loglikelihood.

The Gaussian approach is justified and expanded in Ripatti and Palmgren [126]. Let the random effects have a covariance matrix $\Sigma = \Sigma(\theta)$, where Σ is positive definite. This provides a rich class of models for the random effects; for example, setting $\Sigma = \theta I$ results in a shared frailty model. Ripatti and Palmgren start with the likelihood as a function of β, ω and θ, with λ_0 profiled out. The marginal loglikelihood is

$$L_m(\beta,\theta) = -1/2 \log|\Sigma| + \log\left\{\int \exp[\ell(\beta,\omega) - 1/2\omega'\Sigma^{-1/2}\omega]d\omega\right\}.$$

Following the approach of Breslow and Clayton [23], they use a Laplace approximation to this integral:

$$L_m(\beta,\theta) \approx \ell(\beta,\tilde{\omega}) - 1/2\left(\tilde{\omega}'\Sigma^{-1}\tilde{\omega} + \log|\Sigma| + \log|H(\beta,\tilde{\omega})_{22}|\right), \tag{9.13}$$

where $\tilde{\omega} = \tilde{\omega}(\beta, \theta)$ solves

$$\sum_{i=1}^{n} \int_0^\infty (Z_{ij} - \bar{z}_j(t)) dN_i(t) - \Sigma(\theta)^{-1}\tilde{\omega} = 0.$$

As a result, the first two terms correspond to a penalized partial likelihood with $g(\omega; \theta) = 1/2\tilde{\omega}'\Sigma(\theta)^{-1}\tilde{\omega}$, which can be used as an estimation tool. Ignoring the third term has no impact, as it is constant for fixed θ. The fourth term can influence the estimates. However, the information change as ω varies will be small, and thus the bias introduced by ignoring the term should be small as well.

Maximizing the PPL to obtain $(\hat{\beta}(\theta), \hat{\omega}(\theta))$, substituting them into equation (9.13) to get an approximate profile loglikelihood for θ, and then differentiating with respect to the θ_js gives an estimating equation for θ_j:

$$\text{trace}\left[\Sigma^{-1}\frac{\partial \Sigma}{\partial \theta_j}\right] + \text{trace}\left[(H_{22})^{-1}\frac{\partial \Sigma^{-1}}{\partial \theta_j}\right] - \omega'\Sigma^{-1}\frac{\partial \Sigma}{\partial \theta_j}\Sigma^{-1}\omega = 0, \quad (9.14)$$

with Fisher information that has a jk element of

$$\begin{aligned} &(1/2) \quad \text{trace}\left[\Sigma^{-1}\frac{\partial \Sigma}{\partial \theta_j}\Sigma^{-1}\frac{\partial \Sigma}{\partial \theta_k} + \Sigma^{-1}\frac{\partial^2 \Sigma}{\partial \theta_j \partial \theta_k}\right] + \\ &(1/2) \quad \text{trace}\left[(H_{22})^{-1}\frac{\partial \Sigma^{-1}}{\partial \theta_j}(H_{22})^{-1}\frac{\partial \Sigma^{-1}}{\partial \theta_k} - (H_{22})^{-1}\frac{\partial^2 \Sigma^{-1}}{\partial \theta_j \partial \theta_k}\right] (9.15) \end{aligned}$$

For the shared frailty model the estimating equation (9.14) reduces to

$$\hat{\theta} = \frac{\omega'\omega + \text{trace}[(H_{22})^{-1}]}{q},$$

which is equivalent to the MLE formula of McGilchrist [101].

Yau and McGilchrist [161] display a similar formula for the ML estimate for an arbitrary correlation matrix Σ, and apply the results to the CGD data set using an AR(1) structure for the multiple infections within subject. They also define a REML estimate, which is identical to equations (9.14) and (9.15) above, but with $(H^{-1})_{22}$ replacing $(H_{22})^{-1}$. In addition, their simulations show equation (9.15) to be an overestimate of the actual standard error.

9.6.5 Correspondence of the profile likelihoods

Here we justify equation (9.10). Using the form of the derivatives of the Laplace transform of the gamma density, we can expand equation (9.4) as

$$L_m = \sum_{i=1}^{n} \delta_i \log\left(\int Y_i(t) e^{X_i\beta} d\Lambda_0(t)\right)$$

$$
\begin{aligned}
&+\sum_{j=1}^{q} \log\left[\left(\frac{1}{\nu}\right)^{d_j}\left(1+\frac{A_j}{\nu}\right)^{-(\nu+d_j)}\prod_{k=0}^{d_j-1}(\nu+k)\right] \\
= &\sum_{i=1}^{n} \delta_i \log\left(\int Y_i(t) e^{X_i\beta} d\Lambda_0(t)\right) \\
&+\sum_{j=1}^{q} [-d_j \log\nu - (\nu+d_j)\log(1+A_j/\nu) \\
&\quad + \log\Gamma(\nu+d_j) - \log\Gamma(\nu)].
\end{aligned}
$$

Now let us consider this function restricted to the one-dimensional curve defined by the maximizing values of $\hat\beta(\theta), \hat\omega(\theta), \hat\lambda_0(\theta)$ for each θ, that is, the log profile likelihood for θ. As we have shown (equation (9.7)) on that curve $\hat A_j = (d_j + \nu - \nu e^{\hat\omega_j})/e^{\hat\omega_j}$. Making this substitution into the equation above leads to

$$
\begin{aligned}
L_m(\theta) = &\sum_{i=1}^{n} \delta_i \log\left(\hat\lambda_i e^{X_i\hat\beta}\right) \\
&+\sum_{j=1}^{q} [-d_j \log\nu - \log\Gamma(\nu) - (\nu+d_j)\log(\nu+d_j) \\
&\quad + (\nu+d_j)\log(\nu e^{\hat\omega_j}) + \log\Gamma(\nu+d_j)] \\
= &\sum_{i=1}^{n} \delta_i \log\left(\hat\lambda_i e^{X_i\hat\beta}\right) \\
&+\sum_{j=1}^{q} [-(\nu+d_j)\log(\nu+d_j) + \nu\log(\nu e^{\hat\omega_j}) \\
&\quad + d_j\log(e^{\hat\omega_j}) + \log\Gamma(\nu+d_j) - \log\Gamma(\nu)] \\
= &\sum_{i=1}^{n} \delta_i \log\left(\hat\lambda_i e^{X_i\hat\beta + Z_i\hat\omega}\right) \\
&+\sum_{j=1}^{q} [-(\nu+d_j)\log(\nu+d_j) + \nu\log(\nu e^{\hat\omega_j}) \\
&\quad + \log\Gamma(\nu+d_j) - \log\Gamma(\nu)],
\end{aligned}
$$

where $\hat\lambda_i = \int_0^\infty Y_i(t) d\hat\Lambda_0(t)$ as above.

Subtracting and adding the penalty function $g(\omega;\theta) = -1/\theta \sum_{j=1}^{q} \omega_j - \exp(\omega_j)$, evaluated at $\hat\omega$ results in

$$
L_m(\theta) = \sum_{i=1}^{n} \delta_i \log(\hat\lambda_i e^{X_i\hat\beta + Z_i\hat\omega}) - g(\hat\omega;\theta)
$$

$$
\begin{aligned}
&+\sum_{j=1}^{q}[-\nu\hat{\omega}_j + \nu e^{\hat{\omega}_j} - (\nu + d_j)\log(\nu + d_j) + \nu\log(\nu e^{\hat{\omega}_j}) \\
&\qquad + \log\Gamma(\nu + d_j) - \log\Gamma(\nu)] \\
= &\sum_{j=1}^{q}\left[\nu - (\nu + d_j)\log(\nu + d_j) + \nu\log\nu + \log\left(\frac{\Gamma(\nu + d_j)}{\Gamma(\nu)}\right)\right] \\
&+PPL(\theta),
\end{aligned}
$$

where the last step follows from equation (9.9).

Note that it is computationally advantageous to use

$$
\log\left(\frac{\Gamma(\nu + d_j)}{\Gamma(\nu)}\right) = \sum_{i=0}^{d_j - 1}\log\left(\frac{\nu + i}{\nu + d_j}\right)
$$

instead of

$$
\log\left(\frac{\Gamma(\nu + d_j)}{\Gamma(\nu)}\right) = \log(\Gamma(\nu + d_j)) - \log(\Gamma(\nu)).
$$

Considerable loss of accuracy can occur if one subtracts values of the log–gamma function.

9.7 Sparse computation

When performing estimation with frailty models, memory and time considerations can become an issue. For instance, if there are 300 families, each with their own frailty, and four other variables, then the full information matrix has $304^2 = 92,416$ elements. The Cholesky decomposition must be applied to this matrix with each Newton–Raphson iteration. In our S-Plus implementation, we have applied a technique that can provide significant savings in space and time.

Assume a shared frailty model, with $Z_{ij} = 1$ if subject i is a member of family j, and zero otherwise and with each subject belonging to only one family. If we partition the Cox model's information matrix according to the rows of X and Z,

$$
\mathcal{I} = \begin{pmatrix} \mathcal{I}_{XX} & \mathcal{I}_{XZ} \\ \mathcal{I}_{ZX} & \mathcal{I}_{ZZ} \end{pmatrix},
$$

then the lower right corner will be a diagonally dominant matrix, having almost the form of the variance matrix for a multinomial distribution. For shared frailty models, adding the penalty further increases the dominance of the diagonal. Therefore, using a *sparse* computation option, where only the diagonal of $\mathcal{I}_{ZZ}$ is retained, should not have a large impact on the estimation procedure.

Ignoring a piece of the full information matrix has a number of implications. First, the savings in space can be considerable. If we use the sparse option with the example above, the information matrix consists of only the left-hand "slice" of $304 * 4 = 1,216$ elements along with the 300 element diagonal of the lower corner, a savings of over 95% in memory space. Second, because the score vector and likelihood are not changed, the solution point is identical to the one obtained in the nonsparse case, discounting trivial differences due to distinct iteration paths. Third, the Newton–Raphson iteration may undergo a slight loss of efficiency so that one to two more iterations are required. However, because each N–R iteration requires the Cholesky decomposition of the information matrix, the sparse problem is much faster per iteration than the full matrix version. Finally, the full information matrix is a part of the formulae for the postfit estimates of degrees of freedom and standard error. In a small number of simple examples, the effect of the sparse approximation on these estimates has been surprisingly small.

The sparse routines have some impact on the solution for a Gaussian model, since the REML estimate depends on the matrix H. Using the `sparse=F` option to the frailty function, the routine required 17 Newton–Raphson iterations and gave a solution of $\theta = 0.509$ (but with about three times the total computing time).

We have found two cases where the sparse method does not perform acceptably. The first is if the variance of the random effect is quite large (>5). In this case, each N–R iteration may require a large number (>15) iterations. The second is if one group contains a majority of the observations. The off-diagonal terms are too important to ignore in this case, and the approximate N–R iteration does not converge.

9.8 Concluding remarks

One very important issue that is still not completely resolved is the amount and distribution of information — total number of events, number of groups, and the distribution of events/group — required to produce stable frailty estimates. Ducrocq and Casella [41] give a useful practical example in the context of animal breeding for an inherited trait. The random effect is presumed to have a heritability of 5%, a "typical value," which corresponds to $\theta = .02$. In simulations based on 5,000 dairy cows, both the number of sires and the number of daughters per sire were important; the standard error of $\hat\theta$ was unacceptably large both for 10 sires with 500 daughters each and for 500 sires with 10 daughters each. The biomedical examples given here suggest a smaller number of events for efficacious estimation, but in the context of a larger random effect.

The text has focused on the simple shared frailty model, using either a gamma distribution for the frailty with ML estimation of the frailty variance θ, or a Gaussian distribution with a REML θ estimate. Because it is embedded in a general penalized model framework, however, other extensions are possible. As an example, estimation of a model with nested effects could be based on minimization of the overall AIC. In a data set similar to that of Sastry [127] for instance, there might be both village and familial effects on infant survival. Maximization over both variance parameters would be accomplished by creating a two parameter function

```
tempfun <- function(theta1, theta2) {
    fit <- coxph(Surv(time, status) ~ birth.order + mother.age +
                                  frailty(village, theta=theta1) +
                                  frailty(family, theta=theta2))
    aic <- (fit$loglik[2] - fit$loglik[1]) - sum(fit$df)
    return(2*aic)
    }
```

and using it as the object of `nlminb` or one of the other general maximization routines.

Penalized techniques are a useful estimation tool. The current software has some advantages in terms of speed and extensibility, but is still only a first iteration towards a general and well-rounded tool: likelihood methods of selecting θ are restricted to the shared frailty case (essentially assuming that the covariate is a class variable) and to only two distributions; appropriate residuals for testing the assumptions are unavailable (e.g., a dfbeta that would have immediately revealed the large influence in the kidney data), and the corpus of examples where random effects are both useful and not useful needs to be much broader. Important theoretical issues concerning the comparability of the approximate Wald and integrated likelihood ratio tests of the frailty variance need to be addressed.

The models are still useful and deserve wider use. The ability of a frailty term to "correct" the other coefficients in the hidden covariate example is tantalizing, but should be viewed with caution. In the end, the only truly reliable way to test the question "Is treatment still efficacious for subjects with a treatment failure" is rerandomization of participants, at some midpoint of a trial.

10

Expected Survival

The calculation of an expected survival (based on some reference population) for a cohort of patients under study has a long history. These methods are most familiar when the reference population is census based, for example, the overall survival experience of the United States population by age and sex. Recently, these ideas have been rediscovered and applied to the proportional hazards model. In this case the reference population is the result of a fitted Cox model, with the results of the model applied to a new population of subjects. Many of the computational and interpretation issues with the estimates are particularly clear in the case of population data. Therefore, this chapter elaborates on both population- and model-based techniques.

10.1 Individual survival, population based

The building block for all of the expected survival work is the *individual* expected curve. For instance, what is the expected survival of a 45-year-old US male over the next 10 years, beginning on July 4, 1967? The code below shows that the chance of reaching a 55th birthday is 0.911.

```
> tdata <- data.frame(age= chron('7/4/67') - chron('3/10/22'),
                      sex='male', year= chron('7/4/67'))
> survexp(~1, data=tdata, ratetable=survexp.us,
                      times=(1:5)*730.5)
```

```
Time n.risk survival
 730      1    0.987
1461      1    0.971
2192      1    0.953
2922      1    0.933
3652      1    0.911
```

(The `chron` function accepts a date and returns the number of days since 1/1/60. The equivalent SAS function is `mdy`.) The basic pattern of this code is repeated for both individual and cohort survival, both population-based and Cox model-based: create a data set containing the hypothetical individual(s) for which a curve is desired, and then compute the curve based upon both this data set and a rate table data set. For population rate tables, the `survexp` function expects the age to be in days, the date to be stored as the number of days since 1/1/1960, and the gender to be one of "male" or "female."

The similar result in SAS uses the `%survexp` macro.

```
data temp;
    birth = mdy(3,10, 1922);
    entry = mdy(7, 4, 1967);
    sex   = 'M';
    time =0; status =0;       /* dummy values */
    output;

%survexp(data=temp, pop=US_T, birthdt=birth, firstdt=entry,
                    sex=sex,  method=1, points= 0 to 3650 by 1461,
                    time=time, event=status);
proc print;
```

```
           OBS     TIME      EXP_PT

            1         0     1.00000
            2      1461     0.97102
            3      2922     0.93325
```

The foundational data set for expected survival curves is in a population rate table; several are included with S-Plus and with the SAS macros (see appendix B.) Each rate table is a multiway array of hazard rates, for example, the rate table for the total US, `survexp.us`, is a three way array whose dimensions are age (0–1 days, 1–7, 7–28, 28–365 days and yearly thereafter to age 109), sex M/F, and the seven calendar years 1940, 1950, 1960, 1970, 1980, 1990, and 2000. The data are derived from the decennial US census, with the year 2000 data being an extrapolation. Each cell of the table contains the hazard (per day) of death for a subject of that age and sex in the given calendar year.

The rate tables been compiled over several years by the Section of Biostatistics, Mayo Clinic. As such they are somewhat restricted in number, essentially consisting of populations for which Mayo does significant amounts of patient care. However, given the underlying population data, users can easily construct their own. Further details of the tables' construction and use are found in a series of technical reports [13, 146].

In the published life tables, upon which the rate tables are based, each entry is the probability that a given subject, in a given calendar year, will die before his or her next birthday [150]. The entry for a 20-year-old male in 1950, for instance, contains the probability that a subject who turns 20 years of age in 1950 will not reach his 21st birthday. The log of this survival probability q_i is related to the cumulative hazard $\Lambda(t)$ as

$$-\log(1-q_i) = \Lambda(i+1) - \Lambda(i) = 365.25\,\lambda_i.$$

The rate tables contain daily hazard rates λ_i.

Given the basic data, there are two standard ways to compute an expected survival curve: as a product of conditional survival probabilities $\prod(1-q_i)$ (Kaplan–Meier-like) or as the exponential of a cumulative hazard $\exp(-\sum\lambda_i)$ (Nelson–Aalen-like). If all computations involve only whole years of followup, the results of the two approaches are identical. If there are partial-year computations they will differ slightly; the product-limit approach essentially uses a linear interpolation on the $S(t)$ or survival scale, and the hazard-based approach an interpolation on the $\Lambda(t)$ or cumulative hazard scale. For example, assume that a woman born on August 31, 1942 enters a study on May 11, 1963. The two-year survival involves 112 days (11May63 to 30Aug63) at the "20 years old, 1962" rate ($\lambda_{20,1962}$), 366 days (August to August) at rate $\lambda_{21,1963}$, and 254 days at rate $\lambda_{22,1964}$. The result of the hazard-based and product-limit computations turns out to be .9994115 and .9994103, respectively. The method of computation makes essentially no difference. The internal routines use a hazard-based approach since it is easier: a sum of death rates, each times the number of days at that rate.

10.2 Individual survival, Cox model

The individual survival curve in a population setting depends on both the underlying rate table and on the age, sex, and calendar year values of a hypothetical subject. In a Cox model, the fitted model takes the place of the rate table, and the hypothetical individual is specified in terms of covariates that were part of the model. There are again two main computing variants, which differ in their output somewhat more than in the population case. The variance of the estimate and the handling of time-dependent covariates are two additional issues.

10.2.1 *Natural history of PBC*

In the PBC natural history model discussed earlier, one of the important outcomes of the model is patient-specific survival curves. That is, given the state of a patient's disease at present, what is the expected future or "natural history" survival for this patient. The result is an important input to clinical decision making. Assume that the patient in question is 53 years old, has no edema, and has bilirubin, protime, and albumin values of 2, 12, and 2, respectively. The code to produce a survival curve in SAS is as follows.

```
data temp1; set pbc;
    lbili = log(bili);
    lpro  = log(protime);
    lalb  = log(albumin);

data temp2;
    age =  53;
    edema= 0;
    lbili= log(2);
    lalb = log(2);
    lpro = log(12);
    output;

proc phreg data=temp1;
    model futime * status(2) = age edema lbili lpro lalb;
    baseline output=sfit covariates=temp2
                          survival upper lower/ nomean;
```

The expected survival curve is produced by the `baseline` statement, which in the above code obtains a description of the characteristics of the desired patient from the data set `temp2`. The created data set `sfit` will contain the survival curve along with upper and lower 95% confidence bands. The `nomean` option suppresses creation of a curve for the "mean" subject (more on this later).

The S-Plus result is shown in Figure 10.1, which contains the expected survival curve along with 95% confidence intervals. The odds of this patient living another 10 years are not encouraging. The S-Plus code is similar.

```
> # Fit a Cox model to the original data set
> pbcfit <- coxph(Surv(futime, status==2) ~ age + log(bili) +
                       log(protime) + log(albumin) + edema, pbc)

> # Create a data set corresponding to the hypothetical subject
> temp <- data.frame(age=53, edema=0, bili=2, protime=12,
                                                  albumin=2)
> # Obtain and plot the expected curve
> sfit <- survfit(pbcfit, newdata=temp)
> plot(sfit, xscale=365.24, xlab="Years",ylab="Expected Survival")
```

In both packages we start by creating a separate data set that contains the covariate values of the hypothetical subject. In this case the data set has only one observation, so only a single curve is produced; in general the result will contain a separate curve for each "patient" in the new data set.

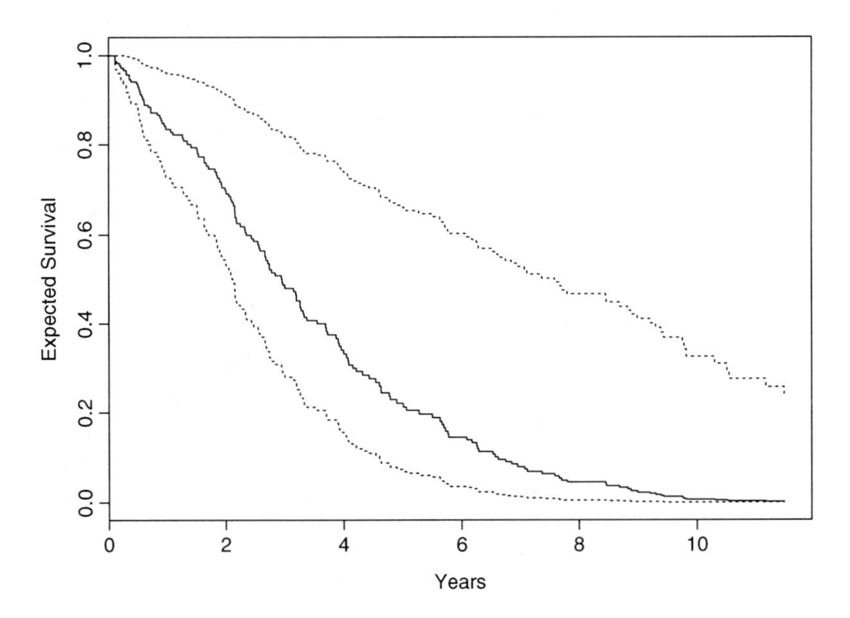

FIGURE 10.1: *Expected survival for a 53-year-old PBC patient with selected laboratory values*

For a stratified Cox model there is a separate baseline hazard for each stratum. For example, if the PBC data had been stratified by enrolling institution there would be a curve for a 53-year-old with bilirubin = 2, protime = 12, etc. who comes from the population at institution 1, another for institution 2, and so on. If the data set of hypothetical subjects had 4 observations, and the Cox model 5 strata, then the output data set would contain 5∗4 = 20 individual curves, which can sometimes be a bit confusing.

```
> xfit <- coxph(Surv(futime, status==2) ~ age + log(bili) +
                              strata(edema), data=pbc)
> temp <- data.frame(age=c(53, 60), bili=c(2, 3))
> curves <- survfit(xfit, newdata=temp)
> print(curves)
              n events mean se(mean) median 0.95LCL 0.95UCL
  edema=0 354    116 2876     71.6   3222    2796    3762
  edema=0 354    116 2194     44.4   2111    1786    2540
edema=0.5  44     26 2381    280.4   3282    1925      NA
edema=0.5  44     26 1711    174.6   1576    1168      NA
  edema=1  20     19 1503    588.6   1434     971      NA
  edema=1  20     19  913    253.3    859     400      NA
```

In the example just shown, the `curves` object contains six survival curves, the projected survival of a 53-year-old, bilirubin = 2, in the edema = 0 stratum, followed by that for a 60-year-old with bilirubin = 3 in the edema = 0 stratum, and so on. If plotted, the curves would appear in this order: `plot(curves[5:6])` would display only the last two. The data set produced by a SAS `baseline` statement is in the same order; 117 observations for the first curve (a first point at `(time=0, survival=1)` followed by the 116 steps for the 116 events), 117 for the second curve, 27 for the third, and so on.

10.2.2 "Mean" survival

If no secondary data set (`newdata`) is provided to the `survfit` function, or the `mean` option is selected in the `phreg baseline` statement, then the curve(s) produced will be that for the "mean" subject, one per stratum of the original model. However, the exact interpretation of this curve is somewhat difficult. As we discuss in the next sections, it is *not* a representative curve for the PBC data set as a whole, but rather for a single hypothetical individual with the following covariate values.

```
> pbcfit$mean
    age edema log(bili) log(protime) log(albumin)
 50.743   0.1     0.571        2.369        1.244
```

These covariate values are the average in the data set, after deletion of any observations with missing values. For a categorical variable such as edema, a value of 0.1 has no real meaning. (It is somewhat like that famous "average family" with 2.3 children.) A better default for the program would have been to use the mean age, the most frequent edema category (0), the median bilirubin value (since it is so highly skewed), and so on, that is, a curve that actually corresponds to an interesting patient. Intelligent guessing at this level is beyond the scope of the software, however, and users should not expect anything really interpretable from the "mean" curve.

10.2.3 Estimators

The Breslow [22] or Nelson–Aalen estimate of the baseline cumulative hazard is a simple extension of the nocovariate formula (2.1) of Chapter 2:

$$\hat\Lambda_0(t,\hat\beta) = \int_0^t \frac{d\bar N(s)}{\sum_{j=1}^n Y_j(s)\hat r_j(s)}, \tag{10.1}$$

with a variance estimate that is also a direct analogue of the simple case

$$\text{var}[\hat\Lambda_0(t,\hat\beta)] = \int_0^t \frac{d\bar N(s)}{\left[\sum_{j=1}^n Y_j(s) r_j(s)\right]^2}. \tag{10.2}$$

The Nelson–Aalen estimate of cumulative hazard for a hypothetical subject with covariates $X^\dagger$ is then

$$\hat\Lambda(t,\hat\beta,X^\dagger) = e^{X^{\dagger}\hat\beta}\hat\Lambda_0(t,\hat\beta), \tag{10.3}$$

with a corresponding Breslow estimate of survival $S(t) = \exp[-\hat{\Lambda}(t, \hat{\beta}, X^{\dagger})]$. The variance of the cumulative hazards was derived in Tsiatis [149] using a delta method argument, and later derived directly from martingale theory by Andersen et al. [4]. A consistent estimator of the variance comprises two terms

$$\begin{aligned} \text{var}[\hat{\Lambda}(t, \hat{\beta}, X^{\dagger})] &= \left(e^{X^{\dagger}\hat{\beta}}\right)^2 \int_0^t \frac{d\overline{N}(s)}{\left[\sum_{j=1}^n Y_j(s)\hat{r}_j(s)\right]^2} \\ &\quad + q'(t)\mathcal{I}^{-1}q'(t), \end{aligned} \tag{10.4}$$

where

$$q(t) = \int_0^t [X^{\dagger} - \bar{x}(s)] \frac{e^{X^{\dagger}\hat{\beta}}\, d\overline{N}(s)}{\sum_{j=1}^n Y_j(s)\hat{r}_j(s)}.$$

In the no-covariate case this reduces the standard Nelson–Aalen estimator and variance. When there are tied event times, an important variation of the estimate is the analogue of the Fleming–Harrington estimate. For example, if observations 1 to 5 were at risk at time t with observations 1 to 2 experiencing an event, then the term for that time point

$$\frac{2}{r_1 + r_2 + r_3 + r_4 + r_5}$$

arising in equation (10.1) would be replaced by

$$\frac{1}{r_1 + r_2 + r_3 + r_4 + r_5} + \frac{1}{.5r_1 + .5r_2 + r_3 + r_4 + r_5}.$$

This is identical to the computations for $\hat{\beta}$ that correspond to the Efron approximation.

The Kalbfleisch–Prentice estimate is of the product-limit form

$$S(t, \hat{\beta}, X*) = \prod_{t_{(k)} \le t} \alpha_k, \tag{10.5}$$

where $t_{(k)}$ are the unique event times, and α_k satisfies the equation

$$\sum_{i=1}^n \Delta N_i(t_{(k)}) \frac{r_i(t_{(k)})}{1 - \alpha_k^{r_i(t_{(k)})}} = \sum_i r_i(t_{(k)}),$$

where $\Delta N_i(t_{(k)})$ is 1 if subject i has an event at time $t_{(k)}$. The left term is thus a sum over the subjects with an event at that time, and the right a sum over all subjects at risk. If there is only one event at time $t_{(k)}$ then the equation can be solved for α_k,

$$\alpha_k = \left(1 - \frac{r_{(k)}}{\sum_i r_i(t_{(k)})}\right)^{-r_{(k)}},$$

with $r_{(k)}$ the risk score of the subject who experienced the event. If there are tied events then the equation is solved by iteration. Since the solution point is known to lie in the interval $(0, 1]$ any of several computational methods will suffice, including binomial search. When there are no covariates, this estimator simplifies to the Kaplan–Meier. The variance of $\log(S)$ is taken to be the variance of the cumulative hazard as shown in equation (10.4), based on the asymptotic equivalence of the two estimators.

The variance of the survival estimate $S(t)$ itself, for either estimator, can be approximated as $S^2(t)\text{var}[\hat{\Lambda}(t)]$. Confidence intervals and standard errors on this scale can be quite inaccurate, however, as discussed earlier in Chapter 2.

As was shown in Chapter 2 for the non-Cox model estimates, the actual difference between the hazard-based and product-limit estimators is usually small except perhaps in the right-hand tail — where the standard errors are often large in any case. SAS defaults to the Kalbfleisch–Prentice estimate; the Breslow estimate can be chosen with the `method=ch` option. S-Plus defaults to the Fleming–Harrington estimate when the Efron approximation for ties is used, and to the Nelson–Aalen estimate when the Breslow approximation is requested; the Kalbfleisch–Prentice estimate is an option.

The hazard-based estimates apply directly to counting process data, and the computer codes for both packages support this estimate for (start, stop] data sets. Extension of the product-limit estimate to counting process data is not as well supported.

10.2.4 Time-dependent covariates

When the model contains time-dependent covariates baseline survival estimates can still be produced, but the results can be quite surprising. As an example we look at a followup data set to the original PBC study. The data set `pbcseq` contains sequential laboratory measurements on the 312 protocol patients of the PBC study. Patients were scheduled to return at 6 months, 12 months, and yearly thereafter; most patients have these visits, and many also have one or two “extra” (in connection to a Mayo Clinic appointment for another indication, for instance). The observations for a particular subject are shown below.

```
id  start  stop  event  drug asites  edema  bili  albumin  ...
4       0   188      0     1     0     0.5   1.8    2.54
4     188   372      0     1     0     0.5   1.6    2.88
4     372   729      0     1     0     0.5   1.7    2.80
4     729  1254      0     1     0     1.0   3.2    2.92
4    1254  1462      0     1     0     1.0   3.7    2.59
4    1462  1824      0     1     0     1.0   4.0    2.59
4    1824  1925      2     1     0     1.0   5.3    1.83
```

In years, the visit times are 0, .5, 1, 2, 3.4, 4, and 5, so other than a delayed visit in year 3 this patient was compliant with the protocol. The subject died after 5.3 years on study (the event variable is 0 = alive, 1 = transplant, 2 = death) preceded by a steady worsening in bilirubin levels.

A time-dependent covariate model is fit to the data as follows, using the same covariates and transforms as were used for the fit to baseline data set pbc.

```
> pbcsfit <- coxph(Surv(start, stop, event==2) ~ age + log(bili) +
                   log(protime) + log(albumin) + edema,
                   data=pbcseq)
> pbcsfit
                 coef exp(coef) se(coef)     z       p
          age   0.046    1.0471  0.00891  5.17 2.4e-07
    log(bili)   1.085    2.9592  0.11112  9.76 0.0e+00
 log(protime)   2.848   17.2604  0.63166  4.51 6.5e-06
 log(albumin)  -3.719    0.0243  0.49528 -7.51 6.0e-14
        edema   0.806    2.2387  0.23270  3.46 5.3e-04

Likelihood ratio test=474  on 5 df, p=0  n= 1945

> rbind(pbcfit$coef, pbcsfit$coef)
       age log(bili) log(protime) log(albumin) edema
old  0.040     0.864        2.387       -2.507 0.896
new  0.046     1.085        2.848       -3.719 0.806
```

Notice that the coefficients for four of the five covariates have become larger in the new model; that is, under more continuous monitoring bilirubin is even more predictive than in the original PBC fit. Medically, this is not surprising.

(An occasional point of confusion with time-dependent covariates is the role of "age," which we now elucidate. The above data set uses "age at enrollment" throughout, but would have produced exactly the same results using current age. The internal computations for the model depend only on hazard ratios; if a_i is the enrollment age then $a_i + t$ will be the current age at time t and the hazard ratio for two subjects i and j will be

$$\frac{\lambda_0(t)e^{\beta(a_i+t)}}{\lambda_0(t)e^{\beta(a_j+t)}} = \frac{e^{\beta a_i}}{e^{\beta a_j}}.$$

As long as age is entered as a linear term in the model, the fit depends only on the age at entry. If there were a quadratic term in age, a spline, or other complex function, this would not be true, but the PBC models have only used a linear term. Now, back to our regular broadcast ...)

Now, compute the survival curve for the mean subject.

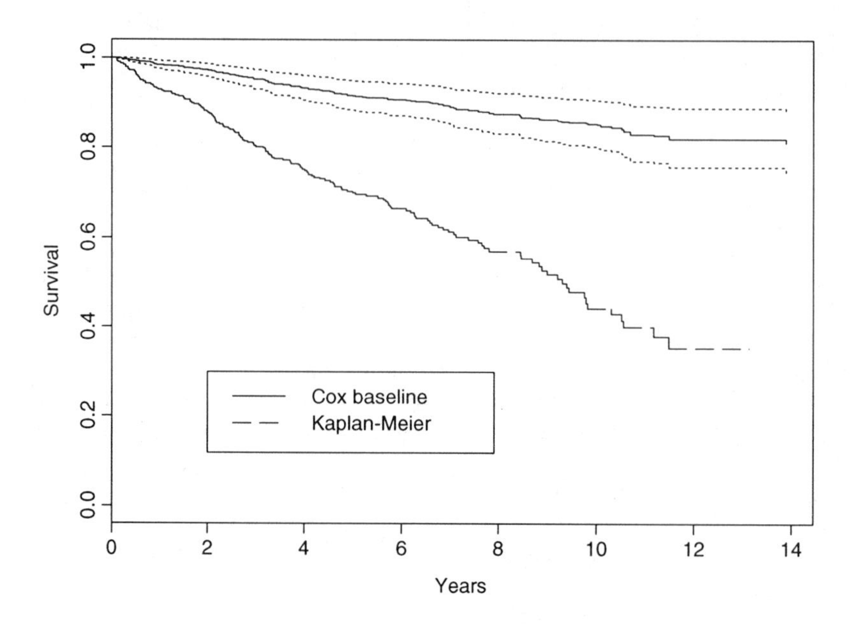

FIGURE 10.2: *Kaplan–Meier survival for the PBC patients, along with the baseline curve for a time-dependent covariate model*

```
> surv1 <- survfit(pbcsfit)                              #Cox baseline
> plot(surv1, xscale=365.24, xlab='Years', ylab='Survival')
> surv2 <- survfit(Surv(futime, status==2)~1, pbc)    #KM curve
> lines(surv2, lty=3, xscale=365.24, mark.time=F)   #add to plot
```

The resulting baseline survival curve along with a Kaplan–Meier curve for the patients is shown in Figure 10.2. Why is the baseline survival so far from the Kaplan–Meier, when it is computed for an "average" subject?

In this disease the normal course is for liver function tests to slowly worsen over several years, but then progress rapidly as the sclerosis and damage near a critical threshold, followed shortly thereafter by liver failure. The model captures this fact, that failure is preceded by large values of bilirubin, edema, and prothrombin time. The "mean" survival curve corresponds, by default, to a fictional patient who starts with fairly average covariate values *and then never changes* in those covariates. The survival for such a subject — if such a person even exists — would be quite good compared to the usual PBC patient.

The fundamental issue with time-dependent covariates is not a computational but a conceptual one: if a time-dependent covariate is in the model, then to produce a baseline survival curve one must specify not just baseline values for the hypothetical subject of the curve, but rather an entire *covariate path* for that subject over time. Creating such a covariate path is difficult; it is all too easy to create baseline hazards that correspond to a subject who is either uninteresting or impossible.

In S-Plus it is possible to obtain a survival curve for an arbitrary covariate path. The hypothetical subject is represented by a multiple observation data set that contains both the predictor and response variables found in the `coxph` model. For instance, assume a PBC patient whose bilirubin

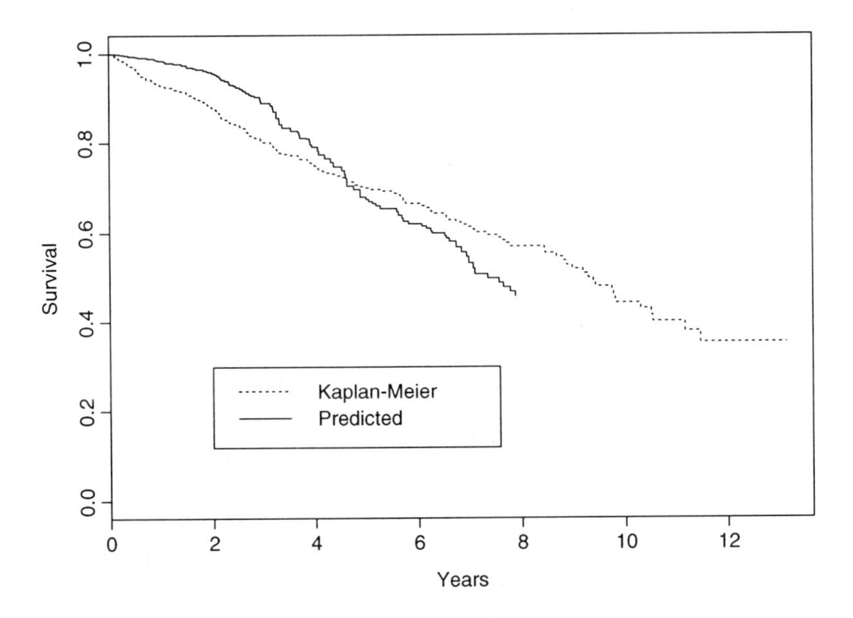

FIGURE 10.3: *Overall PBC survival and that for a hypothetical covariate path*

increased by 1–2 units a year for four years, but whose other covariates remained constant.

```
> temp <- data.frame(start=c(   0,  365,  730, 1095, 1460),
                     stop =c( 365,  730, 1095,1460, 3000),
                     event=c(   0,    0,    0,    0,    0),
                     age  =c(  53,   53,   53,   53,   53),
                     bili =c(   1,    2,    3,    5,    7),
                     edema=c(   1,    1,    1,    1,    1),
                     albumin=c(3.5, 3.5, 3.5,  3.5,  3.5),
                     protime=c(11,   11,   11,   11,   11))
> fit <- survfit(pbcsfit, newdata=temp, individual=T)
```

(The program expects the new data set to have all of the covariates found in the original `coxph` call, even though the `event` variable is not needed for an expected curve.) The keyword `individual=T` in the `survfit` call specifies that this set of five observations should be treated as a single covariate path, rather than used to generate five curves. Figure 10.3 shows this curve superimposed onto the overall Kaplan–Meier of the study. Note that it only extends as far as specified by the data frame, and that it has a shape that may be more indicative of a typical PBC subject. Although SAS will generate the data for Figure 10.2, using the standard `baseline` statement, it does not produce an expected curve for a covariate path.

Some authors have argued that although a hazard function may be mathematically defined for a model such as the one above, that "this hazard bears no relationship to a survivor function" [73, Section 5.3.2]. A basic concern is that in order to have a rising bilirubin the subject must be re-measured and ergo, still alive. We tend to disagree, and could imagine some hypothetical "cohort" of subjects who follow a given path, losing members to death along the way. The population-based curves of the prior section also make use of a covariate path, albeit a much more assured one. In computing the 10-year survival for a 45-year-old subject, say, the rate table entries for age 45, 46, ..., 54 will all be used in turn while the gender value remains constant. The program "knows" the covariate path with respect to age and sex. A proportional hazards model with a nonlinear age effect could make use of similar computations. Examples where the covariate path is guaranteed are the exception, however. A major concern with cases such as the bilirubin example above, still, is whether the hypothetical path represents any patient at all. Survival curves based on a time-dependent covariate must be used with extreme caution.

10.3 Cohort survival, population

10.3.1 Motivation

There are many situations where it is desirable or necessary to estimate an expected number of events or expected time to event for a cohort of subjects. These can occur when measurements have been made on a cohort of study subjects and the question arises as to whether the lifetimes are greater than, less than, or similar to what would be expected in the general population or in some other comparison group. An example is the comparison of postsurgical survival of patients receiving a total hip arthroplasty to that for an age- and sex-matched control [74], to explore the possibility of a long-term general deficit associated with the procedure. The ideal approach in these situations is to have had a randomized study in which subjects from the appropriate comparison population were also enrolled. Unfortunately, this is not always possible or convenient. In these situations, investigators often turn to historical or nonconcurrent controls to estimate an expected event rate in the cohort of interest. A key assumption in such an analysis, of course, is that the historical control is *appropriate*, that is, that the survival experience of the historical group is exactly the survival we would have observed, had a control group actually been recruited. Many of the limitations in the use of nonconcurrent controls have been detailed elsewhere, and a discussion of these is beyond the scope of this overview.

There are four common estimates of cohort expected survival; we deal with each in turn.

10.3.2 Naive estimate

The simplest estimate of cohort survival is to calculate the survival of a single "average" individual from the study group. In the PBC data set, for instance, this might be a subject with the mean age (50.7), female gender (90% of the PBC subjects are female), either the arithmetic (3.2)

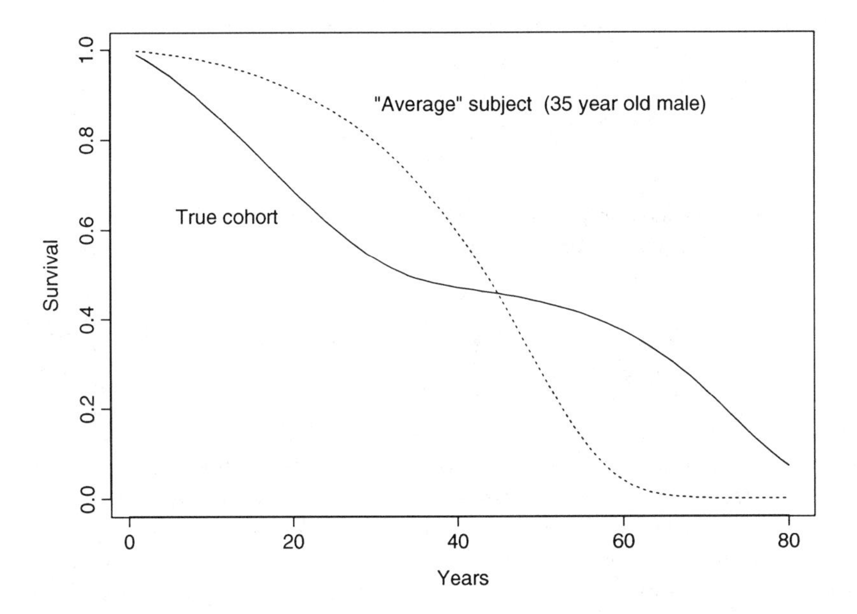

FIGURE 10.4: *Naive versus actual expected survival for the baseball example*

or geometric (1.8) mean of bilirubin (the latter corresponding to the use of log(bili) in the model), and so on. In some situations this might be an acceptable approximation, for example, if there were very little variation among the study subjects. A simple counterexample, however, shows the flaws in the method. Imagine a cohort of 60-year-old grandfathers and 10-year-old grandsons, attending a baseball game together. For some reason we would like to calculate the expected survival of this cohort (perhaps to plan the size of future family reunions). Figure 10.4 shows the true and naive curves for this cohort. The true curve shows the expected two dips, corresponding to the deaths of the grandfathers followed 40 years later by mortality for the grandsons. The naive curve, which is the expected survival of a cohort of 35-year-old males, has no relationship to the actual pattern.

10.3.3 Ederer estimate

Let $\lambda_i(t)$ be the expected hazard function for subject i of the study population, drawn from a population table, and matched with subject i based on age, sex, and other relevant factors. Then

$$\begin{aligned} \Lambda_i(t) &= \int_0^t \lambda_i(s)ds \\ S_i(t) &= \exp(-\Lambda_i(t)) \end{aligned}$$

are the expected cumulative hazard and expected survival curves, respectively, for a hypothetical control subject who matches a study subject i at the start of followup.

The simplest estimate of survival for the matched cohort of control subjects is the *exact* estimate of Ederer et al. [42]

$$S_e(t) = (1/n) \sum_{i=1}^{n} S_i(t). \tag{10.6}$$

(In fact, this was the computation used for the grandfather/grandson example above.) The estimate can also be written as a weighted sum of hazards

$$\begin{aligned} \Lambda_e(t) &= \int_0^t \frac{\sum_{i=1}^n S_i(s)\lambda_i(s)}{\sum_{i=1}^n S_i(s)} ds \\ S_e(t) &= \exp[-\Lambda_e(t)]. \end{aligned}$$

The hazard function at any time is the average of the hazards of those still alive at that time, which can be estimated by a weighted average with weights $S_i(t)$, the probability of being alive and still in the risk set.

The exact method gives the survival curve of a fictional matched control group, assuming complete followup for all of the controls. One technical problem with the exact method is that it often requires population data that are not yet available. For instance assume that a study is open for enrollment from 1985 to 1995, with followup to the analysis date in 1998. If an 11-year expected survival were produced on 1/98, the estimate for the last subject enrolled involves year 2006 US population data.

The word "exact" is a dangerous one in statistics and often misapplied. As with other methods so labeled, the Ederer exact estimate needs to be understood as "exactly calculable" and not as "correct." There is such a thing as the correct calculation of the wrong quantity.

10.3.4 Hakulinen estimate

Several authors have shown that the Ederer method can be misleading if censoring is not independent of age and sex (or whatever the matching factors are for the referent population). Indeed, independence is often not the case. In a long study it is not uncommon to allow older or sicker patients to enroll only after the initial phase. An extreme example of this is demonstrated in Verheul et al. [152], concerning 643 consecutive patients over the age of 20 who had an aortic valve replacement in the Academic Medical Centre, Amsterdam, from 1966 to 1986. The mean age of patients at surgery over the first 10 years was 48, but in the second 10 years it increased to 62, and the proportion of patients over the age of 70 had increased from 1% to 27%. Assume that an analysis of the data were to take place 1 year after the end of the study period. The Kaplan–Meier curve will span 21 years, but the last 10 years of the curve will be computed over a younger cohort than the study as a whole, since the majority of elderly patients have not yet had 10+ years of followup. The Ederer curve for expected survival of an age-matched control group, on the other hand, is computed based on 21 years of followup for each and every subject: its right-hand half incorporates all of the eldest subjects. The Kaplan–Meier is biased upwards (as compared to what it will be when followup is completed), the Ederer is not, and comparison of the two gives a false impression of utility for the surgical treatment.

In Hakulinen's cohort method [58, 59], each study subject is again paired with a fictional referent from the cohort population, but this referent is now treated as though he or she were followed up in the same way as the study patient. Each referent is thus exposed to censoring, and in particular has a maximum *potential* followup, that is, they will become censored at the analysis date. The formula for the estimate is

$$\begin{aligned} \Lambda_h(t) &= \int_0^t \frac{\sum_{i=1}^n S_i(s)C_i(s)\lambda_i(s)}{\sum_{i=1}^n S_i(s)C_i(s)}\, ds \qquad (10.7) \\ S_h(t) &= \exp[-\Lambda_h(t)], \end{aligned}$$

where $C_i(t)$ is a censoring indicator which is 1 during the period of potential followup and 0 thereafter. C_i depends only on the enrollment date for the study subject (and the paired hypothetical control) and the date that subject will become censored, but not on the survival status or event date of the study subject. For observational studies or clinical trials where censoring is induced by the analysis date this is easily computed, but determination of the potential followup could be a problem if there are large numbers lost to followup, that is, censored substantially before the analysis date.

In practice, the program is usually invoked using the actual censoring time for those patients who are censored, and the *maximum* potential followup for those who have died. By the maximum potential followup we mean the difference between enrollment date and the most optimistic last contact date; for example, if patients are contacted every 3 months on average and the study was closed 6 months ago this date would be 7.5 months ago. It may be true that the (hypothetical) matched control for a case who died 30 years ago would have little actual chance of such long followup, but this is not really important. Almost all of the numerical difference between the Ederer and Hakulinen estimates results from censoring those patients who were most recently entered on study.

The formula (10.7) differs somewhat from that presented in Hakulinen [59]. He assumes that the data are grouped in time intervals, and thus develops a modification of the usual actuarial formula.

10.3.5 Conditional expected survival

The conditional estimate was suggested as a computational simplification of the exact method by Ederer and Heise [43]; it is the method advocated by Verheul [152] as a correction for the biases of the exact method, and is also called the "Ederer2" approach. It has the form

$$\begin{aligned} \Lambda_c(t) &= \int_0^t \frac{\sum_{i=1}^n Y_i(s)\lambda_i(s)}{\sum_{i=1}^n Y_i(s)} \, ds \\ S_c(t) &= \exp[-\Lambda_c(t)]. \end{aligned} \tag{10.8}$$

The weight $Y_i(t)$ is 1 if the subject is alive and at risk at time t, and 0 otherwise. If the study group does not in reality differ in survival rate from the comparison population, then the estimate should be closely related to Hakulinen's cohort method, since $\mathcal{E}(Y_i(t)) = S_i(t)C_i(t)$. One advantage of the conditional estimate, shared with Hakulinen's method, is that it remains consistent when there is differential censoring as in the aortic valve example. This advantage was not noted by Ederer and Heise, and the "exact" calculation was adopted as the preferred method [42, 58].

The main problem with the conditional method is one of interpretation; unlike the Ederer and Hakulinen estimators it does not correspond to the hypothetical followup of a control cohort. One wag in our department has suggested calling it the lab-rat estimator, since the control subject is removed from the calculation ("sacrificed") whenever his or her matching case dies. Another issue with the conditional estimator is that it has a larger variance than either the Ederer or Hakulinen estimate. In fact, the variance of these latter two can usually be assumed to be zero, at least in comparison to the variance of the Kaplan–Meier of the sample. Rate tables are normally based on a very large sample size so the individual rates λ_i are very precise, and the censoring indicators $C_i(t)$ are based on the study design rather than on patient outcomes. The conditional estimate $S_c(t)$, however, depends on the observed survival pattern.

Andersen and Væth [7] make the interesting suggestion that the difference between the log of the conditional estimate and the log of the Kaplan–Meier can be viewed as an estimate of an additive hazard model

$$\lambda(t) = \lambda_e(t) + \alpha(t)\,,$$

where λ is the hazard for the study group, λ_e is the expected hazard for the subjects, and α the excess hazard created by the disease or condition. Thus the difference between curves may be interpretable even though the conditional estimate $S_c(t)$ itself is not.

10.3.6 Example

The MGUS study was introduced in Section 8.4.1. Since the condition is a relatively benign one, it is of interest to compare the observed patient survival to an expected curve for the population. Since the patients in the study represent a referral rather than a local population, we use the US total population as a reference.

Because the `survexp` routine deals with two data sets, the study group and the rate table, it is necessary to have matching variable names and definitions in each. Assume that the data set `mgus3` has been created with the necessary conversions: `age` = age in days at diagnosis of MGUS, `sex` = 1

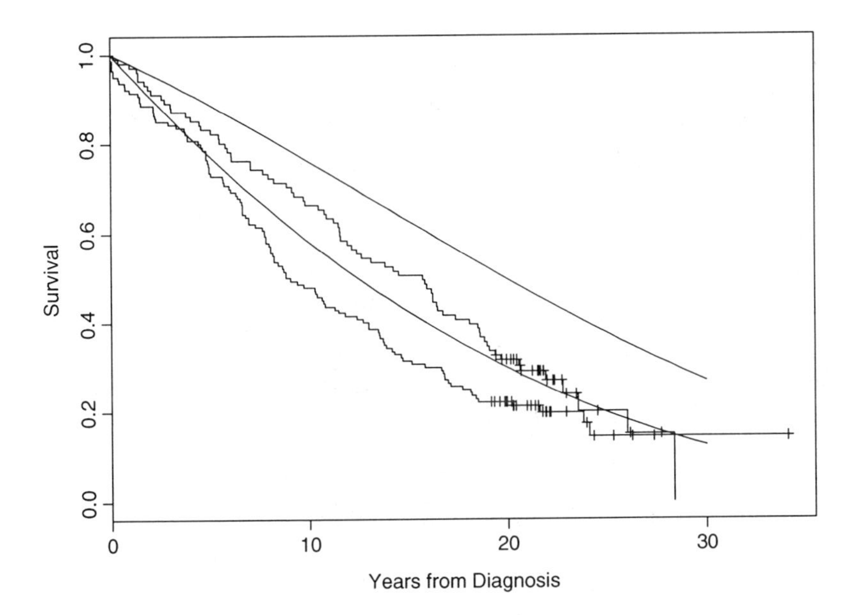

FIGURE 10.5: *Observed and expected survival for MGUS patients, by gender. Step functions are the observed Kaplan–Meier; smooth functions the expected survival. The male curve is below the female curve in each case*

= male/2 = female, `year` = date of diagnosis stored as number of days since 1/1/1960 (the standard SAS format), along with followup time, status, and maximum potential followup for each patient. The data set has 130 events and 111 censored subjects. All subjects were followed up to within 16 months of the analysis cutoff, that is, sometime between January 1990 and April 1991 (between 19 and 34 years of total followup for each patient); no patients were lost to followup. The maximum potential followup time for each subject is taken as the difference between the diagnosis date and August 1, 1990.

The observed and expected survival curves are shown in Figure 10.5, separated by gender. The cluster of + marks on the curves between 17 and 30 years are the patients censored due to the end of followup. Females have a superior survival to males, in both the observed and expected data, which is not surprising given that the median age at diagnosis is 64 years. The curve was produced by the following code.

```
> fitkm0 <- survfit(Surv(time, status) ~sex, data=mgus)  #KM
> plot(fitkm0, xscale=365.25)

> fited <- survexp(~ sex, data=mgus3, ratetable=survexp.us,
                   times= seq(1, 30*365, length=50))     #Ederer
> lines(fited, xscale=365.25)
```

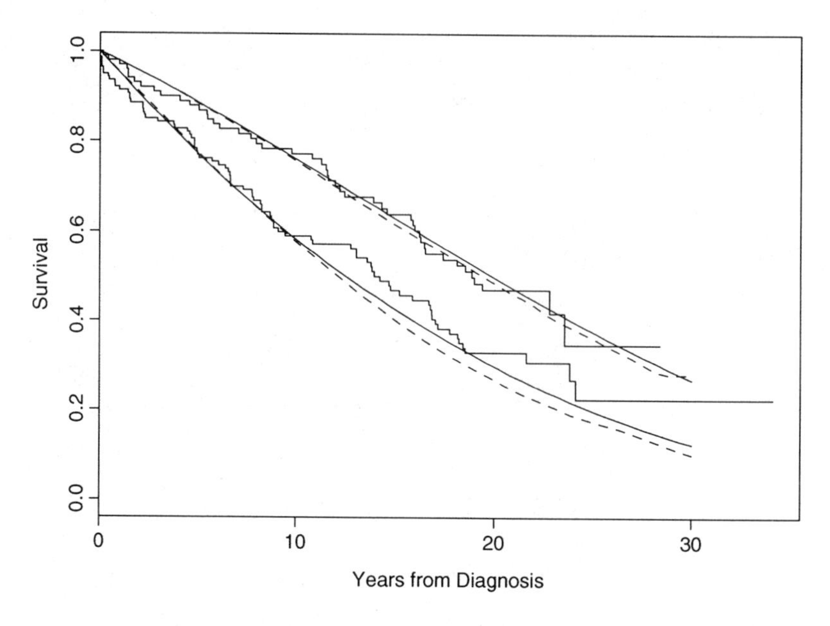

FIGURE 10.6: *MGUS survival, excluding lymphoproliferate disease, along with expected survival*

The `xscale` argument scales the horizontal axis to years; the `times` argument gives the set of x-coordinates for the expected survival computation, 50 points evenly spaced between one day and 30 years.

Here is the SAS macro version. It requires a birth date instead of an age, and has an option to plot the Kaplan–Meier and expected together.

```
%survexp(data=mgus, birthdt =birth, firstdt =dxdate, sex=sex,
         pop='US_T', time=futime, event=status, plottype=3);
```

There is a clear survival deficit associated with the condition. One question is whether the excess death rate is due only to an increased incidence of plasma cell malignancies. This can be approached by a comparison of the expected survival with the Kaplan–Meier curves for "lymphoproliferative disease free" survival, that is, censoring the 59/271 subjects who contracted the disease as of the disease date. The following computes the Kaplan–Meier curve for the modified data, along with the Ederer, Hakulinen, and conditional estimates of expected survival, with `ltime, lstat` containting the modified time.

```
> fitkm <- survfit(Surv(ltime, lstat) ~ sex, data=mgus3)  # KM
> plot(fitkm, xscale=365.25, mark.time=F)
> lines(fited, xscale=365.25)                              # Ederer

> maxtime <- julian(8, 1, 1990) - mgus$dxdate
> fithk <- survexp(maxtime ~sex, data=mgus2, ratetable=survexp.us,
                   conditional=F, times=seq(1, 30*365, length=50))
> lines(fithk, col=3:4, xscale=365.25)                  # Hakulinen

> fitcond<- survexp(ltime ~sex, data=mgus2, ratetable=survexp.us,
                   conditional=T, times=seq(1, 30*365, length=50))
> lines(fitcond, xscale=365.25, lty=3)               # Conditional
```

The result is shown in Figure (10.6). As might be anticipated given the censoring pattern, the Ederer and Hakulinen estimates are almost precisely identical, and completely overlay each other on the plot. The conditional estimate is a small amount lower. Both closely correspond to the observed data. These data would suggest that MGUS does not confer significant mortality, over and above the additional blood cell malignancies for which it is the presumed origin.

10.4 Cohort survival, Cox model

10.4.1 Liver transplantation in PBC

The issues and computations for cohort survival in a Cox model framework are essentially the same as for the population model case. A useful example for all of the methods is the evaluation of liver transplantation in PBC.

Liver transplant is felt to be the only curative procedure available for patients with primary biliary cirrhosis. Due to a variety of factors, however, including the high cost and risk of the procedure and the limited number of donor organs, this premise has never been subjected to a comparative trial. When a donor organ becomes available a liver transplant team, either local to a center or collectively via the procedures of UNOS (United Network for Organ Sharing) must decide which of the multiple needy recipients will receive it. A randomized trial is socially unsalable in this environment, both now and in the conceivable future.

One possible option for evaluating liver transplant would be to compare the posttransplant survival experience of each patient to what "would have happened" to a matched but untransplanted control. The appropriate matching criteria are provided in this instance by the variables of the PBC natural history model, and the "expected" survival is obtained from that source. The data set `olt` contains the survival after orthotopic liver transplant for 215 liver transplants of PBC patients, done at Mayo Clinic, Baylor College of Medicine, and Pittsburgh Medical Center from April of 1985 through September of 1994; see Ricci et al. [125] for a more complete description of the data set. Throughout, we have constrained both the analysis and graphs to the first five years posttransplant. This is easily done by censoring all subjects at five years (those who have not died or been lost to followup before that time).

Thus, just as in the population case studied above, we have need for a cohort survival estimate. How do the transplanted patients as a whole compare to a hypothetical control arm of untransplanted patients?

For the purposes of estimating cohort survival, the choice of estimator for the individual curves is not critical. Most of the difference between them, if any, will come at the tail of the estimate, a point where the variance estimates are particularly large anyway.

10.4.2 Naive estimate

One of the more commonly used estimates, unfortunately, is the naive estimate: compute the mean covariate vector for the subjects, and from this compute a single baseline survival curve. The S-Plus and SAS computations are identical to Section 10.2.1, with creation of a single observation data set followed by a fit of the model.

```
> pbcfit <- coxph(Surv(time, status==2) ~ age + edema + log(bili)+
                              log(protime) + albumin, data=pbc)
> dummy <- data.frame(age = mean(olt$age),
                      bili= mean(olt$bili),
                      protime = mean(olt$protime),
                      albumin = mean(olt$albumin),
                      edema = mean(olt$edema))
> naive <- survfit(pbcfit, newdata=dummy)
```

The problem with this process is the same as with the baseball game example used earlier in the chapter. The average survival of a cohort is not at all the same as the survival of a single "average" member. (Because the original PBC model is based on log(bilirubin), the above dummy data set perhaps should have used the geometric mean `exp(mean(log(olt$bili)))`, but that does not address the fundamental issue.)

The use of this estimate for a Cox model was proposed in Neuberger et al. [112], and is sometimes referred to by that label. Thomsen et al. [147] argue against this estimate for a different reason. However it is considered, the estimate is plainly misguided.

10.4.3 Ederer estimate

The Cox model version of the Ederer estimate is $S_e(t) = 1/n \sum S_i(t)$, where the S_i are the n individual predicted survival curves. This curve is easily computed in SAS.

```
data temp1; set pbc;
    lbili = log(bili);
    lpro  = log(protime);
    lalb  = lob(albumin);
```

```
data temp2; set olt;
    lbili = log(bili);
    lpro  = log(protime);
    lalb  = lob(albumin);

proc phreg data=temp1;
    model  futime*status(0) = age  lbili  lpro  lalb  edema;
    baseline out=curves covariats=temp2 survival /nomean;

proc sort data=curves; by time;
proc means noprint; by time;
    var surv;
    output out=exact mean=surv;
```

The computation in S-Plus uses the `survexp` function.

```
pbcfit <- coxph(Surv(futime, status) ~ age + log(bili) +
                         log(protime) + log(albumin) + edema, pbc)
exact <- survexp( ~1, data=olt, ratetable=pbcfit)

survkm <- survfit(Surv(futime, status) ~1, olt)
plot(survkm, conf.int=F)
lines(exact, lty=2)
```

Figure 10.7 shows the Kaplan–Meier estimate of posttransplant survival along with both the Ederer and Hakulinen expected survival curves.

The Ederer estimate has been proposed in the Cox model context by Chang et al. [30], Makuch [97], and Murphy and Haywood [109]. Gail and Byar [51] provide a rigorous summary of the ideas and compute an appropriate (though complex) variance estimator, referring to the estimate as the "direct-adjusted survival" estimate, which is now the most commonly used label. Neither SAS nor S-Plus currently computes the variance estimate, however.

10.4.4 Hakulinen and conditional estimates

Hakulinen's method has been rediscovered in the Cox model context as well, in work by Bonsel et al. [19]. (The documentation of the method is omitted from the published paper, but is presented in Thomsen et al. [148].) As we can see in Figure 10.7 the exact and cohort curves differ very little, and several authors including Thomsen et al. [147] have commented on this. The conditions under which the two estimates would differ significantly seem to appear only infrequently in the proportional hazards modeling context:

- an extended accrual period;
- subjects accrued early to the study differ from those recruited later, with respect to important covariates in the Cox model which is being used as a control population; and
- analysis at a time point where a substantial fraction of the later arrivals are censored.

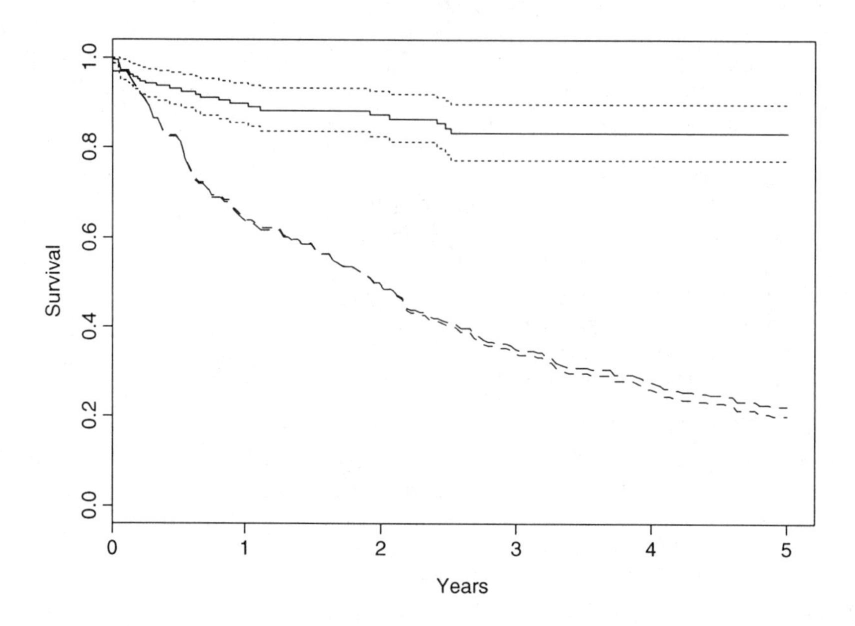

FIGURE 10.7: *Observed and expected survival for PBC patients, posttransplant*

Similar comments apply to the conditional estimator, which is often close in value to the Hakulinen estimate. Thomsen et al. [147] refer to the conditional estimator as the "direct" estimate, but admit that "the interpretation of the estimate is difficult."

In order to compute the Hakulinen estimate a maximal followup time is required. The `olt` data set contains a variable `olt.dt` containing the transplant date. Followup for the data set was complete for each patient through approximately December 1994. If a transplant subject is censored, we assume that the matched control subject would also have been censored on that date, and use the maximal time only for the events.

```
ctime <- ifelse(olt$status==0, olt$futime,
                               chron('12/1/94')- olt$olt.dt )
survhk <- survexp(ctime ~1, data=olt, ratetable=pbcfit)
lines(cohort, lty=3)

conditional <- survexp(futime ~ 1, data=olt, ratetable=pbcfit,
                       conditional=T)
```

There are no facilities to compute the Hakulinen or conditional estimates in SAS. They might be needed quite infrequently, however.

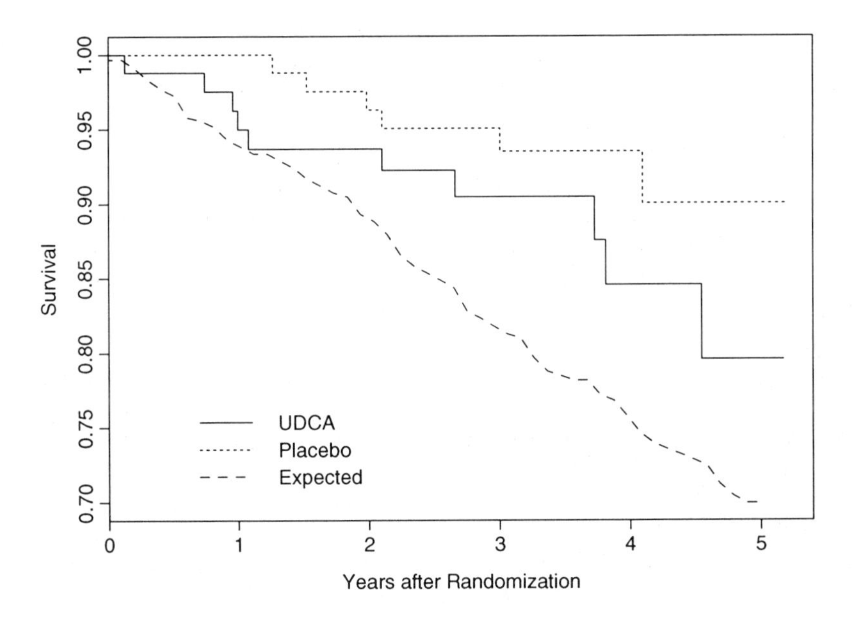

FIGURE 10.8: *Treatment, placebo, and expected survival for the UDCA study*

10.4.5 Comparing observed to expected for the UDCA trial

D-penicillamine, the agent used in the trial for the PBC data set, was shown not to be effective; several other drugs have since been evaluated in this disease. A randomized double-blind trial of a new agent, ursodeoxycholic acid (UDCA), was conducted at the Mayo Clinic from 1988 to 1992 and enrolled 180 patients. The data are reported in Lindor et al. [89]. Figure 10.8 shows a plot of the treatment and control arms, along with the expected survival for both of the arms based on the PBC natural history model. The code below creates the plot, using as input a data set `udca3` which is set up similarly to the `pbc` data set: one observation per subject, and a status variable of 0 = alive, 1 = liver transplant, and 2 = dead. (This data set can easily be created from the `udca2` data set considered earlier.)

```
> risk <- c(pbcfit$x %*% pbcfit$coef)
> fit1 <- coxph(Surv(futime, status==2) ~ pbcrisk, data= pbc)
> sfit1 <- survfit(Surv(futime, status==2) ~ rx, data=udca3)
> expect1 <- survexp( ~ 1, data=udca3, ratetable=fit1)

> plot(sfit1, lty=1:2, ylim=c(.7,1), mark.time=F, xscale=365.24)
> lines(expect1, lty=3, xscale=365.24)
> title(xlab="Years post Randomization", ylab='Survival')
> legend(5,1, c("UDCA", "Placebo", "Expected"), lty=1:3)

> expect1b <- survexp( ~ rx, data=udca3, ratetable=fit)
```

The `udca3` data set was created with the Mayo risk score rather than the individual variables of age, bilirubin, edema, prothrombin time and albumin, so we begin by refitting the `pbc` data using the risk score as the only covariate. (By definition, this fit must have a coefficient of 1, since the risk score was derived on the same data set.) We then fit the survival curves to the udca3 data, and compute the overall expected curve. The computation for expect1b shows how to get expected curves separately for the two treatment arms. However, in this study they are nearly coincident and are not shown on the graph.

The plot shows that UDCA is indeed more effective than placebo at preventing mortality. The expected curve, however, is considerably below that for the placebo arm, whereas we might have anticipated that they would overlap. There are several possible explanations for this, including possible recruitment differences in the two studies, improvement in supportive care, and so on. One likely contributor, though, is the increasing popularity of transplant. In the PBC data set 4% of the patients received OLT within four years of enrollment, versus 8% for the UDCA data. Presumably, with increasing comfort and experience with OLT, patients who once would have died early are being rescued with transplant. A more fair comparison of the old and new series might be in terms of the combined endpoint death/olt.

We still wish to control for the effect of Mayo risk score in the comparison, but need a new estimate of "baseline hazard" corresponding to the combined endpoint. Because of wide experience with the Mayo PBC risk score, however, including numerous validation studies, we fix the coefficients of any new model at their current values, allowing only the baseline hazard estimate to vary.

```
> fit2 <- coxph(Surv(futime, status>0) ~ risk, pbc,
                    iter=0, init=1)

> sfit2 <- survfit(Surv(futime, status>0) ~ rx, udca3)
> expect2 <- survexp( ~ 1, data=udca3,
                                ratetable=fit2)

> plot(sfit2, lty=1:2, ylim=c(.7,1), mark.time=F, xscale=365.24)
> lines(expect2, lty=3, xscale=365.24)
> title(xlab="Years post Randomization", ylab='Death/OLT')
> legend(4.6,1, c("UDCA", "Placebo", "Expected"), lty=1:3)
```

By allowing no iterations (iter=0) we force fit2 to retain the same coefficients as the Mayo model, although it is based on both OLT and death (status>0). The new plot in Figure 10.9 shows much better concordance between the placebo arm and the expected curve.

We can augment this by looking directly at the observed versus expected numbers of death/OLT events in the two groups, divided by groupings of risk score. The results are shown in Table 10.1; the divisions of risk score were chosen to give approximately the same number of subjects in each group. The key step in creating the output is the use of survexp with the cohort=F argument; this gives a vector result containing the expected survival of each individual subject, at the time of the event or last followup.

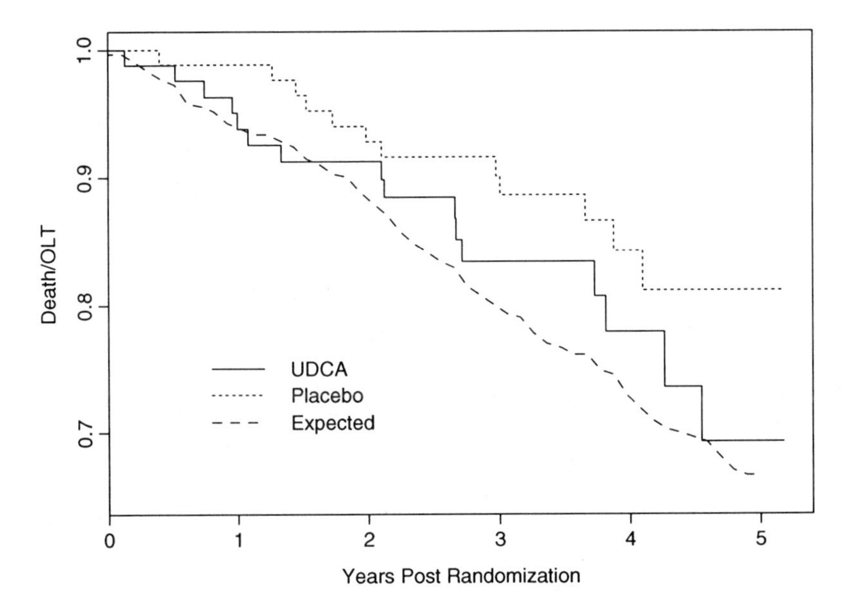

FIGURE 10.9: *UDCA, placebo, and expected survival for the death/OLT endpoint*

```
> tdata <- na.omit(udca3[, c('risk', 'rx', 'status', 'futime')])
> group <- cut(tdata$risk, c(0, 4.4, 5.4, 6.4, 10))
> expect3 <- survexp(futime ~ 1, data=tdata,
                        ratetable=fit2, cohort=F)

> temp1 <- table(group, tdata$rx)
> temp2 <- tapply((tdata$status >0), list(group,tdata$rx), sum)
> temp3 <- tapply(-log(expect3),list(group, tdata$rx), sum)
```

There is one subject in the data set who is missing on the risk score variable. We start by using the `na.omit` function to create a data set that has no missing values for the covariates that will be tabulated. Then `temp1` will be a 4×2 matrix of the number of subjects, by risk group and treatment arm, `temp2` a 4×2 matrix containing the number of death/OLT events, and `temp3` a 4×2 matrix of the expected number of events under the revised Mayo model. These results are found in the first six columns of Table 10.1. The placebo outcome is, as indicated on the earlier graph, in close accord with the expected. There are 13 and 15.4 observed and expected death/OLT events, respectively, and both the observed and expected show an increasing trend with risk score. In the treated group the expected number of events is far larger than the observed count and there is some evidence, although certainly not "significant," for a larger UDCA benefit in the sickest patients.

It was observed that most patients on UDCA have an early positive biochemical response (e.g., lowered bilirubin, alkaline phosphotase, etc. values)

	Placebo			UDCA			After 6 Months UDCA		
Score	n	Obs	Exp	n	Obs	Exp	n	Obs	Exp
≤ 4.4	24	0	1.0	29	2	2.4	52	2	3.0
4.4–5.4	38	5	3.1	26	1	6.4	17	2	3.2
5.4–6.4	20	1	4.3	20	5	10.7	11	6	4.7
> 6.4	9	7	7.1	13	7	21.1	5	3	5.2
Total	91	13	15.4	88	15	40.5	85	13	16

TABLE 10.1: *Observed and expected numbers of death/OLT events*

that stabilizes sometime within the first three to six months. Given that these patients also survive longer, the question arose as to whether a "revised" risk score, based on the lowered laboratory results, would accurately predict their "revised" survival experience. The UDCA data set also contains the risk score at six months. An additional three treated subjects are missing the six-month score due to missing lab values at that time: one is a transplant at 144 days, one a death at 1.3 years and the third still surviving at 6.3 years. All the remaining patients had more than six months of followup and are included in the sums. Computations are essentially identical to those shown above, with a restriction to the treated group.

```
> tdata <-na.omit(udca3[udca3$rx=='Urso',
                        c('risk.6', 'rx', 'status', 'futime')])
> tdata$risk <- tdata$risk.6    #rename
> group2 <- cut(tdata$risk, c(0, 4.4, 5.4, 6.4, 10))
> newtime <-  tdata$futime - 183
> expect4 <- survexp(newtime ~ 1,
                     data=tdata, ratetable=fit2, cohort=F)

> temp4 <- table(group2)
> temp5 <- tapply((tdata$status >0), group2, sum)
> temp6 <- tapply(-log(expect4),  group2, sum)
```

Results are shown in the last three columns of Table 10.1. Looking at death/OLT survival after six months of UDCA therapy, we see that the observed and expected numbers of events, 13 and 16, respectively, now are in reasonably close agreement. More important, there is agreement within each of the four risk subgroups, with an overall chi-square of $\sum(O-E)^2/E = 2.03$ on three degrees of freedom. It appears that the original Mayo model is valid for predicting patient survival after UDCA treatment, and that the amount of survival benefit is roughly proportional to the amount of improvement in a subject's laboratory parameters.

Let us discuss, finally, one area of confusion with the modeling above. Because the Mayo PBC risk score had proven very useful in patient management, and UDCA use has become widespread, the information that the score was still useful post-UDCA administration was well received when reported at scientific meetings. The authors were then asked whether the "new" risk score model (i.e., with a baseline hazard based on death/OLT) should be used in place of the original results. The answer is probably not. In patient counseling, a main use of the original model, one is trying to present a description of the natural course of the disease, that is, what will happen (on average) without major interventions such as liver transplant, and this is what predicted survival curves based on the original model represent. In *assessing* the Mayo PBC model on the UDCA data, however, natural history is not what occurred, transplant did intervene in a nonrandom way by selecting out more ill patients, and the resultant bias needed to be addressed. The revised approach will be useful in evaluation of other PBC treatments.

Appendix A

Introduction to SAS and S-Plus

The examples in the book are shown using two computer packages, SAS (SAS Institute, Cary, NC) and S-Plus (MathSoft, Inc., Seattle, WA). There are several reasons for this, but the primary one is simple:

> these two packages are familiar to the authors.

We suspect that the methods outlined here can be implemented using many other packages, and some of the computations might even be easier. Our focus on SAS and S-Plus should not be taken in any way as evidence that these are the only, or even the best, ways to accomplish the analysis.

One concern with any textbook that contains computer code is that it will quickly become obsolete; we do not think that this should be a particular concern in this case. The first reason for this is that the code we have shown is purposefully simplistic; it was chosen so from a teaching perspective. For instance, any particularly competent SAS programmer will realize that the multiple events example in Section 8.5.4 consisting of multiple `if (...) then do;` constructs, could be considerably shortened by using a `do` loop. Although more compact, it would also make the code much less transparent to those less familiar with the package.

As the packages evolve and new options are added, some of the analyses presented here may indeed become simpler to execute. However, the code shown here will continue to work, and should provide a reference point at least for new keystrokes. For all the analyses presented, the code is reasonably efficient in terms of computer time. In the case of marginal Cox models, for instance, the user may in time not have to invoke the SAS `iml` procedure "by hand," but the matrix multiplication done by the procedure can not be avoided.

The sections below are designed as a quick overview that contrasts the two packages, with the intended audience being a user who is proficient in one of them while wanting an overview of the other. A more complete (and useful) introduction to SAS can be found in Delwich and Slaughter, *The Little SAS Book* [39]. For S-Plus we would recommend Spector, *An Introduction to S and S-plus* [137] or Venables and Ripley, *Modern Applied Statistics with S-PLUS* [151] for a more comprehensive treatment. Both packages are large and full featured. Although each has strengths and weaknesses for certain tasks, the statement that "you cannot do x in SAS, or y in S" is certain to bring forth a stream of protest from dedicated users, along with a collection of working codes. Even the statement "you cannot do x easily in ... " is guaranteed to be controversial. For the record, we find data input, data manipulation, and printed reports (e.g., to give to someone else) to be much easier in SAS, and program development, graphics, and interactive analysis to be much easier in S-Plus, but have done each of these tasks successfully in both packages.

A.1 SAS

SAS is possibly the most widely used statistical analysis package in the world, and is used for data analysis and manipulation well outside the statistical realm. The first edition appeared in the early 1970s, and until their Version 5 it was available only on IBM mainframe computers, but is now sold for a wide variety of hardware platforms. Perhaps as impressive as any other aspect of the package is the tremendous amount of printed documentation available from SAS Institute (well over 10 lineal feet of bookshelf), as well as numerous books by other authors.

The basic unit of operation in SAS is a *data set.* Data sets are rectangular with each row as an observation and variables in the columns. Variables can be numeric or character and the size of the data set is essentially unlimited. The language is case-insensitive; variable names and keywords can be from one to eight characters long, can contain the alphabetic characters, numbers, or the "_" character, but cannot begin with a number. Program statements end in a semicolon (both the names and the ; betray the language's roots in PL/I), except for comments, which can either be a statement beginning with an asterisk and ending with a semicolon, or start with `/*` and end with `*/`. It is still somewhat standard to display SAS code in all upper case, but we do not do so.

In the body of a SAS job the statements can be grouped into four operations, of which the last two are infrequent:

- the `data` step: create a data set by reading in a file, subsetting existing data sets, or combining existing data sets;
- the `procedure` step: pass a data file to an analysis procedure, along with the statements controlling that procedure;
- definition of a macro;
- set global options, such as the length of a printed page or the current page title(s).

Statements that set global options, such as `options`, `goptions`, and `libname`, and macro definitions (if any) are usually placed at the start of a SAS job. Other than these, the statements that follow are processed in groups. Starting with a `data` or `proc` statement, any following statements up to the next `data` or `proc` statement are processed as a batch. Using this block structure, the SAS `data` step provides very powerful and perhaps unmatched capability for data creation and manipulation. These capabilities prove very useful in several of our examples, particularly in the analysis of multiple event data. We here reprise the Stanford heart transplant data example, with annotation.

```
options linesize=80;                                                  1
data temp;                                                            2
    infile 'data.jasa';                                               3
    input id  @6 birth_dt mmddyy8. @16 entry_dt mmddyy8.              4
              @26 tx_dt mmddyy8.   @37 fu_dt mmddyy8.                 5
              fustat  prior_sx ;                                      6

    format birth_dt entry_dt tx_dt fu_dt date7.;                      7
```

Line 1: Set the linesize for all printout to be 80 characters. This would be a standard value if working at a terminal.

Line 2: Create a new data set `temp`, using all of the programming statements found between this line and the next `data` or `proc` statement.

Line 3: Data will be read from the disk file `data.jasa`. (This was done in UNIX. On other operating systems we would have been more likely to name the original data file as `jasa.dat`.) The first three lines of the data file are as follows.

```
1  1 10 37   11 15 67    .          1 3 68    1   0
2  3 2 16    1 2 68      .          1 7 68    1   0
3  9 19 13   1 6 68    1 6 68       1 21 68   1   0
```

Lines 4–6: Input a line of data. The first variable will be called `id`; since the input data contains a blank after the id variable, no positional information is required here; `id 2-3` would also have been valid. The dates are each given as a (starting column, name, format) triple, the last declaring that they are in month/day/year order.

Line 7: The format to be used in any printout of the dates is declared to be of the `12Mar89` type of form. If no format were given, they would print out as integers; each is stored internally as the number of days since January 1, 1960.

```
data stanford;                                                          1
    set temp;                                                           2
    drop fu_dt fustat birth_dt entry_dt tx_dt;                          3

    age =  (entry_dt - birth_dt)/365.25  - 48;                          4
    year = (entry_dt - mdy(10,1,67))/ 365.25;  *time since 1Oct67;
    wait =  tx_dt - entry_dt;                                           6
    if (id = 38) then wait = wait - .1;   *first special case;          7

    if (tx_dt =.) then do;                                              8
        rx = 0;                  * standard therapy;                    9
        start = 0;                                                     10
        stop  = fu_dt - entry_dt;                                      11
        if (id=15) then stop = 0.5;  *the other special case;          12
        status= fustat;                                                13
        output;                                                        14
        end;                                                           15

    else do;                                                           16
        rx =0;          *first an interval on standard treatment;17
        start = 0;                                                     18
        stop  = wait;                                                  19
        status= 0;                                                     20
        output;                                                        21

        rx =1;          *then an interval on surgical treatment; 22
        start = wait;                                                  23
        stop  = fu_dt - entry_dt;                                      24
        status= fustat;                                                25
        output;                                                        26
        end;
```

Lines 1–2: A new data set `stanford` will be created using the data set `temp` as input. One pass through the remaining statements will be made for each line of data in the input.

Line 3: These variables will not be retained in the final data set, but are available for computation throughout the data step code (lines 1–26).

Lines 4–7: Create the age, year, and waiting time variables. The `mdy` function creates a SAS date; it is only one of many date manipulation functions available. Due to the way dates are stored, calculation of a time interval can be done by simple subtraction.

Lines 8–15: If the patient did not receive a transplant, which is indicated by a missing value for transplant date, then one line of output is created with a time interval from 0 to the total number of days of followup. The `output` statement causes an observation to be written to the `stanford` data set, using current values of the variables.

Lines 16–26: If the patient did receive a transplant, two lines of output are written.

```
data temp2; set stanford;
    age_rx   = age * rx;
    prior_rx = prior_sx * rx;
proc phreg data=temp2;
    model (start stop) * status(0) = age prior_sx rx age_rx
                                     prior_rx;
```

Finally, a proportional hazards model is fit. The analysis will use two interaction variables, the age with treatment interaction `age_rx` which equals `age` if `rx=1` and is 0 otherwise, and the interaction of treatment (`rx`) with prior therapy. A new data set is created that contains these temporary variables. Since the following `phreg` procedure expects its input to be contained in a single data set, creation of a new data set containing both the old and new variables was necessary.

The procedure for proportional hazards regression is then invoked. The exact format of a model statement is procedure specific, but an overall structure of

dependent variable(s) = predictor variables / options;

is common. In `phreg` the status variable is followed by a parenthesized list containing the codes to be considered as censored.

The basic survival routines of SAS are summarized below. The routines are

- `lifetest` Computation of Kaplan–Meier curves, and the log–rank, Gehan–Wilcoxon, and other tests,
- `lifereg` accelerated failure time models, and
- `phreg` Cox proportional hazard model.

As well, we make use of several SAS macros:

- `%surv` Computation of Kaplan–Meier survival, with tests and plots,
- `%survtd` survival curves with left-truncated data,
- `%phlev` robust variance for a Cox model,
- `%schoen` resting proportional hazards, and
- `%survexp` expected survival.

A.2 S-Plus

S-Plus is a product of MathSoft, Inc., and is based on the S package first described in Becker and Chambers [12]. The S package itself is an ongoing research project and analysis tool of Bell Laboratories, now Lucent Technologies, and is not generally available. All of the examples in the book were created with S-Plus. The design of S-Plus differs from that of SAS in several significant ways.

- S is designed for interactive use. Each S-Plus statement is executed as soon as it is typed. SAS statements are executed in groups.
- S functions return their entire result back to the S-Plus program for possible further processing or manipulation. Some portions of the result may then be printed. SAS is output-oriented: all of the relevant results are printed, and some portions of the output may then be returned to the SAS job as data sets for further processing. (A new "output delivery system" in SAS promises to eventually make all printed output available, however.)
- S has a much richer data structure (more on this below).
- One of the main design goals of S was extensibility. User-written extensions to S or S-Plus have the same syntax and usage as the base language itself. SAS macros, on the other hand, have a completely different syntax, usage, and creation process from the base SAS language.

The S-Plus language has a rich array of data structures. They include

- single elements: numeric, logical, character, NULL, and language expressions (S-Plus code is itself a data type in the language, and can be manipulated as data);
- vectors, matrices, or arrays of elements of any of the above types;
- data frames: rectangular data objects with variables as columns and observations as rows, very similar to SAS data sets; and
- lists: a collection of any of the legal data elements.

Functions in S-Plus are designed to return all of the results of a calculation back to the package as a single object which is usually a list; some portions of the result may then be printed. The help page for `coxph.object` shows that the result of a Cox model, for instance, is a list with components

- `coefficients` – a vector of length p, the number of variables;
- `var` – a $p \times p$ matrix;

- `loglik` – a vector of length 2, containing the partial likelihood at the initial and final values of the iteration;
- `score` – the value of the efficient score test;
- `iter` – the number of iterations used;
- `linear predictors` – a vector of length n containing the fitted values $X\hat{\beta}$;
- `residuals`– a vector of length n;
- `call` – a copy of the expression that generated the fit;

The main S-Plus functions for survival are as follows.

- `Surv` – A *packaging* function. This is used on the left-hand side of all formulas, and can encompass right-censored, left-censored, interval-censored, and counting process data.
- `coxph` – Cox's proportional hazards model.
- `survreg` – Accelerated failure time models (parametric).
- `survfit` – Create a survival curve, either from raw data or from a model fit.
- `survdiff` – One and two sample tests for equality of survival curves.
- `survexp` – Expected survival curve for a cohort.
- `pyears` – Person years tabulation.
- `cox.zph` – Tests for proportional hazards.

The data manipulation capabilities of S-Plus are generally weaker than those of SAS, and the examples in the book rarely use S-Plus for such a task. Below, we give code that parallels the SAS example above to create the analysis data set for the Stanford heart transplant study. Before running the code the raw data set was modified to use "NA" for the missing transplant dates (which S-Plus prefers) instead of "." for missing (which SAS prefers). We have also left out the command prompt ">" used in the rest of the text to distinguish user-entered text from the S-Plus responses, since the example is all user entered text.

```
temp <- scan("data.jasa", what=list(id=0, b.mo=0, b.d=0, b.y=0,
                                      a.mo=0, a.d=0, a.y=0,
                                      t.mo=0, t.d=0, t.y=0,
                                      f.mo=0, f.d=0, f.y=0,
                                fu.stat=0, surg=0, mismatch=0,
                                hla.a2=0, mscore=0, reject=0))
```

```
temp3 <- julian(temp$b.mo, temp$b.d, temp$b.y)
temp4 <- julian(temp$a.mo, temp$a.d, temp$a.y)
temp5 <- julian(temp$t.mo, temp$t.d, temp$t.y)
temp6 <- julian(temp$f.mo, temp$f.d, temp$f.y)

jasa <- data.frame( id=temp$id,        birth.dt=temp3,
                    accept.dt=temp4, tx.date=temp5,
                    fu.date=temp6,   fustat=temp$fu.stat,
                    surgery = temp$surg,
                    age    =  temp4 - temp3,
                    futime =  temp6 - temp4,
                    wait.time= temp5 - temp4,
                    transplant = 1*(!is.na(temp5)),
                    mismatch=temp$mismatch, hla.a2=temp$hla.a2,
                    mscore = temp$mscore,   reject=temp$reject)
rm(temp, temp3, temp4, temp5, temp6)

stanfun <- function(jasa) ]{
    id <- jasa$id
    tx <-  jasa$transplant
    covar <- cbind(jasa$age/365.25 -48,
                  (jasa$accept.dt - julian(10,1,1967))/365.25,
                  jasa$surgery)
    n <- length(tx)      #number in study
    ntx <- sum(tx)       #number transplanted
    # The patient who died on the day of transplant is
    #   treated differently
    special <- (id ==38)
    wait    <- jasa$wait.time
    wait[special] <- wait[special] - .5

    age <- year <- surgery <- transplant <- id2 <- double(n+ntx)
    start <- stop <- event <- double(n+ntx)
    ii <- 1
    for (i in 1:n) {
        age[ii] <- covar[i,1]
        year[ii] <- covar[i,2]
        surgery[ii] <- covar[i,3]
        transplant[ii] <- 0
        id2[ii] <- id[i]

        if (tx[i])  { #transplanted  - 2 lines if data
            start[ii] <- 0
            stop[ii]  <- wait[i]
            event[ii] <- 0

            ii <- ii+1
            start[ii] <- wait[i]
```

```
            stop[ii]  <- jasa$futime[i]
            event[ii] <- jasa$fustat[i]
            age[ii] <- covar[i,1]
            year[ii] <- covar[i,2]
            surgery[ii] <- covar[i,3]
            transplant[ii] <- 1
            id2[ii] <- id[i]
            }
        else {                              # one line of data
            start[ii] <-0
            if (id[ii] ==15) stop[ii] = .5  #second special case
            else             stop[ii] <- jasa$futime[i]
            event[ii]<- jasa$fustat[i]
            }
        ii <- ii+1
        }

    data.frame(start, stop, event, age, year, surgery,
                transplant=factor(transplant), id=id2)
    }
stanford <- stanfun(jasa)
```

An example model equation in S-Plus is as follows.

```
Surv(futime, fustat) ~ age + sex + log(bili)
```

The $\sim$ can be read as "is modeled as." Parts of the equation are

- `Surv(futime, futstat)` The survival time and status variables. Time must be ≥ 0; the status variable is 0 = censored (alive at last fu), and 1 = uncensored (dead). The status can also be true/false; this allows expressions such as `Surv(futime, stat=='dead')` or `Surv(futime, (stat2==1 | stat2==3))` to be used.
- `age + sex +` ... The predictor variables.
- `log(bili)` Variable transformations can be coded directly in the model formula.
- `ns(age,df=4)` Creates the necessary variables for a natural spline with four degrees of freedom.
- `age:sex` The interaction of age and sex.
- `age *sex` Equivalent to `age + sex + age:sex`.
- `factor(inst)` Treat `inst` as a categorical variable. Character variables are automatically treated as factors.
- `1` The intercept term, included by default. `age + sex -1` is a fit without an intercept.

Throughout the book, we have assumed that two of the global S-Plus options have been reset from their default values. These are the `contrasts` option, which controls how dummy variables are created for factors, and the `na.action` option, which controls how missing values are handled.

```
options(contrasts='contr.treatment')
```

The `contrasts` option controls how factor variables are coded. The default value for this option is `c('contr.helmert', 'contr.poly')`, which specifies polynomial contrasts for ordered factor variables, and Helmert contrasts for all others. (Factors are unordered by default.) Helmert contrasts are very difficult to interpret (our opinion) except in certain orthogonal experimental designs. Using treatment contrasts, the first level of the covariate acts as the reference cell. For instance, if `institute` were Rochester, Jacksonville, or Scottsdale, the dummy variables would be

- instituteRochester= 1 if institute=='Rochester', 0 otherwise
- instituteScottsdale= 1 if institute=='Scottsdale', 0 otherwise

since "Jacksonville" is the smallest value alphabetically. (SAS by default uses the last category of a factor variable as the reference cell.)

```
options(na.action='na.omit')
```

The default action for missing values in S-Plus is `na.fail`, which prints an error message "Missing values not allowed" and exits. The `na.omit` option removes observations with missing values before fitting the model.

The survival functions in S-Plus are derived from code written by the first author over a period of several years. At infrequent intervals this code has been submitted to statlib (`http://lib.stat.cmu.edu`), a statistical software repository maintained by the Statistics Department of Carnegie Mellon University. Table A.1 below gives a chronology of the versions found in S-Plus and statlib; entries further down the list are more recent. The dates listed for the S-Plus distributions are approximate. The statlib versions give users the opportunity to view the actual source code of the package, should they wish to do so, but the distributed code is usually more up to date.

Survival (5/90)	
Survival2 (7/91)	
	S-Plus 2.0
Survival3 (4/93)	
Survival4 (4/94)	
	S-Plus 3.3 (4/95)
	S-Plus 3.4 (8/96)
	S-Plus 4.0 (3/97)
Survival5 (12/98)	
	S-Plus 5.1 (9/99)
	S-Plus 2000 (1/2000)

TABLE A.1: *S-Plus survival code genesis*

Appendix B

SAS Macros

This appendix describes the arguments and purpose of the macros `daspline`, `phlev`, `schoen`, `surv`, and `survtd`, discussed in this book. The actual SAS text of the macros can be found on the web pages for the Section of Biostatistics, Mayo Clinic: www.mayo.edu/hsr/biostat.html. Subsidiary macros needed by these macros can be found there. Examples include macro `dshide`, called by macro `daspline`, and macro `survlrk` which computes the logrank statistics for macro `surv`.

B.1 daspline

The SAS macros for spline fits are used with the kind permission of the author, Frank Harrell, Jr. For a given list of variables, the macro `daspline` generates formulas for dummy variables that allow fitting of Stone and Koo's [140, 139] additive splines constrained to be linear in the tails. If the variables are named `A` and `B`, for example, the generated dummy variables will be `A1, A2, ..., Ap` and `B1, B2, ..., Bq`, where p and q are the number of knots minus 2 (if a variable name is 8 characters long, the last character is ignored when forming dummy variable names). The spline models are then fitted by specifying as independent variables `A`, `A1-Ap`, `B`, and `B1-Bq`. If knot points are not specified, `nk` knots will be selected automatically, where `nk` = 3–7 is a user-specified number of knots. The following quantiles are used according to the number of knots:

nk	Quantiles						
3	.05	.5	.95				
4	.05	.35	.65	.95			
5	.05	.275	.5	.725	.95		
6	.05	.23	.41	.59	.77	.95	
7	.025	.18333	.34166	.5	.65833	.81666	.975

Stone and Koo [139] recommend using the following quantiles if the sample size is n: 0, $1/(1+m)$, .5, $1/(1+1/m)$, 1, where $m = \sqrt{n}$. Instead of letting `daspline` choose knots, knots may be given for up to 20 variables by specifying the knot points for variable i with a `knot` i parameter.

Formulas for the necessary dummy variables are constructed; the formulae for user variable `x` are stored in macro variable `&_x` (the eighth letter of the variable name is truncated if needed). Knot points computed by `daspline` or given by the user are stored in global macro variables named `_knot1_`, `_knot2_`, ...

Example:

```
%daspline(age height, nk=5, data=data1);
data temp; set data1;
    &_age;        *constructs the variables age1, age2, age3;
    &_height;
proc reg;
    model y=age age1 age2 age3 height height1 height2 height3;

%daspline(weight height, knot1=20 50 100 200 250 280,
                         knot2=25 30 40 50 70);
data temp2; set data2;
    &_weight;
    &_height;

%MACRO DASPLINE(x,nk=4,knot1=,knot2=,knot3=,knot4=,
       knot5=,knot6=,knot7=,knot8=,knot9=,knot10=,
       knot11=,knot12=,knot13=,knot14=,knot15=,
       knot16=,knot17=,knot18=,knot19=,knot20=,
       norm=2,data=_LAST_);
```

- List of variables, separated by spaces.
- `nk` Number of knots to use if `knot`i is not given for variable i (default = 4).
- `knot1` At least 3 knot points for the first variable, separated by spaces.
- `knot2` For variable 2, and so on.
- `norm` Normalization:
  - `norm` = 0 (default): no normalization of constructed variables;

- `norm` = 1 : divide by cube of difference in last two knots makes all variables unitless
- `norm` = 2 : (default) divide by square of difference in outer knots; makes all variables in original units of x.

B.2 phlev

This macro uses the dfbeta residuals D from a proportional hazards model to compute the approximate jackknife variance estimate $D'D$. The new variance matrix may be output as a data set, or may be used to create a "new" `phreg` style printout with jackknife standard errors, z-statistics, and p-values. Some data sets, particularly those with recurring events, may contain multiple observations for a single individual. The macro has the option of "collapsing"the matrix of dfbeta residuals before computing the matrix product, to give the approximate grouped-jackknife variance estimate $\widetilde{D}'\widetilde{D}$. This variance is also appropriate when there are correlations within groups (collapsing within group). The macro was developed by E. Bergstralh and J. Kosanke under the direction of T. Therneau.

```
%macro phlev(data=,      time=, event=,      xvars=,
             strata=, id=,     collapse=N, outlev=phlev,
             outvar=phvar,     plot=N,      scaled=N,
             ref=N,            ties=efron);
```

- `data` Input SAS data set name.
- `time` Time variable for survival.
- `event` Event variable for survival; 1 = event, 0 = censored.
- `xvars` List of covariates for Cox model.
- `strata` Stratification variable(one only) for stratified Cox models.
- `id` Name of id variable to be included in the output dataset. It must be numeric.
- `collapse` `Y,N,T,F` If yes or true (`Y,T`), then the residual matrix is collapsed (summed) based on unique values of the id variable. Default is not to collapse (`N`).
- `outlev` Name of the data set containing the dfbeta residuals. The variable names will be the same as the covariate names in the Cox model. The data set will also contain the id variable, if one was specified. Default data set name is `phlev`.

- `outvar` Name of the output data set containing the robust variance estimate. There is one observation and one variable for each covariate. Default data set name is `phvar`.

- `plot` = `Y,N,T,F` If yes or true(`Y,T`), a plot of residuals for each observation or id value (if collapse = `Y`) is produced. A separate plot is created for each covariate. Default is `N`.

- `dfbeta` = `Y,N,T,F` If yes or true (`Y,T`) (default), the dfbeta residuals are plotted. If `N`, the score residuals are used.

- `ref` = `Y,N,T,F` If yes or true (`Y,T`), reference lines are drawn on the plots at +-se(beta). Default is `N`.

- `ties`= efron. The option to be used for ties in the phreg procedure. Legal values are defined in the phreg documentation, this macro uses the Efron approximation by default.

The macro prints the `phreg` output used to fit the Cox model and a summary table including the Cox model betas, se, and chi-square along with the robust se and its associated chi-square. It also includes the global Wald chi-square test based on the leverage residuals. The summary table is available as a SAS data set named `_b_se`.

B.3 schoen

This macro uses the scaled Schoenfeld residuals to produce plots and tests of proportional hazards. The matrix of Schoenfeld residuals, and the plots, have one observation per death. The macro was developed by E. Bergstralh and J. Kosanke under the direction of T. Therneau.

```
%macro schoen(data=_last_,time=,event=,xvars=,vref=yes,
              strata=,outsch=schr,outbt=schbt,plot=r,points=yes,
              df=4,pvars=,alpha=.05,rug=no, ties=efron);
```

- `data` Input SAS data set name; default is last data set created.

- `time` Time variable for survival.

- `event` Event variable for survival; 1 = event, 0 = censored.

- `xvars` List of covariates for Cox model.

- `strata` Stratification variable(one only) for stratified Cox models.

- `outsch` Name of output data set containing Schoenfeld residuals. There is one obs per each event time. The variables containing the residuals have the same name as the covariates (`xvars`). The data set also includes the time variable and the strata variable.

- `outbt` Name of output data set containing the scaled Schoenfeld residuals (Bt). There is one obs per each event time. The variables containing the scaled residuals have the same name as the covariates (`xvars`). The dataset also includes the time variable, the rank of the time(`rtime`) and a variable (`probevt`) which is equal to "1 minus the overall Kaplan–Meier" at the given time.

- `plot` Possible values are t,r,k,n. Indicates that SAS/Graph plots of Bt versus time (t), rank of time (r) or "1 — overall Kaplan–Meier" (`k`) are to be done. Default is r. For no plots use n. The name of the graphics catalogue is `gschbt`.

- `vref` Indicator to control plotting of a vertical reference line at y = 0. Values are yes(default) and no.

- `points` Indicates whether to plot the actual data points. Default is yes.

- `df` Degrees of freedom for smooth spline overlaid on the scatterplot. Possible values are 3 to 7. Default is 4.

- `pvars`Variables to plot. Default is all `xzvars`.

- `alpha` Confidence coefficient for plotting standard error bars. Default is .05. A value of 0 means do not plot se bars.

- `rug` Indicator to control plotting of rug of x values. Values are yes and no(default).

B.4 surv

This macro calculates the survival curve $S(t)$, standard error, confidence limits, and median survival time. It will also computes the k-sample logrank test and produces plots upon request. The macro was developed by Janice Offord. Because of its extensive list of options, the description below has been abbreviated to the major ones.

```
%macro surv  (time= ,event= ,cen_vl=0, printop=1,class= ,by= ,
              data=_last_, out=_survout, points= ,cl=3,
              alpha=.05,plottype=1,plotop=1,scale=1,maxtime= ,
              xdivisor= ,laserprt= ,logrank=1,medtype=1,
              outsum=_survsum);
```

- `time` Variable containing time to event or last follow-up in any units (Required).

- `event` Event variable as a numeric two-valued variable, (0,1), (1,2) etc. The event value must be 1 larger than the censoring value. (Required).

- `cen_vl` Censoring value for the `event` variable as 0,1 etc. Event = Cen_vl + 1. (Default is 0).
- `class` List of classification variables. They may be either character or numeric. Note - Any observations in the input dataset with missing `class` data, are not included in the results.
- `by` List of "by" variables. They may be either character or numeric.
- `out` Output dataset name (Default is `_survout`).
- `outsum` Output summary dataset name (Default is `_survsum`).
- `data` Input dataset name (Default is the last dataset created).
- `printop` printing options (Default is 1):
- `points` Specific time points at which survival statistics are needed, as months, half-years, years. These points are specified by dividing time into intervals as: '0 to 36500 by 365'. The endpoint of each interval will be the time point to be reported. If you have comas within your statement, enclose the entire parameter in quotes, as: '0 to 360 by 30, 0 to 3650 by 182.5'. You may also specify specific points as well as groups of points as: '1,5,10,15,0 to 36500 by 182.5'.
- `cl` Type of confidence limits (Default is 3)

  1 = Greenwood (actual). 2 = Greenwood with modified lower limit. 3 = log-e transformation (log). 4 = log-e transformation with modified lower limit. 5 = log(-log-e) transformation (log(-log)). 6 = log(log-e) transformation with modified lower limit. 7 = logit transformation (logit). 8 =logit transformation with modified lower limit.
- `alpha` Type I error rate for confidence limits (Default is .05).
- `logrank` Option to compute the logrank k-sample test statistics for the groups defined by the variable `class`.
- Other options to control aspects of the plot and/or the output data set.

Examples:

```
%surv(time=fu_time,event=fu_stat,cen_vl=1);

%surv(time=fu_time,event=fu_stat,cen_vl=1,class=arm,
        out=two,data=one,printop=4,logrank=1,cl=6,
        points='0 to 36500 by 182.5');

%surv(time=fu_time, event=fu_stat, cen_vl=1, class=arm,
```

```
        by=course, out=two, data=one, printop=6,
        logrank=2, plottype=2, xdivisor=365,
        points='0 to 360 by 30, 361 to 36500 by 365');
```

B.5 survtd

This macro calculates the survival function $S(t)$, standard error, confidence limits, and median survival time, for the following special cases: 1) Left-truncated survival, and 2) Time dependent calculations where a person can change state (`class`) after time zero.

```
%macro survtd  (strttime= ,stoptime= ,event= ,cen_vl=0, printop=1,
                class= ,by= , mintime=0,
                data=_last_, out=_survout,points= ,cl=3,
                alpha=.05,plottype=1,plotop=1,scale=1,maxtime= ,
                xdivisor= ,laserprt= ,medtype=1,outsum=_survsum);
```

- `strttime` Variable containing the start of the time interval.
- `stoptime` Variable containing the end of the time interval.
- `event` Variable containing the event status at `stoptime`, as a numeric two-valued variable, (0,1), (1,2) etc. The event value must be 1 larger than the censoring value. (Required).
- `cen_vl` Censoring value for the `event` variable as 0,1 etc. Event = Cen_vl + 1. (Default is 0).
- `class` Classification or state variable(s). They may be either character or numeric. Note - Any observations in the input dataset with missing `class` data, are not included in the results.
- `mintime` the beginning time for the suvival calculations and x-axis of the graph (Defualt is 0).
- Remaining parameters are equivalent to those in `%surv`.

Examples:

```
%survtd(strttime=roch_dt, stoptime=fu_time,event=fu_stat,cen_vl=1);

%survtd(strttime=arrtime,stoptime=fu_time,event=fu_stat,cen_vl=1,
          out=two,data=one,printop=4,cl=6, mintime=30,
          points='0 to 36500 by 182.5');


%survtd(strttime=arrtime,stoptime=fu_time,event=fu_stat,cen_vl=1,
           class=chf,out=two,data=one,printop=4,cl=6,
           points='0 to 36500 by 182.5');
```

B.6 survexp

This macro will calculate expected survival probabilities for a group of individuals based on age, calendar year, sex, and race. All calculations are done by interpolation between decades changing hazard values on each birthday. The output may contain: 1. summary table with one-sample logrank test, 2. list of estimates $S(t)$ for the time points, and 3. a graph of the observed and expected curves. The macro presumes the existence of the baseline rate tables in a known directory.

```
%macro survexp(pop=mn_w, method=2, data= ,birthdt= , firstdt= ,
        lastdt= , time= ,sex= , race= ,points=0 to 3650 by 36.5,
        out=_outexp, event= , cen_vl=0, printop=0, plotop=1,
        plottype=1, laserprt= , by= , pop80=n, pvals=y);
```

- `pop` Population to be used.
- `method` Method used to compute the expected survival: 1 = Ederer, 2 = Hakulinen, 3 = conditional.
- `data` Input dataset name.
- `birthdt` Name of the birth data variable.
- `firstdt` Name of the variable containing the date of the start of follow-up.
- `sex` Sex variable recorded as one of m/f, M/F, or 1/2 (1=male).
- `race` Optional race variable
- `time` Time in days to event or censoring.
- `event` Event variable, 0 = censored, 1 = event.
- `lastdt` Last possible follow-up date (required for Hakulinen method).
- Options to control the plots and/or output data set.

Appendix C

S Functions

These are some extra S-Plus functions used in the text that are not part of the standard package. The functions may be found on the web page of the Section of Biostatistics, Mayo Clinic, `www.mayo.edu/hsr/biostat.html`.

C.1 mlowess

Produce a `lowess` smooth, but with automatic removal of missing values.

```
mlowess <- function(x, y, ...) {
    keep <- !(is.na(x) | is.na(y))
    lowess(x[keep], y[keep], ...)
    }
```

C.2 waldtest

Do a Wald test on the requested coefficients.

```
waldtest(fit, cmat, var)
```

The input arguments are

- `fit` Either a vector of coefficients from a model fit, or more commonly, the complete model result (for instance, a `coxph` object).
- `cmat` Either a contrast matrix C or a vector of numbers. In the case of a matrix the test is $(C\beta)'(C'\Sigma C)^{-1}(C\beta)$, treating β as a column

vector, with degrees of freedom equal to the number of columns of C. In the case where a vector of numbers is the argument, the appropriate C matrix is constructed to do a simultaneous test of all selected coefficients equal to zero.

- `var` The variance matrix of the coefficients. If `fit` is the full result of a model fit, this parameter is usually unnecessary.

The result of the function is a vector containing the test statistic, its degrees of freedom, and a p-value.

C.3 gamterms

This function returns individual terms of fit, along with the standard errors, in a way useful for plotting. (It was originally written to aid in plotting `gam` fits, but applies more broadly).

```
gamterms(fit, se.fit=T)
```

The input arguments are

- `fit` The result of an S-Plus fitting function such as `gam` or `coxph`.

- `se.fit` If true, the result will contain standard error calculations, as well as the mean.

The result of the function is a list of data frames. Consider the following example.

```
> fit <- coxph(Surv(time, status) ~ sex + factor(institution)
                                  + ns(age,4), data=mydata)
> gt  <- gamterms(fit)
```

In this fit there are 3 "terms". The 0/1 variable `sex` will be represented by a single coefficient in the output. The categorical variable `institution`, with k levels, will be represented by $k-1$ coefficients (whose coding depends on the global `contrast` option), and the natural spline for `age` by 4 coefficients. The `gamterms` result `gt` is a list with 4 elements, `gt$constant` is a single number containing the overall average of the linear predictor $X\hat{\beta}$ for the observations in the data set, and `gt$sex`, `gt$institution`, and `gt$age` are each a data frame. Each of the data frames has 3 variables `x`, `y` and `se`. The dataframe `gt$sex` contains 2 rows, that for `institution` has k rows, and the dataframe `gt$age` has one row for each unique value of `age` in the data, the dataframes are sorted in order of x.

C.4 plotterm

The `plotterm` function is a fairly simple one, consisting of a call to `gamterms` followed by the creation of a line plot with the function and its pointwise standard errors.

```
plotterm(fit, term=1, se=T, p=0.95, rug=T, ...)
```

The input arguments are

- `fit` The result of an S-Plus fitting function such as `gam` or `coxph`.
- `term` Which term of the model should be plotted.
- `se` If true, standard errors are also plotted.
- `p` The confidence level for the standard error bands, with a default of 95%.
- `rug` Should a rug be added to the plot.
- ... Any other arguments given are passed forward to the plotting routine, line type or colors for example.

Appendix D

Data Sets

We describe here some of the data sets used in the book. A more complete collection is availale at `http://www.mayo.edu/hsr/biostat.html`, the Mayo Biostatistics Web site.

D.1 Advanced lung cancer

This data set is derived from a study of prognostic variables in advanced cancer patients, conducted by the North Central Cancer Treatment Group ([95]). The subset used here contains 228 lung cancer patients. The variables in the data set are:

enrolling instituion

survival time

status: 1 = alive, 2 = dead

age

sex: 1 = male, 2 = female

physician's estimate of the ECOG performance score (0–4)

physician's estimate of the Karnofsky score, a competitor to the ECOG performance score. Legal values are 20, 30, ..., 100.

patient's estimate of his/her Karnofsky score

calories consumed at meals, excluding beverages and snacks

weight loss in the last six months

The data set is included with S-Plus, as it forms part of the test suite for the survival routines. There are several missing values.

D.2 Primary biliary cirrhosis

This is almost identical to the data set found in Appendix D of Fleming and Harrington [50]; the only differences are: age is in days, status is coded differently, and the sex and stage variables are not missing for obs 313–418.

The data are from the Mayo Clinic trial in primary biliary cirrhosis (PBC) of the liver conducted between 1974 and 1984. PBC is a progressive disease thought to be of an autoimmune origin; the subsequent inflammatory process eventually leads to cirrhosis and destruction of the liver's bile ducts and death of the patient. A more extended discussion can be found in Dickson, et al. [40] and in Markus, et al. [100]. A total of 424 PBC patients, referred to Mayo Clinic during that 10-year interval, met eligibility criteria for the randomized placebo-controlled trial of the drug D-penicillamine. The first 312 cases in the data set participated in the randomized trial and contain largely complete data. The additional 112 cases did not participate in the clinical trial, but consented to have basic measurements recorded and to be followed for survival. Six of those cases were lost to followup shortly after diagnosis, so the data here are on an additional 106 cases as well as the 312 randomized participants. Missing data items are denoted by ".".

The important variables are:

case number;

number of days between registration and the earlier of death, transplantation, or study analysis time in July, 1986;

status: 0 = alive at last contact, 1 = liver transplant, 2 = death;

drug: 1 = D-penicillamine, 2 = placebo;

age in days;

sex: 0 = male, 1 = female;

presence of ascites: 0 = no, 1 = yes;

presence of hepatomegaly: 0 = no, 1 = yes;

presence of spiders: 0 = no, 1 = yes;

presence of edema: 0 = no edema and no diuretic therapy for edema; .5 = edema present without diuretics, or edema resolved by diuretics; 1 = edema despite diuretic therapy;

serum bilirubin in mg/dl;

serum cholesterol in mg/dl;

albumin in gm/dl;

urine copper in ug/day;

alkaline phosphatase in U/liter;

SGOT in U/ml;

triglycerides in mg/dl;

platelets per cubic ml/1000;

prothrombin time in seconds; and

histologic stage of disease.

Here is a listing of the first 20 observations.

ID	FU_DAYS	STATUS	DRUG	AGE	SEX	ASCITES	HEPATOM	SPIDERS	EDEMA	BILI	CHOL
1	400	2	1	1464	1	1	1	1	1.0	14.5	261
2	4500	0	1	20617	1	0	1	1	0.0	1.1	302
3	1012	2	1	25594	0	0	0	0	0.5	1.4	176
4	1925	2	1	19994	1	0	1	1	0.5	1.8	244
5	1504	1	2	13918	1	0	1	1	0.0	3.4	279
6	2503	2	2	24201	1	0	1	0	0.0	0.8	248
7	1832	0	2	20284	1	0	1	0	0.0	1.0	322
8	2466	2	2	19379	1	0	0	0	0.0	0.3	280
9	2400	2	1	15526	1	0	0	1	0.0	3.2	562
10	51	2	2	25772	1	1	0	1	1.0	12.6	200
11	3762	2	2	19619	1	0	1	1	0.0	1.4	259
12	304	2	2	21600	1	0	0	1	0.0	3.6	236
13	3577	0	2	16688	1	0	0	0	0.0	0.7	281
14	1217	2	2	20535	0	1	1	0	1.0	0.8	.
15	3584	2	1	23612	1	0	0	0	0.0	0.8	231
16	3672	0	2	14772	1	0	0	0	0.0	0.7	204
17	769	2	2	19060	1	0	1	0	0.0	2.7	274
18	131	2	1	19698	1	0	1	1	1.0	11.4	178
19	4232	0	1	18102	1	0	1	0	0.5	0.7	235
20	1356	2	2	21898	1	0	1	0	0.0	5.1	374

ID	ALBUMIN	COPPER	ALK_PHOS	SGOT	TRIG	PLATELET	PROTIME	STAGE
1	2.60	156	1718.0	137.95	172	190	12.2	4
2	4.14	54	7394.8	113.52	88	221	10.6	3
3	3.48	210	516.0	96.10	55	151	12.0	4
4	2.54	64	6121.8	60.63	92	183	10.3	4
5	3.53	143	671.0	113.15	72	136	10.9	3
6	3.98	50	944.0	93.00	63	.	11.0	3
7	4.09	52	824.0	60.45	213	204	9.7	3
8	4.00	52	4651.2	28.38	189	373	11.0	3
9	3.08	79	2276.0	144.15	88	251	11.0	2
10	2.74	140	918.0	147.25	143	302	11.5	4
11	4.16	46	1104.0	79.05	79	258	12.0	4
12	3.52	94	591.0	82.15	95	71	13.6	4
13	3.85	40	1181.0	88.35	130	244	10.6	3
14	2.27	43	728.0	71.00	.	156	11.0	4
15	3.87	173	9009.8	127.71	96	295	11.0	3
16	3.66	28	685.0	72.85	58	198	10.8	3
17	3.15	159	1533.0	117.80	128	224	10.5	4
18	2.80	588	961.0	280.55	200	283	12.4	4
19	3.56	39	1881.0	93.00	123	209	11.0	3
20	3.51	140	1919.0	122.45	135	322	13.0	4

D.3 Sequential PBC

This data set is a followup to the original PBC data set, which contains the baseline measurements and survival of 426 subjects, 312 formal study participants, and 106 eligible nonenrolled subjects. The data set contains multiple laboratory results, but only on the first 312 patients. Some baseline data values in this file differ from the original PBC file, for instance, the data errors in prothrombin time and age which were discovered after the original analysis, during research work on dfbeta residuals. (These two data points are discussed in Fleming and Harrington, [50] Figure 4.6.7.) Another major difference is that there was significantly more followup for many of the patients at the time this data set was assembled.

One "feature" of the data deserves special comment. The last observation before death or liver transplant often has many more missing covariates than other data rows. The original clinical protocol for these patients specified visits at six months, one year, and annually thereafter. At these protocol visits lab values were obtained for a large prespecified battery of tests. "Extra" visits, often undertaken because of worsening medical condition, did not necessarily have all this lab work. The missing values are thus potentially informative, and violate the usual "missing at random" assumptions that are assumed in analyses. Because of the earlier published results on the Mayo PBC risk score, however, the five variables involved in that computation were usually obtained, that is, age, bilirubin, albumin, prothrombin time, and edema score.

The variables in the data set are:

case number;

number of days between registration and the earlier of death, transplantation, or study analysis time;

status: 0 = alive, 1 = transplanted, 2 = dead;

drug: 1 = D-penicillamine, 0 = placebo;

age in days, at registration;

sex: 0 = male, 1 = female;

day: number of days between enrollment and this visit date; remaining values on the line of data refer to this visit;

presence of ascites: 0 = no 1 = yes;

presence of hepatomegaly: 0 = no, 1 = yes;

presence of spiders: 0 = no, 1=yes;

presence of edema: 0 = no edema and no diuretic therapy for edema; .5 = edema present without diuretics, or edema resolved by diuretics; 1 = edema despite diuretic therapy;

serum bilirubin in mg/dl;

serum cholesterol in mg/dl;

albumin in gm/dl;

alkaline phosphatase in U/liter;

SGOT in U/ml (serum glutamic-oxaloacetic transaminase, the enzyme name has subsequently changed to "ALT" in the medical literature);

platelets per cubic ml/1000;

prothrombin time in seconds; and

histologic stage of disease.

A listing of the first 22 observations (four subjects) follows. The first five variables of the PBC data set (`fu_days, status, drug, sex, age` have been suppressed from the printout.

ID	DAYS	ASCITES	HEPATOM	SPIDERS	EDEMA	BILI	CHOL	ALBUMIN	ALK_PHOS	SGOT	PLATELET	PROTIME	STAGE
1	0	1	1	1	1.0	14.5	261	2.60	1718	138.0	190	12.2	4
1	192	1	1	1	1.0	21.3	.	2.94	1612	6.2	183	11.2	4
2	0	0	1	1	0.0	1.1	302	4.14	7395	113.5	221	10.6	3
2	182	0	1	1	0.0	0.8	.	3.60	2107	139.5	188	11.0	3
2	365	0	1	1	0.0	1.0	.	3.55	1711	144.2	161	11.6	3
2	768	0	1	1	0.0	1.9	.	3.92	1365	144.2	122	10.6	3
2	1790	1	1	1	0.5	2.6	230	3.32	1110	131.8	135	11.3	3
2	2151	1	1	1	1.0	3.6	.	2.92	996	131.8	100	11.5	3
2	2515	1	1	1	1.0	4.2	.	2.73	860	145.7	103	11.5	3
2	2882	1	1	1	1.0	3.6	244	2.80	779	119.0	113	11.5	3
2	3226	1	1	1	1.0	4.6	237	2.67	669	88.0	100	11.5	3
3	0	0	0	0	0.5	1.4	176	3.48	516	96.1	151	12.0	4
3	176	0	1	1	0.0	1.1	.	3.29	353	69.8	160	12.0	4
3	364	0	0	0	0.5	1.5	233	3.57	218	57.4	107	12.0	4
3	743	0	0	1	0.5	1.8	185	3.25	447	88.4	109	13.3	4
4	0	0	1	1	0.5	1.8	244	2.54	6122	60.6	183	10.3	4
4	188	0	1	1	0.5	1.6	.	2.88	1175	169.0	240	19.0	4
4	372	0	1	1	0.5	1.7	.	2.80	1157	165.9	251	11.6	4
4	729	0	1	1	1.0	3.2	.	2.92	1178	167.4	220	10.8	4
4	1254	0	0	1	1.0	3.7	293	2.59	1067	204.6	338	13.7	4
4	1462	0	1	1	1.0	4.0	.	2.59	1035	162.8	200	12.8	4
4	1824	1	1	1	1.0	5.3	140	1.83	623	131.8	101	17.0	4

D.4 rIFN-g in patients with chronic granulomatous disease

Chronic granulomatous disease (CGD) is a heterogenous group of uncommon inherited disorders characterized by recurrent pyogenic infections that usually begin early in life and may lead to death in childhood. Interferon gamma is a principal macrophage-activating factor shown to partially correct the metabolic defect in phagocytes. It was hypothesized that treatment with interferon might reduce the frequency of serious infections in patients with CGD. In 1986, Genentech, Inc. conducted a randomized, double-blind, placebo-controlled trial in 128 CGD patients who received Genentech's humanized interferon gamma (rIFN-g) or placebo three times daily for a year. The primary endpoint of the study was the time to the first serious infection. However, data were collected on all serious infections until the end of followup, which occurred before day 400 for most patients. Thirty of the

65 patients in the placebo group and 14 of the 63 patients in the rIFN-g group had at least one serious infection. The total number of infections was 56 and 20 in the placebo and treatment groups, respectively. One patient was taken off on the day of his last infection; all others have some followup after their last episode.

Variables are:

Subject id, (128 subjects, max id = 135);

Center	174	Harvard Medical School
	204	Scripps Institute
	222	Copenhagen, Denmark
	238	NIH
	242	L.A. Children's Hospital
	243	Mott Children's Hospital
	245	Univ. of Utah
	246	Children's Hospital of PA
	248	Univ. of Washington
	249	Univ. of Minnesota
	328	Univ. of Zurich, Switzerland
	331	Texas Children's Hospital
	332	Amsterdam, Netherlands
	336	Mt. Sinai Medical Center;

Randomization date month/day/year;

Treatment arm: 0 = placebo, 1 = rIFN-g;

Sex: 1 = Male, 2 = Female;

Age (in years) at time of study entry;

Height (in cm) at time of study entry;

Weight (in kg) at time of study entry;

Pattern of inheritance (stratification factor): 1 = X-linked; 2 = autosomal recessive;

Use of corticosteroids at time of study entry: 1 = used corticosteroids; 2 = did not use corticosteroids;

Use of prophylactic antibiotics at time of study entry: 1 = used prophylactic antibiotics; 2 = did not use prophylactic antibiotics;

Institution category: 1 = US — NIH; 2 = US — other; 3 = Europe — Amsterdam; 4 = Europe — other;

Time from randomization to last followup; and

Event times: time(s) from randomization until infection. The maximum number of infections observed was seven.

Below are the first 15 observations, but with the listing trunctated beyond the fourth infection.

```
204 082888 1 2 12 147.0  62.0 2 2 2 2 414 219 373   .   .
204 082888 0 1 15 159.0  47.5 2 2 1 2 439   8  26 152 241
204 082988 1 1 19 171.0  72.7 1 2 1 2 382   .   .   .   .
204 091388 1 1 12 142.0  34.0 1 2 1 2 388   .   .   .   .
238 092888 0 1 17 162.5  52.7 1 2 1 1 383 246 253   .   .
245 093088 1 2 44 153.3  45.0 2 2 2 2 364   .   .   .   .
245 093088 0 1 22 175.0  59.7 1 2 1 2 364 292   .   .   .
245 093088 1 1  7 111.0  17.4 1 2 1 2 363   .   .   .   .
238 100488 0 1 27 176.0  82.8 2 2 1 1 349 294   .   .   .
238 100488 1 1  5 113.0  19.5 1 2 1 1 371   .   .   .   .
238 100488 0 1  2  93.0  13.2 1 2 1 1 102  19   .   .   .
238 101088 1 1  8 124.0  25.4 1 2 1 1 388 373   .   .   .
238 101088 1 1 12 144.0  36.9 1 2 1 1 388   .   .   .   .
204 101188 0 1  1  79.0  10.5 1 2 1 2 363 211 260 265 269
204 101788 1 1  9 134.5  32.7 2 2 1 2 367  82 114 337   .
```

D.5 rhDNase for the treatment of cystic fibrosis

In patients with cystic fibrosis, extracellular DNA is released by leukocytes that accumulate in the airways in response to chronic bacterial infection. This excess DNA thickens the mucus, which then cannot be cleared from the lung by the cilia. The accumulation leads to exacerbations of respiratory symptoms and progressive deterioration of lung function. More than 90% of cystic fibrosis patients eventually die of lung disease.

Deoxyribonuclease I (DNase I) is a human enzyme normally present in the mucus of human lungs that digests extracellular DNA. Genentech, Inc. has cloned a highly purified recombinant DNase I (rhDNase or Pulmozyme) which when delivered to the lungs in an aerosolized form cuts extracellular DNA, reducing the viscoelasticity of airway secretions and improving clearance. In 1992 the company conducted a randomized double-blind trial comparing rhDNase to placebo. Patients were then monitored for pulmonary exacerbations, along with measures of lung volume and flow. The primary endpoint was the time until first pulmonary exacerbation; however, data on all exacerbations were collected for 169 days.

The variables are:

subject id;

treatment arm: 0 = placebo, 1 = rhDNase;

FEV: "forced expiratory volume," a measure of lung capacity;

FEV2: a second measurement of FEV;

randomization date;

last followup date on study; and

infections: there are up to five infections; each is a pair of numbers, (e.g., "0 104" shows that a patient had a lung infection and was on antibiotic therapy from day 90 to 104).

Note! A few subjects were infected at the time of enrollment; 951317 for instance has a first infection interval of −21 to 7. We do not count this first infection as an "event," and the subject first enters the risk set at day 7. This data does not exactly reproduce the numbers in Therneau and Hamilton [144]. There are multiple ways to define an infection; the number of infections and exact timing of them changed at times during the analysis, and this is not exactly the 1997 data set. (For instance, does an infection start with oral antibiotic or is IV antibiotic required?) None of the substantive conclusions is changed, however.

Below are the first 20 lines of the data set.

```
493301 1  28.8  28.1 20MAR92 04SEP92
493303 1  64.0  63.0 24MAR92 09SEP92
493305 0  67.2  68.7 24MAR92 08SEP92 65 75
493309 1  57.6  56.5 26MAR92 10SEP92
493310 0  57.6  56.3 24MAR92 11SEP92
493311 1  25.6  25.3 27MAR92 09SEP92
493312 0  86.4  85.4 27MAR92 11SEP92
493313 0  32.0  32.4 28MAR92 10SEP92 90 104
589301 1  86.4  86.0 27FEB92 14AUG92
589302 0  28.8  29.2 06MAR92 22AUG92 8 22   63 88
589303 0 112.0 110.7 28FEB92 15AUG92 60 74   83 124
589305 0  70.4  71.7 04MAR92 20AUG92 50 68
589307 1  96.0  94.5 05MAR92 21AUG92
589309 0  44.8  44.6 05MAR92 21AUG92 99 114
589310 1  70.4  70.1 06MAR92 22AUG92 35 64   71 108
589311 1  54.4  53.8 11MAR92 27AUG92
589312 0  73.6  73.2 12MAR92 24SEP92 8 13
589313 1  96.0  97.2 12MAR92 28AUG92
589314 0 105.6 107.0 12MAR92 28AUG92
589316 1  80.0  79.4 19MAR92 02SEP92
```

Appendix E

Test Data

It is useful to have a set of test data where the results have been worked out in detail, both to illuminate the computations and to form a test case for software programs. The data sets below are quite simple, but have proven useful in this regard.

E.1 Test data 1

In this data set x is a 0/1 treatment covariate, with $n = 6$ subjects. There is one tied death time, one time with a death and a censoring, one with only a death, and one with only a censoring. (This is as small as a data set can be and still cover the four cases.) Let $r = \exp(\beta)$ be the risk score for a subject with $x = 1$. Table E.1 shows the data set along with the mean and increment to the hazard at each point.

E.1.1 Breslow estimates

The loglikelihood has a term for each event; each term is the log of the ratio of the score for the subject who had an event over the sum of scores

			$\bar{x}(t)$		$d\hat{\Lambda}_0(t)$	
Time	Status	x	Breslow	Efron	Breslow	Efron
1	1	1	$r/(r+1)$	$r/(r+1)$	$1/(3r+3)$	$1/(3r+3)$
1	0	1				
6	1	1	$r/(r+3)$	$r/(r+3)$	$2/(r+3)$	$1/(r+3)$
6	1	0		$r/(r+5)$		$2/(r+5)$
8	0	0				
9	1	0	0	0	1	1

TABLE E.1: *Test data 1*

for those who did not.

$$\begin{aligned} LL &= \{\beta - \log(3r+3)\} + \{\beta - \log(r+3)\} + \{0 - \log(r+3)\} + \{0-0\} \\ &= 2\beta - \log(3r+3) - 2\log(r+3). \end{aligned}$$

$$\begin{aligned} U &= \left(1 - \frac{r}{r+1}\right) + \left(1 - \frac{r}{r+3}\right) + \left(0 - \frac{r}{r+3}\right) + (0-0) \\ &= \frac{-r^2+3r+6}{(r+1)(r+3)}. \end{aligned}$$

$$\begin{aligned} \mathcal{I} &= \left\{\frac{r}{r+1} - \left(\frac{r}{r+1}\right)^2\right\} + 2\left\{\frac{r}{r+3} - \left(\frac{r}{r+3}\right)^2\right\} + (0-0) \\ &= \frac{r}{(r+1)^2} + \frac{6r}{(r+3)^2}. \end{aligned}$$

The actual solution corresponds to $U(\beta) = 0$, which from the quadratic formula is $r = (1/2)(3+\sqrt{33}) \approx 4.372281$, or $\hat\beta = \log(r) \approx 1.475285$. Then

$$\begin{array}{ll} LL(0) = -4.564348 & LL(\hat\beta) = -3.824750 \\ U(0) = 1 & U(\hat\beta) = 0 \\ \mathcal{I}(0) = 5/8 = 0.625 & \mathcal{I}(\hat\beta) = 0.634168\,. \end{array}$$

Newton–Raphson iteration has increments of $-\mathcal{I}^{-1}U$. Starting with the usual initial estimate of $\beta = 0$, the N–R iterates are 0, 8/5, 1.4727236, 1.4752838, 1.4752849, ... S-Plus considers the algorithm to have converged after three iterations, SAS after four (using the default convergence criteria in each package).

The martingale residuals are a simple function of the cumulative hazard, $M_i = \delta_i - r\hat\Lambda(t_i)$.

Subject	Λ_0	$\widehat{M}(0)$	$\widehat{M}(\hat\beta)$
1	$1/(3r+3)$	5/6	.728714
2	$1/(3r+3)$	–1/6	–.271286
3	$1/(3r+3) + 2/(r+3)$	1/3	–.457427
4	$1/(3r+3) + 2/(r+3)$	1/3	.666667
5	$1/(3r+3) + 2/(r+3)$	–2/3	–.333333
6	$1/(3r+3) + 2/(r+3) + 1$	–2/3	–.333333

The score residual L_i can be calculated from the entries in Table E.1. For subject number 3, for instance, we have

$$\begin{aligned} L_3 &= \int_0^6 \{1 - \bar{x}(t)\} d\widehat{M}_i(t) \\ &= \left(1 - \frac{r}{r+1}\right)\frac{r}{3r+3} + \left(1 - \frac{r}{r+3}\right)\left(1 - \frac{2r}{r+3}\right). \end{aligned}$$

Let $a = (r+1)(3r+3)$ and $b = (r+3)^2$; then the residuals are as follows.

Subject	L	$L(0)$	$L(\hat{\beta})$
1	$(2r+3)/a$	5/12	.135643
2	$-r/a$	-1/12	-.050497
3	$-r/a + 3(3-r)/b$	7/24	-.126244
4	$r/a + r(r+1)/b$	-1/24	-.381681
5	$r/a + 2r/b$	5/24	.211389
6	$r/a + 2r/b$	5/24	.211389

The Schoenfeld residuals are defined at the three unique death times, and have values of $1 - r/(r+1) = 1/(r+1)$, $\{1 - r/(r+3)\} + \{0 - r/(r+3)\} = (3-r)/(3+r)$, and 0 at times 1, 6, and 9, respectively. For convenience in plotting and use, however, the programs return one residual for each event rather than one per unique event time. The two values returned for time 6 are $3/(r+3)$ and $-r/(r+3)$.

The Nelson–Aalen estimate of the hazard is closely related to the Breslow approximation for ties. The baseline hazard is shown as the column Λ_0 above. The hazard estimate for a subject with covariate x_i is $\Lambda_i(t) = \exp(x_i\beta)\Lambda_0(t)$ and the survival estimate is $S_i(t) = \exp(-\Lambda_i(t))$.

The variance of the cumulative hazard is the sum of two terms. Term 1 is a natural extension of the Nelson–Aalen estimator to the case where there are weights. It is a running sum, with an increment at each death time of $dN(t)/(\sum Y_i(t)r_i(t))^2$. For a subject with covariate x_i this term is multiplied by $[\exp(x_i\beta)]^2$.

The second term is $d\mathcal{I}^{-1}d'$, where $\mathcal{I}$ is the variance–covariance matrix of the Cox model, and d is a vector. The second term accounts for the fact that the weights themselves have a variance; d is the derivative of $S(t)$ with respect to β and can be formally written as

$$\exp(x\beta)\int_0^t (\bar{x}(s) - x_i)d\hat{\Lambda}_0(s)\,.$$

This can be recognized as -1 times the score residual process for a subject with x_i as covariates and no events; it measures leverage of a particular observation on the estimate of β. It is intuitive that a small score residual — an obs with such covariates has little influence on β — results in a small added variance; that is, β has little influence on the estimated survival.

Time	Term 1
1	$1/(3r+3)^2$
6	$1/(3r+3)^2 + 2/(r+3)^2$
9	$1/(3r+3)^2 + 2/(r+3)^2 + 1/1^2$

Time	d
1	$(r/(r+1)) * 1/(3r+3)$
6	$(r/(r+1)) * 1/(3r+3) + (r/(r+3)) * 2/(r+3)$
9	$(r/(r+1)) * 1/(3r+3) + (r/(r+3)) * 2/(r+3) + 0 * 1$

For $\beta = 0$, $x = 0$:

Time	Variance		
1	$1/36$	$+ 1.6 * (1/12)^2$	$= 7/180$
6	$(1/36 + 2/16)$	$+ 1.6 * (1/12 + 2/16)^2$	$= 2/9$
9	$(1/36 + 2/16 + 1)$	$+ 1.6 * (1/12 + 2/16 + 0)^2$	$= 11/9$

For $\beta = 1.4752849$, $x = 0$

Time	Variance		
1	0.0038498	+ .004021	= 0.007871
2	0.040648	+ .0704631	= 0.111111
4	1.040648	+ .0704631	= 1.111111

E.1.2 Efron approximation

The Efron approximation [45] differs from the Breslow only at day 6, where two deaths occur. A useful way to think about the approximation is this: assume that if the data had been measured with higher accuracy that the deaths would not have been tied, that is two cases died on day 6 but they did not perish at the same instant on that day. There are thus two separate events on day 6. Four subjects were alive and at risk for the first of the events. Three subjects were at risk for the second event, either subjects 3, 5, and 6 or subjects 2, 5, and 6, but we do not know which. In some sense then, subjects 3 and 4 each have ".5" probability of being at risk for the second event at time $2 + \epsilon$. In the computation, we treat the two deaths as two separate times (two terms in the loglik), with subjects 3 and 4 each having a case weight of 1/2 for the second event. The mean covariate for the second event is then

$$\frac{1 * r/2 + 0 * 1/2 + 0 * 1 + 0 * 1}{r/2 + 1/2 + 1 + 1} = \frac{r}{r+5}$$

and the main quantities are

$$\begin{aligned} LL &= \{\beta - \log(3r+3)\} + \{\beta - \log(r+3)\} + \{0 - \log(r+5)\} + \{0 - 0\} \\ &= 2\beta - \log(3r+3) - \log(r+5) - \log(r+3). \end{aligned}$$

$$\begin{aligned}
U &= \left(1-\frac{r}{r+1}\right)+\left(1-\frac{r}{r+3}\right)+\left(0-\frac{r}{r+5}\right)+(0-0)\\
&= \frac{-r^3+23r+30}{(r+1)(r+3)(r+5)}.\\
I &= \left\{\frac{r}{r+1}-\left(\frac{r}{r+1}\right)^2\right\}+\left\{\frac{r}{r+3}-\left(\frac{r}{r+3}\right)^2\right\}\\
&\quad+\left\{\frac{r}{r+5}-\left(\frac{r}{r+5}\right)^2\right\}
\end{aligned}$$

The solution corresponds to the one positive root of $U(\beta) = 0$, which can be written as $\phi = \arccos\{(45/23)\sqrt{3/23}\}$, $r = 2\sqrt{23/3}\cos(\phi/3) \approx 5.348721$, or $\hat\beta = \log(r) \approx 1.676858$.

Then

$$\begin{array}{ll}
LL(0) = -4.276666 & LL(\hat\beta) = -3.358979\\
U(0) = 52/48 & U(\hat\beta) = 0\\
\mathcal{I}(0) = 83/144 & \mathcal{I}(\hat\beta) = 0.652077.
\end{array}$$

The cumulative hazard now has a jump of size $1/(r+3)+2/(r+5)$ at time 6. Efron [45] did not discuss estimation of the cumulative hazard, but it follows directly from the same argument as that used for the loglikelihood so we refer to it as the "Efron" estimate of the hazard. In S-Plus this hazard is the default whenever the Efron approximation for ties is used; the estimate is not available in SAS. For simple survival curves (i.e., the no-covariate case), the estimate is explored by Fleming and Harrington [49] as an alternative to the Kaplan–Meier.

The variance formula for the baseline hazard function is extended in the same way, and is the sum of (hazard increment)^2, treating a tied death as d separate hazard increments. In term 1 of the variance, the increment at time 6 is now $1/(r+3)^2+4/(r+5)^2$ rather than $2/(r+3)^2$. The increment to d at time 6 is $(r/(r+3))*1/(r+3)+(r/(r+5))*2/(r+5)$. (Numerically, the result of this computation is intermediate between the Nelson–Aalen variance and the Greenwood variance used in the Kaplan–Meier, which is an increment of

$$\frac{dN(t)}{[\sum Y_i(t)r_i(t)][\sum Y_i(t)r_i(t)-\sum dN_i(t)Y_i(t)r_i(t)]}.$$

The denominator for the Greenwood formula is the sum over those at risk, times that sum *without* the deaths. At time 6 this latter is $2/[(r+3)(3)]$.)

For $\beta = 0$, $x = 0$, let $v = \mathcal{I}^{-1} = 144/83$.

Time	Variance	
1	$1/36$	
	$+ v(1/12)^2$	$= 119/2988$
6	$(1/36 + 1/16 + 4/25)$	
	$+ v(1/12 + 1/16 + 1/18)^2$	$= 1996/6225$
9	$(1/36 + 1/16 + 4/25 + 1)$	
	$+ v(1/12 + 1/16 + 1/18 + 0)^2$	$= 8221/6225$

For $\beta = 1.676857$, $x = 0$.

Time	Variance	
1	0.00275667 + .00319386	= 0.0059505
2	0.05445330 + .0796212	= 0.134075
4	1.05445330 + .0796212	= 1.134075

Given the cumulative hazard, the martingale and score residuals follow directly using similar computations. Subject 3, for instance, experiences a total hazard of $1/(3r + 3)$ at the first death time, $1/(r + 3)$ at the "first" death on day 6, and $(1/2) * 2/(r + 5)$ at the "second" death on day 6 — notice the case weight of $1/2$ on the last term. Subjects 5 and 6 experience the full hazard of $1/(r + 3) + 2/(r + 5)$ on day 6. Let $a = r + 1$, $b = r + 3$, and $c = r + 5$; then the values of the martingale residuals are as follows.

Subject	$\widehat{M}(0)$	$\widehat{M}(\hat{\beta})$
1	5/6	.719171
2	–1/6	–.280829
3	5/12	–.438341
4	5/12	.731087
5	–3/4	–.365543
6	–3/4	–.365543

The score residuals are

Subject	Score	$L(0)$	$L(\hat{\beta})$
1	$2b/3a^2$	5/12	.113278
2	$-r/3a^2$	–1/12	–.044234
3	$\frac{675+1305r+756r^2-4r^3-79r^4-13r^5}{3a^2b^2c^2}$	55/144	–.102920
4	$\frac{147r-9r^2-200r^3-140r^4-35r^5-3r^6}{3a^2b^2c^2}$	–5/144	–.407840
5	$\frac{2r(177+282r+182r^2+50r^3+5r^4)}{3a^2b^2c^2}$	29/144	.220858
6	same	29/144	.220858

For subject 3, the score residual was computed as

$$\left(1 - \frac{r}{r+1}\right)\left(0 - \frac{1}{3r+3}\right) + \left(1 - \frac{r}{r+3}\right)\left(\frac{1}{2} - \frac{1}{r+3}\right) + \left(1 - \frac{r}{r+5}\right)\left(\frac{1}{2} - \frac{1}{r+5}\right);$$

the single death is counted as $1/2$ event for each of the two day 6 events. Another equivalent approach is to actually form a second data set in which subjects 3 and 4 are each represented by two observations, one at time 6 and the other at time $6 + \epsilon$, each with a case weight of 1/2. Then a computation using the Breslow approximation will give this score residual as the weighted sum of the score residuals for the two psuedo-observations.

The Schoenfeld residuals for the first and last events are identical to the Breslow estimates, that is, $1/(r+1)$ and 0, respectively. The residuals for time 6 are $1 - c$ and $0 - c$, where $c = (1/2)\{r/(r+3) + r/(r+5)\}$, the "average" $\bar{x}$ over the deaths.

It is quite possible to combine the Efron approximation for $\hat{\beta}$ along with the Breslow (or Nelson–Aalen) estimate of $\hat{\Lambda}$, and in fact this is the behavior used in SAS. That is, if the `ties=efron` option is chosen the formulas for LL, U, and $\mathcal{I}$ are those shown in this section, while the hazard and residuals all use the formulas of the prior section. Although this is not perfectly consistent the numerical effect on the residuals is minor, and it does not appear to affect their utility.

E.1.3 Exact partial likelihood

At the tied death time the exact partial likelihood will have a single term. The numerator is a product of the risk scores of the subjects with an event, and the denominator is a sum of such products, where the sum is over all possible choices of two subjects from the four who were at risk at the time. (If there were 10 tied deaths from a pool of 60 available, the sum would be over all $\binom{60}{10}$ subsets, a truly formidable computation!) In our case, three of the four subjects at risk at time 6 have a risk score of $\exp(0x) = 1$ and one a risk score of r, and the sum has six terms $\{r, r, r, 1, 1, 1\}$.

$$\begin{aligned} LL &= \{\beta - \log(3r+3)\} + \{\beta - \log(3r+3)\} + \{0 - 0\} \\ &= 2\{\beta - \log(3r+3)\}. \end{aligned}$$

$$\begin{aligned} U &= \left(1 - \frac{r}{r+1}\right) + \left(1 - \frac{r}{r+1}\right) + (0 - 0) \\ &= \frac{2}{r+1}. \end{aligned}$$

$$\mathcal{I} = \frac{2r}{(r+1)^2}.$$

The solution $U(\beta) = 0$ corresponds to $r = \infty$, with a loglikelihood that asymptotes to $-2\log(3)$. The Newton–Raphson iteration has increments of $(r+1)/r$, so $\hat{\beta} = 0$, 2, 3.1, 4.2, 5.2, and so on. A solution at $\hat{\beta} = 15$ is hardly different in likelihood from the true maximum, however, and most programs will stop iterating shortly after reaching this point. The information matrix,

Time	Status	x	Number at Risk	$\bar{x}$	$d\hat{\Lambda}$
(1,2]	1	1	2	$r/(r+1)$	$1/(r+1)$
(2,3]	1	0	3	$r/(r+2)$	$1/(r+2)$
(5,6]	1	0	5	$3r/(3r+2)$	$1/(3r+2)$
(2,7]	1	1	4	$3r/(3r+1)$	$1/(3r+1)$
(1,8]	1	0	4	$3r/(3r+1)$	$1/(3r+1)$
(7,9]	1	1	5	$3r/(3r+2)$	$2/(3r+2)$
(3,9]	1	1			
(4,9]	0	1			
(8,14]	0	0	2	0	0
(8,17]	0	0	1	0	0

TABLE E.2: *Test data 2*

which measures the curvature of the likelihood function, rapidly goes to zero as β grows.

Both SAS and S-Plus use the Nelson–Aalen estimate of hazard after fitting an exact model, so the formulae of Table E.1 apply. All residuals at $\hat{\beta} = 0$ are thus identical to those for a Breslow approximation. At $\hat{\beta} = \infty$ the martingale residuals are still well defined. Subjects 1 to 3, those with a covariate of 1, experience a hazard of $r/(3r+3) = 1/3$ at time 1. Subject 3 accumulates a hazard of 1/3 at time 1 and a further hazard of 2 at time 6. The remaining subjects are at an infinitely lower risk during days 1 to 6 and accumulate no hazard then, with subject 6 being credited with 1 unit of hazard at the last event. The residuals are thus $1 - 1/3 = 2/3$, $0 - 1/3$, $1 - 7/3 = -4/3$, $1 - 0$, 0, and 0, respectively, for the six subjects.

Values for the score and Schoenfeld residuals can be derived similarly as the limit as $r \to \infty$ of the formulae in Section E.1.1.

E.2 Test data 2

This data set also has a single covariate, but in this case a (start, stop] style of input is employed. Table E.2 shows the data sorted by the end time of the risk intervals. The columns for $\bar{x}$ and hazard are the values at the event times; events occur at the end of each interval for which status = 1.

E.2.1 Breslow approximation

For the Breslow approximation we have

$$\begin{aligned} LL &= \log\left(\frac{r}{r+1}\right) + \log\left(\frac{1}{r+2}\right) + \log\left(\frac{1}{3r+2}\right) + \\ & \quad \log\left(\frac{r}{3r+1}\right) + \log\left(\frac{1}{3r+1}\right) + 2\log\left(\frac{r}{3r+2}\right) \\ &= 4\beta - \log(r+1) - \log(r+3) - 3\log(3r+2) - 2\log(3r+1). \end{aligned}$$

$$\begin{aligned}
U &= \left(1 - \frac{r}{r+1}\right) + \left(0 - \frac{r}{r+2}\right) + \left(0 - \frac{3r}{3r+2}\right) + \\
&\quad \left(1 - \frac{3r}{3r+1}\right) + \left(0 - \frac{3r}{3r+1}\right) + 2\left(1 - \frac{3r}{3r+2}\right) \\
&= 4 - \frac{63s^4 + 201s^3 + 184s^2 + 48s}{9s^4 + 36s^3 + 47s^2 + 24s + 4}.
\end{aligned}$$

$$\begin{aligned}
\mathcal{I} &= \frac{r}{(r+1)^2} + \frac{2r}{(r+2)^2} + \frac{6r}{(3r+2)^2} + \frac{3r}{(3r+1)^2} \\
&\quad \frac{3r}{(3r+2)^2} + \frac{12r}{(3r+2)^2}.
\end{aligned}$$

The solution is at $U(\hat\beta) = 0$ or $r \approx .9189477$; $\hat\beta = \log(r) \approx -.084529$. Then

$$\begin{array}{ll}
LL(0) = -9.392662 & LL(\hat\beta) = -9.387015 \\
U(0) = -2/15 & U(\hat\beta) = 0 \\
\mathcal{I}(0) = 2821/1800 & \mathcal{I}(\hat\beta) = 1.586935.
\end{array}$$

The martingale residuals are (status–cumulative hazard) or $O - E = \delta_i - \int Y_i(s) r_i d\hat\Lambda(s)$. Let $\hat\lambda_1, \ldots, \hat\lambda_6$ be the six increments to the cumulative hazard listed in Table E.2. Then the cumulative hazards and martingale residuals for the subjects are as follows.

Subject	Λ_0	$\widehat{M}(0)$	$\widehat{M}(\hat\beta)$
1	$r\hat\lambda_1$	1–30/60	0.521119
2	$\hat\lambda_2$	1–20/60	0.657411
3	$\hat\lambda_3$	1–12/60	0.789777
4	$r(\hat\lambda_2 + \hat\lambda_3 + \hat\lambda_4)$	1–47/60	0.247388
5	$\hat\lambda_1 + \hat\lambda_2 + \hat\lambda_3 + \hat\lambda_4 + \hat\lambda_5$	1–92/60	-0.606293
6	$r * (\hat\lambda_5 + \hat\lambda_6)$	1–39/60	0.369025
7	$r * (\hat\lambda_3 + \hat\lambda_4 + \hat\lambda_5 + \hat\lambda_6)$	1–66/60	-0.068766
8	$r * (\hat\lambda_3 + \hat\lambda_4 + \hat\lambda_5 + \hat\lambda_6)$	0–66/60	-1.068766
9	$\hat\lambda_6$	0–24/60	-0.420447
10	$\hat\lambda_6$	0–24/60	-0.420447

The score and Schoenfeld residuals can be laid out in a tabular fashion. Each entry in the table is the value of $\{x_i - \bar{x}(t_j)\} d\widehat{M}_i(t_j)$ for subject i and event time t_j. The row sums of the table are the score residuals for the subject; the column sums are the Schoenfeld residuals at each event time. Below is the table for $\beta = \log(2)$ $(r = 2)$. This is a slightly more stringent test than the table for $\beta = 0$, since in this latter case a program could be missing a factor of $r = \exp(\beta) = 1$ and give the correct answer. However, the results are much more compact than those for $\hat\beta$, since the solutions are exact fractions.

	Event Time						Score
Id	2	3	6	7	8	9	Resid
1	$\frac{1}{6}$						$\frac{1}{9}$
2		$-\frac{3}{8}$					$-\frac{3}{8}$
3			$-\frac{21}{32}$				$-\frac{21}{32}$
4		$-\frac{1}{4}$	$-\frac{1}{16}$	$\frac{5}{49}$			$-\frac{165}{784}$
5	$\frac{2}{9}$	$\frac{1}{8}$	$\frac{1}{32}$	$\frac{6}{49}$	$-\frac{36}{49}$		$-\frac{2417}{14112}$
6					$-\frac{2}{49}$	$\frac{1}{8}$	$\frac{33}{392}$
7			$-\frac{1}{16}$	$-\frac{2}{49}$	$-\frac{2}{49}$	$\frac{1}{8}$	$-\frac{15}{784}$
8			$-\frac{1}{16}$	$-\frac{2}{49}$	$-\frac{2}{49}$	$-\frac{1}{8}$	$-\frac{211}{784}$
9						$\frac{3}{16}$	$\frac{3}{16}$
10						$\frac{3}{16}$	$\frac{3}{16}$
	$\frac{1}{3}$	$-\frac{1}{2}$	$-\frac{3}{4}$	$\frac{1}{7}$	$-\frac{6}{7}$	$\frac{1}{2}$	$-\frac{95}{84}$
	$\frac{1}{r+1}$	$\frac{-r}{r+2}$	$\frac{-3r}{r+2}$	$\frac{1}{3r+1}$	$\frac{3r}{3r+1}$	$\frac{4}{3r+2}$	

Both the Schoenfeld and score residuals sum to the score statistic $U(\beta)$. As discussed further above, programs will return two Schoenfeld residuals at time 7, one for each subject who had an event at that time.

E.2.2 Efron approximation

This example has only one tied death time, so only the term(s) for the event at time 9 change. The main quantities at that time point are as follows.

	Breslow	Efron
LL	$2\log\left(\frac{r}{3r+2}\right)$	$\log\left(\frac{r}{3r+2}\right) + \log\left(\frac{r}{2r+2}\right)$
U	$\frac{2}{3r+2}$	$\frac{1}{3r+2} + \frac{1}{2r+2}$
$\mathcal{I}$	$2\frac{6r}{(3r+2)^2}$	$\frac{6r}{(3r+2)^2} + \frac{4r}{(2r+2)^2}$
$d\hat{\Lambda}$	$\frac{2}{3r+2}$	$\frac{1}{3r+2} + \frac{1}{2r+2}$

References

[1] O. O. Aalen. Heterogeneity in survival analysis. *Stat. in Medicine*, 7:1121–1137, 1988.

[2] O. O. Aalen. A linear regression model for the analysis of life times. *Stat. in Medicine*, 8:907–925, 1989.

[3] O. O. Aalen. Further results on the non-parametric linear regression model in survival analysis. *Stat. in Medicine*, 12:1569–1588, 1993.

[4] P. K. Andersen, Ø. Borgan, R. D. Gill, and N. Keiding. *Statistical Models Based on Counting Processes.* Springer-Verlag, New York, 1993.

[5] P. K. Andersen, S. Esbjerg, and T.I.A. Sørensen. Multi-state models for bleeding episodes and morality in lever cirrhosis. *Stat. in Medicine*, 19:587–599, 2000.

[6] P. K. Andersen and R. D Gill. Cox's regression model for counting processes: A large sample study. *Annals of Stat.*, 10:1100–1120, 1982.

[7] P. K. Andersen and M. Væth. Simple parametric and nonparametric models for excess and relative mortality. *Biometrics*, 45:523–535, 1989.

[8] V. E Anderson, H. O. Goodman, and S. Reed. *Variables Related to Human Breast Cancer.* University of Minnesota Press, Minneapolis, 1958.

[9] W. E. Barlow. Robust variance estimation for the case-cohort design. *Biometrics*, 50:1064–1072, 1994.

[10] W. E. Barlow and R. L. Prentice. Residuals for relative risk regression. *Biometrika*, 75:65–74, 1988.

[11] A. A. Bartolucci and M. D. Fraser. Comparative step-up and composite tests for selecting prognostic indicators associated with survival. *Biometrical J.*, 19:437–448, 1977.

[12] R. A. Becker and J. M. Chambers. *S: An Interactive Environment for Data Analysis and Graphics.* Wadsworth, Belmont, CA, 1984.

[13] E. J. Bergstralh and K. P. Offord. Conditional probabilities used in calculating cohort expected survival. Technical Report 37, Department of Health Sciences Research, Mayo Clinic, 1988.

[14] D. Berstein and S. W. Lagakos. Sample size and power determination for stratified clinical trials. *J Stat. Comput. Simul.*, 8:65–73, 1978.

[15] O. Bie, O. Borgan, and K. Liestoel. Confidence intervals and confidence bands for the cumulative hazard rate function and their small sample properties. *Scandinavian J. Stat.*, 14:221–233, 1987.

[16] P. Billingsley. *Convergence of Probability Measures.* Wiley, New York, 1968.

[17] D. A. Binder. Fitting Cox's proportional hazards models from survey data. *Biometrika*, 79:139–147, 1992.

[18] H. W. Block, W. S. Borges, and T. H. Savits. Age-dependent minimal repair. *J. Applied Probability*, 22:370–385, 1985.

[19] G. J. Bonsel, I. J. Klompmaker, F. van't Veer, J. D. F. Habbema, and M. J. H. Slooff. Use of prognostic models for assessment of value of liver transplantation in primary biliary cirrhosis. *Lancet*, 335:493–497, 1990.

[20] L. Breiman, J. H. Friedman, R. A. Olshen, and C. J. Stone. *Classification and Regression Trees.* Wadsworth, Belmont, CA, 1984.

[21] N. E. Breslow. Discussion of Professor Cox's paper. *J. Royal Stat. Soc. B*, 34:216–217, 1972.

[22] N. E. Breslow. Covariance analysis of censored survival data. *Biometrics*, 30:89–99, 1974.

[23] N. E. Breslow and D. G. Clayton. Approximate inference in generalized linear mixed models. *J. Amer. Stat. Assoc.*, 88:9–25, 1993.

[24] N. E. Breslow, L. Edler, and J. Berger. A two-sample censored-data rank test for acceleration. *Biometrics*, 40:1049–1062, 1984.

[25] P. P. Broca. *Traites de Tumerus, volumes 1 and 2.* Asselin, Paris, 1866.

[26] M. C. Bryson and M. E Johnson. The incidence of monotone likelihood in the Cox model. *Technometrics*, 23:381–383, 1981.

[27] K. C. Cain and N. T. Lange. Approximate case influence for the proportional hazards regression model with censored data. *Biometrics*, 40:493–499, 1984.

[28] J. M. Chambers, W. S. Cleveland, B. Kleiner, and P. A. Tukey. *Graphical Methods for Data Analysis.* Wasdworth, Belmont, CA, 1983.

[29] J. M. Chambers and T. J. Hastie. *Statistical Models in S.* Wadsworth, Pacific Grove, CA, 1992.

[30] I. M. Chang, R. Gelman, and M. Pagano. Corrected group prognostic curves and summary statistics. *J. Chronic Diseases*, 35:669–674, 1982.

[31] R. Chappell. A note on linear rank tests and Gill and Schumacher's tests of proportionality. *Biometrika*, 79:199–201, 1992.

[32] C. H. Chen and P. C. Wang. Diagnostic plots in Cox's regression model. *Biometrics*, 47:841–850, 1991.

[33] D. B. Clarkson. Computing extended maximum likelihood estimates in monotone likelihood Cox proportional-hazards models. In *Computer Science and Statistics: Proceedings of the 21st Symposium on the Interface*, pages 464–469, Alexandria, Virginia, 1989. American Statistical Association.

[34] R. D. Cook and S. Weisberg. *Residuals and Influence in Regression.* Chapman and Hall, London, 1982.

[35] D. R. Cox. Regression models and life-tables (with discussion). *J. Royal Stat. Soc. B*, 34:187–220, 1972.

[36] D. R. Cox and D. O. Oakes. *Analysis of Survival Data.* Chapman and Hall, London, 1984.

[37] J. Crowley and M. Hu. Covariance analysis of heart transplant survival data. *J. Amer. Stat. Assoc.*, 72:27–36, 1977.

[38] D. M. DeLong, G. H. Guirguis, and Y. C. So. Efficient computation of subset selection probabilities with application to Cox regression. *Biometrika*, 81:607–611, 1994.

[39] L. D. Delwiche and S. J. Slaughter. *The Little SAS Book.* SAS Institute, Cary, NC, 1998.

[40] E. R. Dickson, P. M. Grambsch, T. R Fleming, L. D. Fisher, and A. Langworthy. Prognosis in primary biliary cirrhosis: Model for decision making. *Hepatology*, 10:1–7, 1989.

[41] V. Ducrocq and G. Casella. A Bayesian analysis of mixed survival models. *Genet. Sel. Evol.*, 28:505–529, 1996.

[42] F. Ederer, L. M. Axtell, and S. J. Cutler. The relative survival rate: A statistical methodology. *National Cancer Inst. Monographs*, 6:101–121, 1961.

[43] F. Ederer and H. Heise. Instructions to IBM 650 programmers in processing survival computations. Methodological Note No. 10, End Results Evaluation Section, National Cancer Institute, 1977.

[44] J. H. Edmonson, T. R. Fleming, D. G. Decker, G. D. Malkasian, E. O. Jorgensen, J. A. Jefferies, M. J. Webb, and L. K. Kvols. Different chemotherapeutic sensitivities and host factors affecting prognosis in advanced ovarian carcinoma versus minimal residual disease. *Cancer Treatment Reports*, 63:241–247, 1979.

[45] B. Efron. The efficiency of Cox's likelihood function for censored data. *J. Amer. Stat. Assoc.*, 72:557–565, 1977.

[46] B. Efron. *The Jackknife, the Bootstrap and Other Resampling Plans.* SIAM, Philadelphia, 1982.

[47] P. H. C. Eilers and B. D. Marx. Flexible smoothing with B-splines and penalties. *Stat. Science*, 11:89–121, 1996.

[48] M. Ezekiel. A method for handling curvilinear correlation for any number of variables. *J. Amer. Stat. Assoc.*, 19:431–453, 1924.

[49] T. R. Fleming and D. P. Harrington. Nonparametric estimation of the survival distribution in censored data. *Comm. Stat. Theory Methods*, 13:2469–2486, 1984.

[50] T. R. Fleming and D. P. Harrington. *Counting Processes and Survival Analysis.* Wiley, New York, 1991.

[51] M. H. Gail and D. P. Byar. Variance calculations for direct adjusted survival curves, with applications to testing for no treatment effect. *Biometrical J.*, 28:587–599, 1986.

[52] M. H. Gail, J. H. Lubin, and L. V. Rubinstein. Likelihood calculations for matched case-control studies and survival studies with tied death times. *Biometrika*, 68:703–707, 1981.

[53] R. Gill and M. Schumacher. A simple test of the proportional hazards assumption. *Biometrika*, 74:289–300, 1987.

[54] P. M. Grambsch and T. M. Therneau. Proportional hazards tests and diagnostics based on weighted residuals. *Biometrika*, 81:515–526, 1994.

[55] P. M. Grambsch, T. M. Therneau, and T. R. Fleming. Diagnostic plots to reveal functional form for covariates in multiplicative intensity models. *Biometrics*, 51:1469–1482, 1995.

[56] R. J. Gray. Flexible methods for analyzing survival data using splines, with applications to breast cancer prognosis. *J. Amer. Stat. Assoc.*, 87:942–951, 1992.

[57] G. Guo and G. Rodríguez. Estimating a multivariate proportional hazards model for clustered data using the EM algorithm, with an application to child survival in Guatemala. *J. Amer. Stat. Assoc.*, 87:969–976, 1992.

[58] T. Hakulinen. Cancer survival corrected for heterogeneity in patient withdrawal. *Biometrics*, 38:933–942, 1982.

[59] T. Hakulinen and K. H. Abeywickrama. A computer program package for relative survival analysis. *Computer Programs in Biomedicine*, 19:197–207, 1985.

[60] C. B. Hall, S. L. Zeger, and K. J. Bandeen-Roche. Adjusted variable plots for Cox's proportional hazards regression model. Technical report, The John's Hopkins University, School of Hygiene and Public Health, Department of Biostatistics, 1995.

[61] F. Harrell. The phglm procedure. In *SAS Supplemental Library User's Guide, Version 5.* SAS Institute Inc, Cary, NC, 1986.

[62] T. J. Hastie. Pseudosplines. *J. Royal Stat. Soc. B*, 58:379–396, 1996.

[63] T. J. Hastie and R. J. Tibshirani. *Generalized Additive Models.* Chapman and Hall, London, 1990.

[64] R. Henderson and P. Oman. Effect of frailty on marginal regression estimates in survival analysis. *J. Royal Stat. Soc. B*, 61:367–379, 1999.

[65] T. Hettmansperger. Median. In P. Armitage and T. Colton, editors, *Encyclopedia of Biostatics*, volume 4, pages 2525–2526. Wiley, New York, 1998.

[66] J. S. Hodges and D. J. Sargent. Counting degrees of freedom in hierarchical and other richly-parameterized models. Research Report 98-004, University of Minnesota, Division of Biostatistics, 1998.

[67] P. Hougaard. Survival models for heterogeneous populations derived from stable distributions. *Biometrika*, 73:387–396, 1986.

[68] P. J. Huber. *Robust Statistics.* Wiley, New York, 1981.

[69] C. M. Hurvich, J. S. Simonoff, and C.-L. Tsai. Smoothing parameter selection in nonparametric regression using an improved Akaike information criterion. *J. Royal Stat. Soc. B*, 60:271–293, 1998.

[70] W. J. Huster, R. Brookmeyer, and S. G. Self. Modelling paired survival data with covariates. *Biometrics*, 45:145–156, 1989.

[71] L. Jaeckel. The infinitesimal jackknife. Memorandum MM 72-1215-11, Bell Laboratories, 1972.

[72] S. Johansen. An extension of Cox's regression model. *Int. Stat. Review*, 51:165–174, 1983.

[73] J. D. Kalbfleisch and R. L. Prentice. *The Statistical Analysis of Failure Time Data.* Wiley, New York, 1980.

[74] B. F. Kavanagh, S. Wallrichs, M. Dewitz, D. Berry, B. Currier, D. Ilstrup, and M. B. Coventry. Charnley low-friction arthroplasty of the hip. Twenty-year results with cement. *J. Arthroplasty*, 9:229–234, 1994.

[75] J. P. Klein. Small sample moments of some estimators of the variance of the Kaplan–Meier and Nelson–Aalen estimators. *Scandinavian J. Stat.*, 18:333–340, 1991.

[76] J. P. Klein. Semiparametric estimation of random effects using the Cox model based on the EM algorithm. *Biometrics*, 48:795–806, 1992.

[77] R. A. Kyle. "Benign" monoclonal gammopathy — after 20 to 35 years of follow-up. *Mayo Clinic Proceedings*, 68:26–36, 1993.

[78] R. A. Kyle. Moncolonal gammopathy of undetermined significance and solitary plasmacytoma. Implications for progression to overt multiple myeloma. *Hematology/Oncology Clinics N. Amer.*, 11:71–87, 1997.

[79] S. W. Lagakos and D. A. Schoenfeld. Properties of proportional-hazards score tests under misspecified regression models. *Biometrics*, 40:1037–1048, 1984.

[80] N. Laird and D. Olivier. Covariance analysis of censored survival data using log-linear analysis techniques. *J. Amer. Stat. Assoc.*, 76:231–240, 1981.

[81] J. A. Laurie, C. G. Moertel, T. R. Fleming, H. S. Wieand, J. E. Leigh, J. Rubin, G. W. McCormack, J. B. Gerstner, J. E. Krook, and J. Malliard. Surgical adjuvant therapy of large-bowel carcinoma: An evaluation of levamisole and the combination of levamisole and fluorouracil: The North Central Cancer Treatment Group and the Mayo Clinic. *J. Clinical Oncology*, 7:1447–1456, 1989.

[82] M. LeBlanc and J. Crowley. Relative risk trees for censored survival data. *Biometrics*, 48:411–425, 1992.

[83] E. W. Lee, L. J. Wei, and D. Amato. Cox-type regression analysis for large number of small groups of correlated failure time observations. In J. P. Klein and P. K. Goel, editors, *Survival Analysis, State of the Art*, pages 237–247. Kluwer, Netherlands, 1992.

[84] K. L. Lee, F. E. Harrell, Jr., H. D. Tolley, and R. A. Rosati. A comparison of test statistics for assessing the effects of concomitant variables in survival analysis. *Biometrics*, 39:341–350, 1983.

[85] D. Y. Lin. Goodness-of-fit analysis for the Cox regression model based on a class of parameter estimators. *J. Amer. Stat. Assoc.*, 86:725–728, 1991.

[86] D. Y. Lin. Cox regression analysis of multivariate failure time data: the marginal approach. *Stat. in Medicine*, 13:2233–2247, 1994.

[87] D. Y. Lin and L. J. Wei. The robust inference for the Cox proportional hazards model. *J. Amer. Stat. Assoc.*, 84:1074–1078, 1989.

[88] D. Y. Lin, L. J. Wei, and Z. Ying. Checking the Cox model with cumulative sums of martingale-based residuals. *Biometrika*, 80:557–572, 1993.

[89] K. D. Lindor, E. R. Dickson, W. P. Baldus, R. A. Jorgensen, J. Ludwig, P. A. Murtaugh, J. M. Harrison, R. H. Wiesner, M. L. Anderson, S. M. Lange, G. LeSage, S. S. Rossi, and A. F. Hofman. Ursodeoxycholic acid in the treatment of primary biliary cirrhosis. *Gastroenterology*, 106:1284–1290, 1994.

[90] C. L. Link. Confidence intervals for the survival function using Cox's proportional-hazard model with covariates. *Biometrics*, 40:601–610, 1984.

[91] C. L. Link. Response to J. O'Quigley, correspondence section. *Biometrics*, 42:219–220, 1986.

[92] S. R. Lipsitz, K. B .G. Dear, and L. Zhao. Jackknife estimators of variance for parameter estimates from estimating equations with applications to clustered survival data. *Biometrics*, 50:842–846, 1994.

[93] S. R. Lipsitz, N. M. Laird, and D. P. Harrington. Using the jackknife to estimate the variance of regression estimators from repeated measures studies. *Comm. Stat. Theory Methods*, 19:821–845, 1990.

[94] R. J. Little. Missing data. In P. Armitage and T. Colton, editors, *Encyclopedia of Biostatics*, volume 4, pages 2622–2635. Wiley, 1998.

[95] C. L. Loprinzi, J. A. Laurie, H. S. Wieand, J. E. Krook, P. J. Novotny, J. W. Kugler, J. Bartel, M. Law, M. Bateman, N. E. Klatt, A. M. Dose, P. S. Etzell, R. A. Nelimark, J. A. Mailliard, and C. G. Moertel. Prospective evaluation of prognostic variables from patient-completed questionnaires. *J. Clinical Oncol.*, 12:601–607, 1994.

[96] M. Lunn and D. McNeil. Applying Cox regression to competing risks. *Biometrics*, 51:524–532, 1995.

[97] R. W. Makuch. Adjusted survival curve estimation using covariates. *J. Chronic Disease*, 35:437–443, 1982.

[98] C. L. Mallows. Augmented partial residuals. *Technometrics*, 28:313–319, 1986.

[99] N. Mantel, N. R. Bohidar, and J. L. Ciminera. Mantel–Haenszel analyses of litter-matched time-to-response data with modifications for recovery of interlitter information. *Cancer Research*, 37:3863–3868, 1977.

[100] B. H. Markus, E. R. Dickson, P. M. Grambsch, T. R. Fleming, V. Mazzaferro, G. B .G. Klintmalm, R. H. Wiesner, D. H. VanThiel, and T. E. Starzl. Efficiency of liver transplantation in patients with primary biliary cirrhosis. *New England J. Medicine*, 320:1709–1713, 1989.

[101] C. A. McGilchrist. REML estimation for survival models with frailty. *Biometrics*, 49:221–225, 1993.

[102] C. A. McGilchrist and C. W. Aisbett. Regression with frailty in survival analysis. *Biometrics*, 47:461–466, 1991.

[103] R. G. Miller, Jr. *Survival Analysis.* Wiley, New York, 1981.

[104] R.G. Miller, Jr. What price Kaplan–Meier? *Biometrics*, 39:1077–1081, 1983.

[105] T. Moreau, J. O'Quigley, and M. Mesbah. A global goodness-of-fit statistic for the proportional hazards model. *Applied Stat.*, 34:212–218, 1985.

[106] A. J. Moss and the Multicenter Diltiazem Postinfarction Trial Research Group. The effect of diltiazem on mortality and reinfarction after myocardial infarction. *New England J. Medicine*, 319:385–392, 1988.

[107] A. J. Moss and the Multicenter Postinfarction Research Group. Risk stratification and survival after myocardial infarction. *New England J. Medicine*, 309:331–336, 1983.

[108] F. Mosteller and J. W. Tukey. *Data Analysis and Regression.* Addison-Wesley, Reading, MA, 1977.

[109] V. K. Murphy and L. J. Haywood. Survival analysis by sex, age group and hemotype in sickle cell disease. *J. Chronic Diseases*, 34:313–319, 1981.

[110] N. J. D. Nagelkerke, J. Oosting, and A. A. M. Hart. A simple test for goodness of fit of Cox's proportional hazards model. *Biometrics*, 40:483–486, 1984.

[111] W. Nelson. Hazard plotting for incomplete failure data. *J. Quality Technology*, 1:27–52, 1969.

[112] J. Neuberger, D. G. Altman, E. Christensen, N. Tygstrup, and R. Williams. Use of a prognostic index in evaluation of liver transplantation for primary biliary cirrhosis. *Transplantation*, 41:713–716, 1986.

[113] G. G. Nielsen, R. D. Gill, P. K. Andersen, and T. I. Sørensen. A counting process approach to maximum likelihood estimation of frailty models. *Scandinavian J. Stat.*, 19:25–43, 1992.

[114] D. Oakes. Frailty models for multiple event times. In J. P. Klein and P. K. Goel, editors, *Survival Analysis, State of the Art.* Kluwer, Netherlands, 1992.

[115] Y. Omori and R. A. Johnson. The influence of random effects on the unconditional hazard rate and survival functions. *Biometrika*, 80:910–914, 1993.

[116] J. O'Quigley and F. Pessione. Score tests for homogeneity of regression effect in the proportional hazards model. *Biometrics*, 45:135–144, 1989.

[117] E. Parner. *Inference in semiparametric frailty models.* PhD thesis, University of Aarhus, Denmark, 1997.

[118] R. Peto. Discussion of Professor Cox's paper. *J. Royal Stat. Soc. B*, 34:205–207, 1972.

[119] A. N. Pettitt and I. Bin Daud. Investigating time dependence in Cox's proportional hazards model. *Applied Stat.*, 39:313–329, 1990.

[120] R. L. Prentice and J. Cai. Covariance and survivor function estimation using censored multivariate failure time data. *Biometrika*, 79:495–512, 1992.

[121] R. L. Prentice and L. A. Gloeckler. Regression analysis of grouped survival data with application to breast cancer data. *Biometrics*, 34:57–67, 1978.

[122] R. L. Prentice, B. J. Williams, and A. V. Peterson. On the regression analysis of multivariate failure time data. *Biometrika*, 68:373–379, 1981.

[123] M. Pugh, J. Robbins, S. Lipsitz, and D. Harrington. Inference in the Cox proportional hazards model with missing covariates. Technical Report 758Z, Department of Biostatistics, Harvard School of Public Health, Boston, 1992.

[124] N. Reid and H. Crépeau. Influence functions for proportional hazards regression. *Biometrika*, 72:1–9, 1985.

[125] P. Ricci, T. M. Therneau, M. Malinchoc, J. T. Benson, J. L. Petz, G. B. Klintmalm, J. S. Crippin, R. H. Wiesner, J. L. Steers, J. Rakela, T. E. Starzl, and E. R. Dickson. A prognostic model for the outcome of liver transplantation in patients with cholestatic liver disease. *Hepatology*, 25:672–677, 1997.

[126] S. Ripatti and J. Palmgren. Estimation of multivariate frailty models using penalized partial likelihood. Research Report 99/1, Department of Biostatistics, University of Copenhagen, 1999.

[127] N. Sastry. A nested frailty model for survival data, with an application to the study of child survival in northesat brazil. *J. Amer. Stat. Assoc.*, 92:426–435, 1997.

[128] D. Schoenfeld. Chi-squared goodness-of-fit tests for the proportional hazards regression model. *Biometrika*, 67:145–153, 1980.

[129] D. Schoenfeld. The asymptotic properties of nonparametric tests for comparing survival distributions. *Biometrika*, 68:316–319, 1981.

[130] D. A. Schoenfeld. Sample-size formula for the proportional-hazards regression model. *Biometrics*, 39:499–503, 1983.

[131] M. Schumacher, M. Olschewski, and C. Schmoor. The impact of heterogeneity on the comparison of survival times. *Stat. in Medicine*, 6:773–784, 1987.

[132] S. G. Self and R. L. Prentice. Asymptotic distribution theory and efficiency results for case-cohort studies. *Annals of Stat.*, 16:64–81, 1988.

[133] T. A Sellers, V. E. Anderson, J. D. Potter, S. A. Bartow, P. L. Chen, L. Everson, R. A. King, C. C. Kuni, L. H. Kushi, P. G. McGovern, S. S. Rich, J. F. Whitbeck, and G. L. Wiesner. Epidemiologic and genetic follow-up study of 544 minnesota breast cancer families: Design and methods. *Genetic Epidemiology*, 12:417–429, 1995.

[134] M. D. Silverstein, E. V. Loftus, Jr., W. J. Sandborn, W. J. Tremaine, B. G. Feagan, P. J. Nietert, W. S. Harmsen, and A. R. Zinsmeister. Clinical course and costs of care for Crohn's disease: Markov model analysis of a population-based cohort. *Gastroenterology*, 117:49–57, 1999.

[135] P. J. Solomon. Effect of misspecification of regression models in the analysis of survival data. *Biometrika*, 71:291–298, 1984.

[136] P. J. Solomon. Amendments and corrections. *Biometrika*, 73:245–245, 1986.

[137] P. Spector. *An Introduction to S and S-Plus.* Wadsworth, Pacific Grove, CA, 1994.

[138] D. M. Stablein, W. H. Carter, Jr., and J. W. Novak. Analysis of survival data with nonproportional hazard functions. *Controlled Clinical Trials*, 2:149–159, 1981.

[139] C. J. Stone. Comment to paper by Hastie and Tibshirani. *Stat. Science*, 1:312–314, 1986.

[140] C. J. Stone and C. Y. Koo. Additive splines in statistics. In *Computational Statistics Section*, pages 646–651, Alexandria, Virginia, 1985. American Statistical Association.

[141] C. A. Struthers and J. D. Kalbfleisch. Misspecified proportional hazard models. *Biometrika*, 73:363–369, 1986.

[142] Surveillance, epidemiology, and end results: Incidence and mortality data, 1973–77. National Cancer Institute Monograph 57, U.S. Department of Health and Human Services, Public Health Service, National Cancer Institute, Bethesda, MD, 1981. NIH Publication No. 81-2330.

[143] T. M. Therneau, P. M. Grambsch, and T. R. Fleming. Martingale based residuals for survival models. *Biometrika*, 77:147–160, 1990.

[144] T. M. Therneau and S. A. Hamilton. rhDNase as an example of recurrent event analysis. *Stat. in Medicine*, 16:2029–2047, 1997.

[145] T. M. Therneau and H. Li. Computing the Cox model for case-cohort designs. *Lifetime Data Analysis*, 5:99–112, 1999.

[146] T. M. Therneau, J. Sicks, E. Bergstralh, and J. Offord. Expected survival based on hazard rates. Technical Report 52, Department of Health Sciences Research, Mayo Clinic, 1994.

[147] B. L. Thomsen, N. Keiding, and D. G. Altman. A note on the calculation of expected survival, illustrated by the survival of liver transplant patients. *Stat. in Medicine*, 10:733–738, 1991.

[148] B. L. Thomsen, N. Keiding, and D. G. Altman. Reply to a letter to the editor. *Stat. in Medicine*, 11:1528–1530, 1992.

[149] A. A. Tsiatis. A large sample study of Cox's regression model. *Annals of Stat.*, 9:93–108, 1981.

[150] Life tables for the geographic divisions of the United States: 1959–61. National Center for Health Statistics, Public Health Service, Washington, U.S. Government Printing Office, May 1965. Vol. 1, number 3.

[151] W. N. Venables and B. D. Ripley. *Modern Applied Statistics with S-PLUS, second edition.* Springer-Verlag, New York, 1997.

[152] H. A. Verheul, E. Dekker, P. Bossuyt, A. C. Moulijn, and A. J. Dunning. Background mortality in clinical survival studies. *Lancet*, 341:872–875, 1993.

[153] P. J .M. Verweij and H. C. Van Houwlingen. Penalized likelihood in Cox regression. *Stat. in Medicine*, 13:2427–2436, 1994.

[154] G. Wahba. Bayesian "confidence intervals" for the cross-validated smoothing spline. *J. Royal Stat. Soc. B*, 45:133–150, 1983.

[155] L. J. Wei, D. Y. Lin, and L. Weissfeld. Regression analysis of multivariate incomplete failure time data by modeling marginal distributions. *J. Amer. Stat. Assoc.*, 84:1065–1073, 1989.

[156] L. J. Wei, Z. Ying, and D. Y. Lin. Linear regression analysis of censored survival data based on rank tests. *Biometrika*, 77:845–851, 1990.

[157] H. White. A heteroskedasticity-consistent covariance matrix estimator and a direct test for heteroskedasticity. *Econometrica*, 48:817–838, 1980.

[158] H. White. Maximum likelihood estimation of misspecified models. *Econometrica*, 50:1–26, 1982.

[159] J. Whitehead. Fitting Cox's regression model to survival data using GLIM. *Applied Stat.*, 29:268–275, 1980.

[160] H. Z. Winkler, L. M. Rainwater, R. P. Myers, G. M. Farrow, T. M. Therneau, H. Zincke, and M. M. Lieber. Stage D1 prostatic adenocarcinoma: Significance of nuclear DNA ploidy patterns studied by flow cytometry. *Mayo Clinic Proceedings*, 63:103–112, 1988.

[161] K. K .W. Yau and C. A. McGilchrist. ML and REML estimation in survival analysis with time dependent correlated frailty. *Stat. in Medicine*, 17:1201–1213, 1998.

[162] S. L. Zeger and K. Y. Liang. Longitudinal data analysis for discrete and continuous outcomes. *Biometrics*, 42:121–130, 1986.

[163] S. L. Zeger, K. Y. Liang, and P. S. Albert. Models for longitudinal data: A generalized estimating equation approach. *Biometrics*, 44:1049–1060, 1988.

Index